THE MOST EFFECTIVE WAYS TO Live LONGER COOKBOOK

THE MOST EFFECTIVE WAYS TO Live LONGER COOKBOOK

THE SURPRISING, UNBIASED TRUTH ABOUT GREAT-TASTING FOOD THAT PREVENTS DISEASE AND GIVES YOU OPTIMAL HEALTH AND LONGEVITY

Jonny Bowden, Ph.D., C.N.S., and Jeannette Bessinger, C.H.H.C.

Best-selling author of **The 150 Healthiest Foods on Earth** and **The Most Effective Ways to Live Longer**

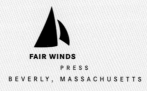

FAIR WINDS
PRESS
BEVERLY, MASSACHUSETTS

First published in the USA in 2010 by
Fair Winds Press, a member of
Quayside Publishing Group
100 Cummings Center
Suite 406-L
Beverly, MA 01915-6101
www.fairwindspress.com

12 11 10 09 08   1 2 3 4 5

ISBN-13: 978-1-59233-445-2
ISBN-10: 1-59233-445-8

Library of Congress Cataloging-in-Publication Data
Bowden, Jonny.
 The most effective ways to live longer cookbook : the surprising, unbiased truth about what to eat to prevent disease, feel great, and have optimal health and longevity / Jonny Bowden, Jeannette Bessinger.
    p. cm.
 Includes index.
 ISBN-13: 978-1-59233-445-2
 ISBN-10: 1-59233-445-8
 1. Natural foods. 2. Nutrition. 3. Longevity. I. Bessinger, Jeannette. II. Title.
 TX369.B69 2010
 641.3'02—dc22

                                                          2010028366

Photography: Richard Fleischman
Food Stylist: Rachel Sherwood
Book design: doublemranch.com

Printed and bound in China

The information in this book is for educational purposes only. It is not intended to replace the advice of a physician or medical practitioner. Please see your health-care provider before beginning any new health program.

From Jonny

*"I dedicate this book to Robert Crayhon: humanitarian, teacher, and friend.
Were it not for you, I would not be doing what I'm doing."*

From Jeannette

*"I dedicate this book with love and deep gratitude to my mom, Judie Porter,
my dad, Frank Knapp, to Pam Knapp, and to Peter Thoms.
May you all live long and healthy lives."*

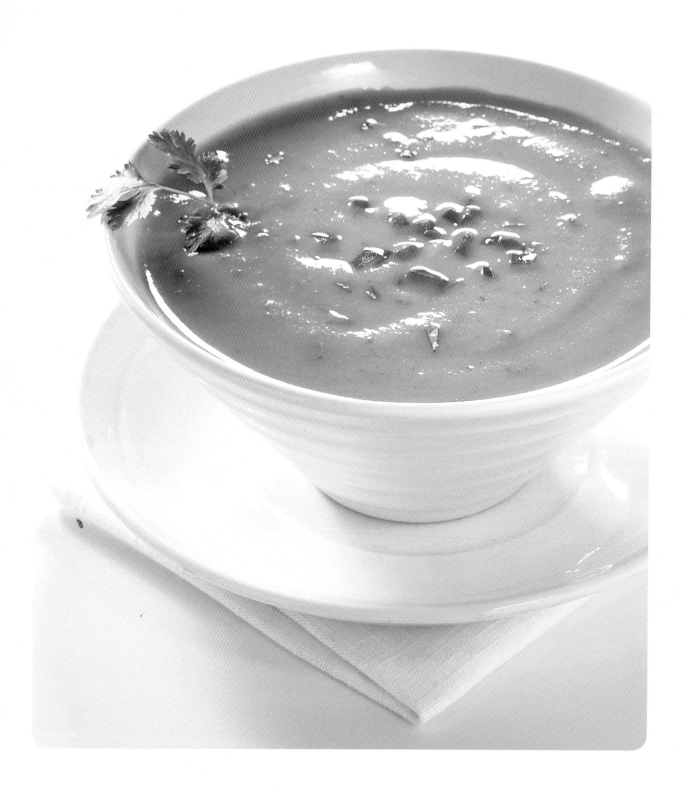

Contents

INTRODUCTION

Whenever I speak to audiences, I can always count on getting a laugh with the following line: Depression is not a Prozac deficiency.

People smile when they hear this because they instinctively recognize the larger truth: We don't get sick because of a dietary deficiency of pharmaceutical drugs. We don't get heart disease, for example, because there's not enough Lipitor in our diet. But we do get sick—very sick—when our diet doesn't provide the vitamins, minerals, phytochemicals, flavonoids, phenols, fiber, protein, fat, and carbohydrates that our body needs to run smoothly and efficiently for decades on end. "Give the body what it needs," I frequently tell audiences, "and it will almost always reward you by making everything you need to feel great."

Which brings us to this book.

While I'm certainly not naive enough to think that you can cure or prevent every disease in the world with food, or that a crummy diet is the cause of every medical misfortune in the world, I'm pretty sure you could prevent a high percentage of the diseases of aging by eating differently. And if you couldn't completely prevent or cure a disease with food, you could almost always make it better. You could shorten its duration, decrease its severity, or, at the very least, improve some other aspect of health even if the primary disease was unaffected. This is what Hippocrates, the father of modern medicine, meant when he said, "Let food be thy medicine and medicine be thy food."

Hippocrates was also credited with another great mantra of modern medicine: "First do no harm." The recipes and eating style in this book meet both of Hippocrates' criteria. No foods or recipes in this book will harm you in any way, and, in my humble opinion, all of them will fuel your body like high-octane gas in a Ferrari, allowing you to perform your best, live life to the fullest, and have boundless energy for decades and decades.

THE FOUR HORSEMEN OF AGING

I wrote a book titled *The Most Effective Ways to Live Longer*. (Shameless plug: I hope you run out and get it immediately!) One of the things I talk about in the book is something I call the Four Horsemen of Aging. These are four basic processes whose deadly handiwork can be seen in virtually every condition we know as a disease of aging. In some cases they directly *cause* the disease and in almost all they either make it worse or make healing it more difficult.

This book is about how to use food to combat them. Let me explain.

The First Horseman of Aging is *oxidative damage*. You've undoubtedly seen the results of oxidative damage even if you don't know what it is. All you have to do is look at what happens to metal when it's left outside in the rain to rust, or watch an apple slice turn brown in the sun. What you're seeing in the rusting or browning is the result of rogue oxygen molecules called *free radicals*, which do the same thing to your cells and DNA that they do to the rusting metal or browning apple slices. These free radicals "rust" you on the inside and age you from the outside (contributing to aging skin, for example).

What to do, what to do?

Once again, food comes to the rescue; this time as a delivery system for one of the most powerful groups of oxidative damage fighters ever assembled anywhere. The collective name for this raging army of disease fighters is, appropriately, *antioxidants*. The best known among them are vitamins C and E, but the minerals zinc and selenium are also powerful antioxidants. So are the pigments called *anthocyanins*, which make blueberries blue and raspberries red. The compound that makes wild salmon pink is a powerful antioxidant known as *astaxanthin*. Literally thousands of flavonoids and phenols and other members of the plant kingdom are powerful antioxidants.

You'll find them all in these deliciously imaginative recipes.

The Second Horseman of Aging is *inflammation*. Chronic inflammation flies under the radar of our perception, unlike the acute inflammation we've all experienced when we stub our toe, develop a tooth infection, experience an asthma attack, or bang our shins. Chronic inflammation—or "silent" inflammation—damages the vascular system, the network of blood vessels that crisscross the whole body; this can lead to strokes and heart attacks. Inflammation damages the nerve cells in the brain, which can lead to all sorts of problems from memory loss to Alzheimer's. Inflammation even depresses your immune system. "The secret to maintaining wellness," says Barry Sears, Ph.D., "is controlling silent inflammation the best you can over a lifetime."

And the best place to start is with food.

Foods have natural anti-inflammatory chemicals that are the equal of almost any drug on the planet. Quercetin, a flavonoid found in apples and onions. Resveratrol, an almost-magical anti-aging compound found in the skins of dark grapes. And the granddaddy of all anti-inflammatories, the omega-3 fatty acids found in cold-water fish and, to some extent, plant foods such as flax. You'll find them all here in abundance. These recipes were put together partly because they taste amazing, but also because they are rich in precisely the chemical compounds known to calm inflammation and cut off the diseases it creates before they even get started.

The Third Horseman of Aging is something called *glycation*. This happens when there's too much sugar in the bloodstream and some of it gloms onto proteins. These sugar-coated proteins become sticky and gum up the works, leading to circulatory problems, kidney problems, and vision difficulties. This is only one of the huge problems with a high-sugar diet (or even a diet high in processed carbs). Another is the oversecretion of insulin, a hormone known both as the "hunger hormone" and the "fat storage" hormone. A chronically elevated level of insulin increases blood pressure, makes it easy to put on weight (and almost impossible to take it off), and contributes to all sorts of medical problems. This is one reason you'll find the recipes in this book to be extremely low in sugar and processed carbs, which raise blood sugar just as much as the white stuff in the sugar bowl.

Yet, amazingly, you'll never miss them. While some of the recipes do indeed use sweeteners (after all, this is a cookbook!), they're used judiciously and always in the context of real food. (Example: Gingered Mango and Green Tea Freeze.) You won't find a single dessert here whose ingredients start with sugar, butter, and white flour. What you *will* find is a selection of desserts that are absolutely delicious and, unlike desserts in most cookbooks, will *add* to your longevity, not subtract from it.

The Fourth Horseman of Aging is *stress*. I won't go into all the ways stress kills (although I talk about it at length in *The Most Effective Ways to Live Longer*), and I won't promise you that food can lower your stress levels. But, stress is a complicated thing with a large hormonal component. Many things can be seen as stressors in the body, from a fight with your mate to a junk food–filled diet. Stress also eats up certain nutrients (such as vitamin B5 and vitamin C). And the main stress hormone, cortisol, has a codependent relationship with the aforementioned fat storage hormone, insulin. So what you eat actually can have an effect, albeit an indirect one, on stress levels. Food, as we all know, can also reduce stress just by being comforting and familiar (which is why we call some foods *comfort foods*).

Each recipe is accompanied by an icon or showing which of the Four Horsemen it helps fight.

The trick is not to remove comfort foods from your diet, but to create comfort foods that actually lengthen your life rather than shorten it! It's a trick I think we've achieved quite nicely in the recipes that follow. For instance, Chef Jeannette uses whole-grain panko bread crumbs and tofu in a classic "chicken parmigiana" recipe to increase the fiber and protein but keep the total calorie count and fat count very low. She also suggests substituting spaghetti squash for the traditional pasta for a super-low glycemic load (sugar hit) and more micronutrients. Traditional mac and cheese gets a makeover with whole-grain pasta, flaxseed, and creamy butternut squash, again to lighten the calorie load and increase the dish's nutrients without compromising on the taste.

IT'S NOT JUST BRAIN FOOD

The book is organized into five sections: heart; brain; bones, muscles, and joints; immune system; and liver. Each section features foods that provide special value for the organs or systems in that section that will support your longevity. So, for example, you'll find heart-healthy foods in the heart section; bone-strengthening foods in the bones, joints, and muscles section; and so on.

I can almost hear you asking yourself, "Why just those five sections? What about the kidneys? The lungs? The eyes? Or any other organ or system in the body? Certainly these important structures are subject to aging and breakdown—why is there nothing about the best foods and recipes to support them as well?"

Good question, and here's the answer: We chose the heart, brain, bones/joints/muscles, immune system, and liver because they get the lion's share of attention when it comes to aging and breakdown. After all, heart disease remains the number-one killer of Americans, virtually every baby boomer is worried about memory and brain health, arthritis and joint issues affect nearly everyone, the liver is the central detoxification organ in the body, and everyone who has ever gotten sick understands the importance of a strong immune system. (The second part of the answer is that we had to make the book shorter than *War and Peace*, so something had to be left out!)

But the good news is that virtually everything that is "good" for one of the systems we chose to concentrate on will also benefit the systems we didn't feature. And sharp-eyed readers will almost certainly realize very quickly that foods and recipes that benefit one of the systems we talk about in the book (say, the heart) also benefit others (say, the brain). These foods and recipes also benefit the organs we *didn't* talk about.

Omega-3 fatty acids from fish, for example, support circulation (heart), reduce inflammation (joints), and protect delicate cell membranes in the neurons (brain). Antioxidants from the fruits and vegetables and salmon featured in the heart section also protect the liver (as well as the eyes and the lungs). Probiotics from yogurt and fermented foods such as sauerkraut are great for the immune system, but also support the liver.

While finding the appropriate categories to put these foods in might have been a challenge for the authors, it's certainly not a problem for you, the reader (and the eater). As I said above, virtually every important food in every recipe in this book does double, perhaps triple, duty. Foods and nutrients are like the Pashtun tribes in the Near East—

they don't really recognize artificially imposed national boundaries and simply move freely between country and country. Nutrients are like that—they don't fit neatly into categories such as "heart-healthy" and "good for the brain." That's actually what makes them so cool. Good food filled with powerful nutrients helps virtually every part of the body (and frequently the mind as well) to function better.

Nonetheless, we did the best we could with sticking these guys into categories even though it sometimes felt a bit like herding cats. The liver section, for example, is filled with foods such as broccoli that contain nutrients such as *sulforaphane*, which actually stimulate detoxification pathways in the liver. And the heart (and brain) sections are filled with foods such as salmon, which contain tons of omega-3 fatty acids. Just rest assured that anything you eat in this book, regardless of the section you find it in, will be good for you—now and as you age—in myriad ways.

And, just as a reference, we give you a quick reminder of why (and how) each recipe is working its magic on your health and longevity. You'll find this info in the short intro Jonny wrote to each recipe Jeannette created. (Feel free to use it to dazzle your dinner guests with little factoids about why what you've prepared is so darn good for them!)

I talked earlier about the Four Horsemen of Aging, and spent a bit of time explaining the negative consequences of too much stress in the body. Stress comes from so many places in our lives that a full discussion of stress and its health consequences could easily fill a book. And this may not come as much of a shock to you, but food is often one of those significant sources of stress for many people. For example: How many people stress out just over what to eat? Or what to feed their family?

We hope this book goes a long way toward reducing that very concern. There isn't a recipe in this book that isn't good for you and, speaking personally, there isn't one that doesn't taste delicious. You can feed your family (or yourself) using these recipes and be confident in the fact that you're providing yourself and your loved ones with amazing nutrition, the right balance of nutrients, good fats (including some healthy saturated ones!), plenty of fiber, very low sugar, and a veritable array of natural antioxidants and anti-inflammatories that will tame the aging fires within and guarantee you a long, productive, energetic life.

Remember, when you take care of yourself, you make it possible to function at the highest level possible, to make the most of your natural gifts, fulfill your potential, and contribute to the world.

That's what we wish for you.

Enjoy the journey.

—**Jonny Bowden**

A WORD ABOUT THE BLUE ZONES FROM CHEF JEANNETTE

In the book that inspired this cookbook, *The Most Effective Ways to Live Longer*, Dr. Jonny discusses at length areas around the globe known as the Blue Zones. These are places such as Sardinia, Okinawa, and several others, where people routinely live to the age of one hundred, in vibrant good health. Writers including Dan Buettner, who has done extensive research on the Blue Zones, looked at what kinds of foods the inhabitants of these regions routinely consume.

While the diets of each of these regions are different, we found several factors in common. One is the consumption of beans. Another is the inclusion of lots of fresh vegetables. A third is the absence of processed foods. The recipes in our book try to incorporate as many of the principles of Blue Zone eating as possible, and to adapt them to modern living (and modern supermarkets). You may not be able to live in the Blue Zones, but you can sure emulate many of their dietary principles, and whenever possible, that's what we tried to do in this book.

Eat to fuel your body, not to fill your belly.

HOW TO EAT FOR LONGEVITY

The simplest technique for eating for logevity can be summed up in one short sentence: Eat to fuel your body, not to fill your belly. Although it is undeniably true that the foods you choose are crucial to your long-term health, how and how much you eat may be as important as what you eat.

As Jonny discusses at length in *The Most Effective Ways to Live Longer*, consuming fewer calories seems to be one of the keys to extending life. Okinawans, one of the longest-lived people on the planet, eat an average of five hundred fewer calories per day than Americans do.

Eating fewer calories is simple, but for many of us, it is not easy. I'm a personal chef and health educator, so I've had a front-row seat for this challenge. Over the years, I've worked with hundreds of people at different ages and stages trying to change their eating and lifestyle habits. Some are successful, many are not. As evidenced by the growing obesity epidemic in many Western countries (and sadly, more and more Eastern countries), overeating has become a lifestyle that seems normal.

The people who have been the most successful in disrupting this habit have changed their fundamental style of eating. Okinawans have a saying that many of the older generation use as a kind of grace before eating: *hara hachi bu*. It means eat until you are 80 percent full, or just sated.

This is a foreign concept for many of us in the West, where not only do we eat until we're 100 percent full at nearly every meal, but where being full means having to loosen your belt to bend over and pick up your napkin.

Hara hachi bu means to eat until the gnawing edge of hunger goes away, but not until our stomachs are actually filled. A normal, healthy stomach is about the size of two closed fists together. Look at your hands like that and imagine the amount of chewed food that would take up 80 percent of that volume. Not very much, is it?

The stomach is an involuntary muscle, and part of the way it digests your food is to roll it around in there to mix the food particles with digestive acids. If it's packed to the max it's harder to do that, which means your system will break down (and thus absorb) fewer nutrients from what you are eating. When you regularly eat to 80 percent fullness, you optimize the conditions for healthy digestion. Which means your whole digestive system has to do less work, which means a lot less wear and tear on your body over several decades, which means, in short: It will last longer.

In the following pages, you will find numerous ideas for nutrient-rich meals, snacks, and drinks designed to prime five key organ systems for optimal performance and stave off the Four Horsemen of Aging. You'll see very little animal meat, more omega-3-rich seafoods, more nuts and seeds, and lots of fruits and veggies. Eating these types of meals and snacks, slowly and moderately, at only four sittings, will have you well on your way to adding quality years to your precious and wonderful life.

Blessings on you and yours,

—**Jeannette Bessinger**

BEFORE YOU COOK

The Surprising Truth about What Nutrition Labels Aren't Telling You

When Jeannette and I published our first cookbook, *The Healthiest Meals on Earth*, we were gratified by the almost uniformly positive feedback we received. But several people were disappointed that we hadn't included nutritional values for the recipes.

It wasn't that we were being lazy. It's that the issue of nutritional "facts" is not as simple as it sounds.

See, the standard nutritional facts label does not begin to tell the whole story about food and health. There's a lot more to food (and recipes) than can be gleaned by a cursory glance at how much fat they contain, or even how many calories. We want you to get the most out of the nutrition facts that we've included in this book, so bear with us for a moment and let's clear up a few basics.

The only things that are required by the U.S. Food and Drug Administration to be on the nutrition facts label are the following:

- Serving size
- Servings per container
- Calories (per serving)
- Calories from fat
- Total fat
- Saturated fat
- Trans fat
- Total carbohydrates
- Dietary fiber
- Sugars
- Protein
- Vitamin A
- Vitamin C
- Calcium
- Iron

You might think all that data tells you a lot, but it actually tells you a lot less than you'd imagine.

It also perpetuates a lot of wrongheaded notions about food.

Let me explain.

While calories, for example, are certainly important, they are very far from the whole picture when it comes to losing, gaining, or maintaining weight. Different foods have significantly different effects on hormones that create fat storage (or fat loss). This is where concepts such as the glycemic index (or glycemic load) come into play, and there is nothing on the nutrition facts label that tells you about that.

Similarly, while vitamin C, vitamin A, calcium, and iron are certainly important, there are no fewer than thirteen vitamins, thirteen major minerals, many more trace minerals, and literally thousands of healthy plant compounds known as phytochemicals, all of which have potential health benefits, some of them enormous. And that's not counting the at least twenty amino acids, all of which perform important functions in the body.

The Skinny on Fat

Then there's the problem with fat.

As I have written countless times—in eight books and hundreds of articles—fat is a terribly misunderstood macronutrient. People think foods with high amounts of fat cause them to gain weight. And the belief that saturated fat is always a bad thing continues to persist despite copious research questioning that concept.

Just a quick example: The fat in coconut is technically a saturated fat, but the body prefers to use it for energy rather than storage, and coconut fat has antiviral and antimicrobial properties to boot. The fat in eggs is mostly in the yolks, but those yolks are also a source of some of the most important and valuable carotenoids for eye health (lutein and zeaxanthin) not to mention the B-vitamin relative choline, which is used to build healthy brain chemicals important for thinking, memory, attention, and longevity.

The moral of the story:
Don't fear fat, and don't recoil if a recipe has what you think is a high fat content.

So sure, a fabulous recipe such as the Chocolate Mixed Nuts for Heart Health on page 61 is high in fat (because of the nuts). But, it's great fat, and nuts are a staple of the diets of every single one of the long-lived societies on Earth. And studies from Harvard show that people who eat nuts—fat and all!—on a regular basis have significantly lower risk for heart disease! So don't worry!

Butter, when it comes from grass-fed cows (see page18), has a particular kind of fat called CLA (conjugated linoleic acid), which has been shown to have anticancer and antiobesity properties. Yet, it shows up on nutritional labels as having saturated fat, with the implication that you should avoid it.

You shouldn't.

So, if you focus only on fat, even saturated fat, you are missing the big picture.

And for those who remain skeptical, let me quote Walter Willett, M.D., Ph.D., chairman of the nutrition department at the Harvard School of Public Health. Willett is the lead researcher on two of the longest-running studies in the history of nutrition, The Nurses' Health Study, in which the dietary habits of more than 100,000 women have been studied for more than 30 years, and the Health Professionals Follow-Up Study, which studied more than 51,000 men since 1986. That's a total of more than 150,000 humans studied for more than five decades. As you can imagine, that kind of research produces an awful lot of valuable data about the effects of diet. Let's see what Willett has to say about his findings. This is what he told Harvard's *World Health News*:

"The relation of fat intake to health is one of the areas that we have examined in detail over the last 20 years in our two large cohort studies: the Nurses' Health Study and the Health Professionals Follow-Up Study. *We have found virtually no relationship between the percentage of calories from fat and any important health outcome.*"

Please read that carefully, because it probably contradicts most of what you read in the popular media. But it is 100 percent true. The percentage of fat in your diet makes absolutely no difference to anything you care about, including weight, cancer, and heart disease. Total calories? Sure. Type of fat? Yup. (The healthy level of consumption for trans fats is exactly zero!) Type of carbs? Yes again. High-sugar carbs, a.k.a. high-glycemic carbs—those that make your blood sugar soar and raise levels of the fat-storing hormone insulin—are definitely a no-no.

Yet, the nutrition facts label masks this important data. It scares you away from foods that have "too much fat" (even though no one has ever successfully defined how much too much fat is).

Remember, fat has more calories than protein and carbohydrates: 9 calories per gram for fat (as compared to 4 per gram for carbs and protein). So recipes with a lot of nuts, which are high in fat, are going to tend to be high in calories. Recipes with salmon will be high in fat. Or with avocado. Or olive oil. Or coconut. Should you avoid these recipes? Absolutely not. These foods will nourish your heart and brain, reduce inflammation, and in many cases, are associated with longer, healthier lives. (They're found in copious amounts in the diets of folks living in the Blue Zones.) The moral of the story: Don't fear fat, and don't recoil if a recipe has what you think is a high fat content.

If I haven't completely convinced you—or even if I have but you want to opt for lower-calorie versions of some of these recipes—you can always choose low-fat versions of some of the ingredients (low-fat yogurt, for example). I'm not a fan of no-fat products for three simple reasons: One, artificially created no-fat foods make up for the removal of fat by adding more sugar, which is far, far more dangerous to your health and longevity than fat is. Two, the fat in foods is satisfying and keeps you full longer, making it less likely that you will overeat. And three, nature designed certain foods to have fat for a very good reason. Important vitamins such as A, E, and K, and important nutrients like the carotenoids (beta-carotene, etc.) are absorbed better with fat.

That said, you can certainly substitute low-fat versions of foods in these recipes (though both Chef Jeannette and I strongly recommend not using fat-free products). You can also eat smaller portions. (Never a bad idea from a longevity point of view! See Jeannette's p.s. about this on page 16). We just urge you to look beyond the obvious listings of calories and fat and consider the vast array of life-extending nutrients that fly beneath the label of a standard nutrition facts label.

Remember, God is in the details—and the details are buried far beneath the surface of the superficial facts label.

A Word on Specific Foods

That said, I'd like to address a few of the choices we've made throughout this book so you can better understand them.

Eggs: The only reason people avoid whole eggs is that they are afraid of the extra fat. Don't be. The yolk contains valuable nutrients that help the brain and the eyes. The cholesterol in eggs has virtually no effect on your blood cholesterol.

Fruit juices: I've written many times that most commercial fruit juices are little more than sugar water with a little extra vitamins. Yet we've included some smoothies and juices here that are largely made of fruit. So what's the deal? Simple. While eating whole fruit is almost always better, juicing, especially when of the homemade variety, is a great vehicle for the delivery of concentrated nutrients. Beet and carrot juice in particular are very good for the liver. But the downside is that even these healthy juices do have the ability to raise your blood sugar rather quickly. If you're not sugar sensitive or struggling with any metabolic issues that involve sugar or insulin metabolism (diabetes, metabolic syndrome), the occasional fruit juice or blended drink won't be a problem.

Sugar: Okay, in a perfect world, we wouldn't eat sugar. (Actually, that's not even true, because I'm pretty sure it wouldn't be a perfect world if we could never, ever have dessert!) So we've compromised. We tried to keep sugar very low in all these recipes, choosing foods that have

God is in the details—
and the details are buried far beneath the surface
of the superficial facts label.

Food is meant to be enjoyed, cherished, and appreciated. The experience of preparing and eating nutritious longevity food is more than the sum of its parts.

a nice even impact on your blood sugar and don't send you off on a craving binge. But let's be honest—this is a cookbook, and this is the real world. A few recipes call for some sweetening, and we made our best effort at damage control. Enough sweetener to make it palatable, but not so much as to be a health hazard. And the foods we did sweeten still have so much redeeming nutritional value that we thought you'd forgive us!

Nuts and oils: All oils, whether they are the cheapest, crummiest, processed corn oil from the supermarket or the finest extra-virgin olive oil imported from Italy, have about 110 to 120 calories per tablespoon. There's just no getting around it. But despite their equality on the calorie scale, all oils are far from being created equal. We used the ones we feel have the most health benefits. Nuts are also high in calories, but are one of the healthiest longevity foods on the planet, as we point out throughout this book. Don't be afraid to eat them. Just eat smaller portions if you're modifying your calories.

A final word: Food is meant to be enjoyed, cherished, and appreciated. The experience of preparing and eating nutritious longevity food is more than the sum of its parts—at least we hope it is! We included the nutrition facts information because you asked for it. But, just like knowing how much money a person makes doesn't begin to tell you the whole story about that person, knowing how many calories and fat are in a food doesn't begin to tell you the whole story about what's on your plate.

—**Dr. Jonny**

P.S. Chef Jeannette on "Standard" Portion Sizes
There is simply no way to pick one appropriate portion size for a general audience made up of different genders, ages, weights, activity levels, and so on. You get the picture. If a given portion size looks like too many calories or too much fat or too many carbs for you, just go smaller. But please remember Dr. Jonny's advice and know that these recipes have been carefully crafted for their overall health value and positive impact on longevity.

Conversely, if you're a 225-pound male athlete, for instance, and you don't feel satisfied after eating one standard portion slowly and mindfully, have a little more. As a culture we need to relearn how to listen carefully to our bodies for those hunger and satisfaction signals that, when in balance, can be our perfect portion guide.

Food Safety and Selection Tips to Help You Live Longer

You know the old computer saying "GIGO"? No? Well, it means "garbage in, garbage out"! In other words, the computer can only work with what you give it, and if you give it bad "input"—that is, misspelled words, incorrect numbers—you're not going to get great "output."

Well, it's the same with recipes and food!

The best recipes in the world are only as good as the ingredients you use to make them. So rather than mentioning them multiple times throughout the recipes, in this section you'll find a compiled set of cool tips for choosing the best ingredients and preparing them in the safest ways. Happy cooking!

FROM CHEF JEANNETTE

Wash Those Fruits and Veggies

Rinse all produce thoroughly before using, even organics. To remove the grit from leafy greens and fresh herbs, submerge them in a large bowl or clean sink full of cold water. If your greens are looking a little wilted, add a splash of white vinegar to the water to replump. Gently swirl to loosen any stuck grime, rinse, and drain or spin in a salad spinner.

Bite-Size Lettuce

In general, lettuce should be torn rather than chopped, but if you're eating the salad shortly after preparing, it's easier to chop it into bite-size pieces with a chef's knife.

Sautéing Onion and Garlic

In most of these recipes, I recommend sautéing onions for 5 minutes. This is shorthand for "sauté until the onions soften and turn translucent, anywhere from 3 to 6 minutes, depending on how much onion is in the pan and how hot your burner runs." Unless the recipe specifies a color, onions shouldn't cook to the point of brownness. In most recipes, I suggest a minute for garlic. This is to give it time to heat and release its flavors, but not to brown. Browning garlic gives it a slightly bitter flavor.

Stevia

I recommend liquid stevia extract as opposed to the powdered form in most of these recipes. Stevia is so sweet that it's easier to control with single drops of the liquid, and I find the distinctive aftertaste milder in the liquid versus powdered form. If you prefer packets, my favorite brand for mild flavor is KAL Pure Stevia Extract Plus Luo Han. For the liquid product, try NuNaturals' Stevia Extract. Both are usually available at a good natural food store.

Salt

We're not big fans of table salt. It's highly processed and stripped of most of its naturally occurring minerals, with a few thrown back in, along with an anti-caking agent. Although it contains traces of hard-to-get iodine, we'd prefer to get that in its naturally occurring form from seafood and sea vegetables.

My favorite everyday salt is "si" sea salt. One of my macrobiotics teachers, salt guru Lino Stanchich, recommended it as among the cleanest and most mineral-loaded varieties out there. It's also inexpensive. It's naturally produced (sun dried and stone ground) in the Southern California/Baja region from a remote area of the Pacific. You can find it in some natural food stores and macrobiotic stores or order it online.

My favorite salt for use when it really counts, such as to finish a great dressing or as an accompaniment to amazing chocolate, is Himalayan pink salt. This is readily available in most natural food stores and all the big raw-food outlets online.

FROM DR. JONNY

Which Produce to Buy Organic

Compared to the arguments over organic versus nonorganic, the U.S. Congress almost sounds civilized. Some studies show organic food has more nutrients than nonorganic; some studies show no such thing. And the folks arguing over these issues are not exactly objective, disinterested parties. Big Food clearly wants you to think there's no special advantage to organic foods, and the organic

(continued on page 18)

people want you to think there's a reason you should be spending so much more money on their stuff. Both have studies to confirm their positions. What's the truth?

Let's take a commonsense approach. Whether or not the nutritional value of organic is higher, one thing's for sure: Organic produce has not been treated with chemicals. Now there are those who will tell you that pesticides and other chemicals that food is sprayed with are safe, but regardless, I'd just as soon not have them in my body. However, the desire to consume minimal pesticides and sprays with my apples has to be balanced against the considerably higher cost of organically grown food.

So, here's my personal solution. The Environmental Working Group, a nonprofit organization devoted to consumer protection, has ranked a hundred or so crops in order of how contaminated they are. The worst of the lot are called the Dirty Dozen, and those are the ones that I'd consider buying in only organic form. The 2009 list of the most contaminated crops (starting with the worst) contains peaches, apples, sweet bell peppers, celery, nectarines, strawberries, cherries, kale, lettuce, imported grapes, carrots, and pears.

On a personal note I'd also buy only organic milk and meat.

Grass–Fed versus Grain–Fed Cows
There's a saying making the rounds in the nutrition world these days that goes like this: Your food is only as good as your *food's* food. Cows that are raised (if you can call it that) on feedlots (also known as factory farms) have a pretty horrible life. They're kept in pens; they never see sunlight; they have high levels of stress hormones in their bloodstream; they're fed grain (more on that in a moment); and they're shot up with antiobiotics, steroids, and hormones, all of which have a 100 percent chance of being passed on to you.

That's what we're eating when we eat factory-farmed, feedlot meat— at home, in restaurants, in fast-food outlets, and everywhere else that we don't eat grass-fed meat.

A cow's digestive system was meant to run on grass. The acidic grain diet fattens them up quickly and gets them to the slaughter-house sooner; plus feeding them grain is more cost-effective for the factory farms that don't have to provide tons of grazing pasture. But it's absolutely horrible for the cows, and therefore, for you. The grain makes them sick, requiring even more antibiotics, and because they get their omega-3 fats from grass, their meat is strikingly low in anti-inflammatory omega-3s and strikingly high in inflammatory omega-6s.

So, I feel strongly about grass-fed meat. And by the way, "grass-fed" and "organic" are not the same thing. Organically raised meat does not necessarily mean that the cow was grass-fed; it just means the cow was fed organic grain, but that's like feeding my family organic gasoline. Gasoline isn't the right food for my family, and grain isn't the right food for cows.

Grass-fed meat is terribly expensive. The good news is that it's easier to obtain these days, even online. (My website, www .jonnybowden.com, has a link to U.S. Wellness Meats under "healthy food.") Farmers who actually raise cows on pasture are, for the most part, incredibly conscientious about their animals' living and eating conditions. Because the cows eat their natural diet of grass, they don't get gastrointestinal sicknesses. Because they're not in crowded pens, they tend to not get sick as much. Because of both of these reasons, they don't have to be (and aren't routinely) shot up with massive antibiotics.

And while grass-fed doesn't always meet the rigorous standards for organic (though it usually does), it doesn't matter too much, because farmers who raise grass-fed animals use minimal chemicals and aren't the types to shoot their cattle up with steroids and hormones.

So, grass-fed is healthier. A *lot* healthier. And for what it's worth, here's my personal motto for dealing with the considerably greater cost: Don't eat it as much. Maybe have a half-pound burger of grass-fed meat once a week instead of seven fast-food burgers. It might be five times as expensive as "mystery" meat, but if you eat it one fifth as often, which is a good nutritional strategy anyway, the price won't make a difference.

Raw organic milk is one of the great health foods of all time.

The Truth about Cow's Milk

Full disclosure (and no surprise to anyone who's read my other books): I'm not a fan of milk. Well, that's not entirely true. I'm a huge fan, a rabid fan, an ecstatic fan of raw organic milk (which we are lucky enough to be able to buy in California supermarkets). Raw organic milk is one of the great health foods of all time. Homogenized, pasteurized milk … not so much.

This is a controversial topic, and I urge you to look into it for yourself. There will be no problem finding smart, credible sources on both sides of the "pro-raw milk" and "anti-raw milk" debate. (For the most thorough and convincing arguments for raw milk, begin with www.realmilk.com and the Weston A. Price Foundation, www.westonaprice.org. For a more establishment view, try the Harvard School of Public Health website and search The Nutrition Source: Calcium and Milk.)

To my mind, the raw-milk people have a stronger argument.

Pasteurization destroys all the enzymes in milk—in fact, the test for successful pasteurization is whether there is an absence of enzymes. These enzymes help the body assimilate all body-building factors, including calcium. That is why those who drink pasteurized milk may suffer, nevertheless, from osteoporosis. Lipase in raw milk helps the body digest and utilize butterfat.

About 20 percent of the proteins in milk are whey proteins, easy to digest but very heat sensitive. They include key enzymes, specialized proteins and enzyme inhibitors, immunoglobulins (antibodies), metal-binding proteins, vitamin-binding proteins, and several growth factors.

There's a very complex class of milk proteins known as immunoglobulins (a.k.a. antibodies), which provide resistance to many viruses, bacteria, and bacterial toxins and may help reduce the severity of asthma symptoms. Studies have shown significant loss of these important disease fighters when milk is heated to normal processing temperatures.

One reason people who are lactose intolerant often do just fine with raw organic milk is that it contains lactose-digesting *Lactobacilli* bacteria. And the end result of lactose digestion is lactic acid, a substance that boosts absorption of calcium, phosphorus, and iron and makes milk proteins more digestible in the bargain.

So, that's how I feel about milk.

But I recognize that not everyone is going to share my enthusiasm.

We've included milk in a lot of the recipes because it's traditional, people will use it anyway, and because even though I'm not a fan of it, the small amounts in these recipes will hardly kill you.

And if raw milk doesn't float your boat, I urge you to at least investigate some of the very tasty vegan milk alternatives such as almond milk and rice milk.

Addendum Note from Chef Jeannette: Though rice milk is the mildest and most easily digested of all the vegan milks, I don't suggest it as an option in the recipes because it has a fairly high glycemic load, and you can do better. My all-around favorite for ingredients, taste, and protein/carb ratio is almond milk. My favorite for nutrition and "whole food" integrity is hemp milk (read more about hemp milk on page 56), but the flavor is heavy. My favorite for high protein is soy milk, but many people are understandably leery of too much soy, especially processed soy. Pick your milk based on your priorities. For all of them, organic versions will be cleaner, and always look for unsweetened: Nobody needs a sweetener added to their milk!

(continued on page 20)

The Best Oils for the Job

OIL	HEAT	PRIMARY TYPE OF OIL	SMOKE POINT	FLAVOR	IDEAL FOR	HEALTH BENEFITS
Almond	High	Monounsaturated	430°F (221°C)	Nutty	Sautéing, stir-frying, searing, baking	High in omega-3 essential fatty acids
Avocado	High	Monounsaturated	510°F (226°C)	Mild, Neutral	Making popcorn	High in Vitamins A, B_1, B_2, D, and E
Clarified Butter (ghee)	Medium-high	Saturated	350°F (180°C)	Slightly nutty flavor	Any type of cooking	Enhances digestion
Coconut	Medium-high	90 percent saturated	350°F (180°C)	Mild, distinct odor	Baking	Antiviral, antibacterial properties
Fish	No	Polyunsaturated	n/a	Fishy	Protein shakes	Reduces cholestrol and inflammation
Flaxseed	Low/no	Polyunsaturated	225°F (107°C)	Nutty	Drizzle on salads or vegetables	Highest plant source of omega-3s
Hempseed	Medium	Polyunsaturated	330°F (165°C)	Mild, nutty	Salads, protein shakes, and vegetable juices	Rich in essential fatty acids
Macadamia Nut	Medium-high	Monounsaturated	390°F (195°C)	Mellow, nutty flavor	Salads	High in antioxidants and vitamin D
Olive	Medium	Monounsaturated	Unrefined extra-virgin 320°F (160°C)	Neutral	Salads, cooking	High in antioxidants
Peanut	High	Monounsaturated some polyunsaturated and saturated	Refined, 450°F (230°C) Unrefined, 320°F (160°C)	Peanut	Stir-frying, sautéing	Resistant to rancidity
Sesame	High	Monounsaturated and polyunsaturated	Refined, 410°F (210°C) Unrefined, 350°F (180°C)	Sesame	Stir-frying, Asian salads	High in vitamin E, detoxifying properties
Walnut	Medium	Polyunsaturated	320°F (160°C)	Walnut	Drizzle on salads and vegetables	High in omega-3 fatty acids

Extra-Virgin Olive Oil

We recommend extra-virgin olive oil exclusively, for two reasons. One, the flavor is way better. Two, so is the nutrition.

Virgin olive oil is obtained only from the olive, the fruit of the olive tree, using solely mechanical or other physical means that don't alter the oil in any way. It has not undergone any treatment other than washing, decanting, centrifuging, and filtering. It hasn't undergone chemical processing or high heat, which can destroy flavor and, equally important, vitamins, minerals, and the delicate and rich array of polyphenols that are largely responsible for the health benefits of olive oil in the first place.

The "extra" in extra-virgin means that the oil undergoes extensive lab and taste testing to meet certain standards that ensure only the highest-quality olive oils are labeled "extra virgin." Plain old (nonvirgin) olive oil is usually a blend of refined and virgin oils, has been chemically treated, and is probably significantly lower in all the good stuff we use olive oil for. Refined olive oil is utterly useless for anything but greasing the garage door.

Use the good stuff. It tastes better and it's better for you.

Cooking Oil Spray

You'll see references to "cooking oil spray" throughout the recipes. This is called for when the recipe requires a superlight, all-over coating of oil, usually for nonstick purposes in a baking pan or on a grill. Most of the commercially available spray oils are made with canola oil, and some use aerosols, both of which we frown on. You can find high-quality organic olive oil sprays in nonaerosol cans, so those can work well for savory dishes that require medium heat or lower.

For a neutrally flavored or high-heat oil, however, we recommend that you buy your own high-quality oils and put them into an oil mister yourself. A stainless steel oil mister is pretty inexpensive to purchase at a kitchen supply store or a bed and bath store (they generally range from $10 to $15), is reusable, and has a pump that allows you to prime for each spray without any harmful pressurized gases.

Good oils for high-heat spraying include peanut and almond oils. For neutrally flavored high-heat dishes, we recommend rice bran oil or avocado oil. Coconut oil solidifies in cooler temperatures, so it does not do well in a mister.

If you don't wish to purchase a mister, you can get away with wiping a light coating of oil on your cooking surface with a paper towel. But if you cook a lot, we recommend investing in a mister or two to save a few trees.

Wild-Caught Salmon

There are a lot of reasons to choose wild salmon over farm-raised. Wild salmon grows naturally, free of artificial diets and chemicals. It gets its pink color from dining on nutritious crustaceans known as krill, which contain high levels of the powerful antioxidant astaxanthin. Farm-raised salmon get their color from dyes and chemicals in their artificial salmon chow.

Farm-raised salmon are fed grain and other stuff that isn't in their natural diet, creating higher inflammatory omega-6 content in their meat. They live their entire lives in cramped quarters. Farmed salmon has a devastating impact on the fragile marine ecosystems, as they use huge open net-cages, exposing the surrounding waters to enormous amounts of chemicals and diseases that harm marine life.

And get this: According to a 2003 report from the Environmental Working Group, farmed salmon in the United States have the highest levels of PCBs (toxic, man-made chemicals). A study in the journal *Science* in January 2004 also suggested that farmed Atlantic salmon had higher levels of PCBs and other toxins than wild Pacific salmon.

We're big fans of Vital Choice for all our wild salmon (not to mention tuna and some other goodies). Other experts, for example Dr. Andrew Weil and Dr. Christianne Northrup, agree with me. I can give Vital Choice a shameless plug because I have no financial interest in the company. You'll find a link on my website, www.jonnybowden.com, under "healthy foods" in the online store. Once you've tasted its amazing fish, flash-frozen and overnighted to you, you'll never go back to regular. Same with its canned tuna!

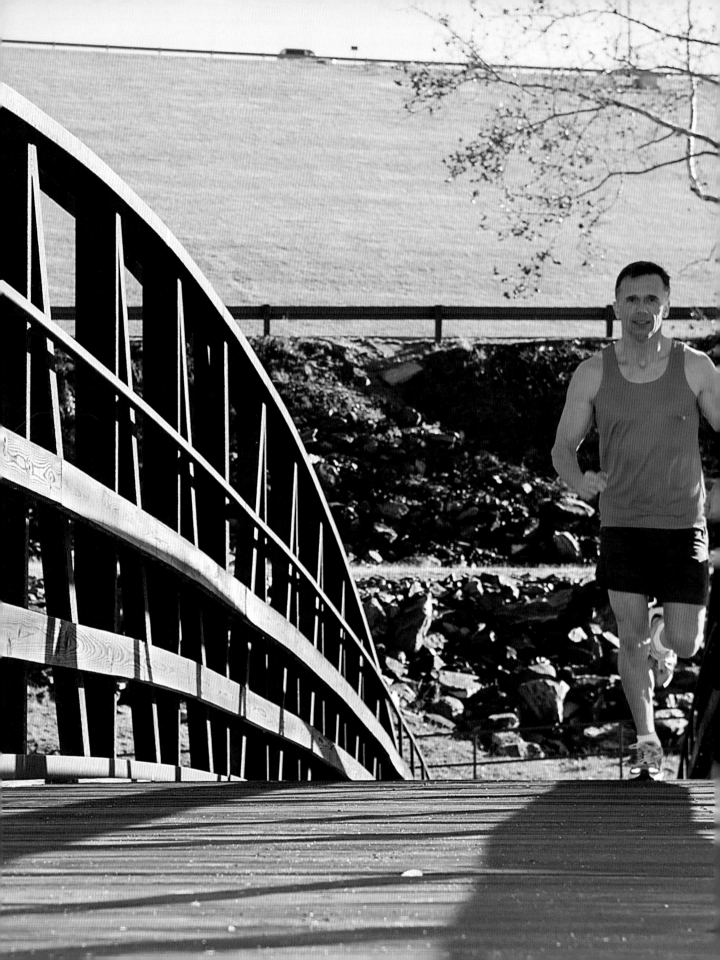

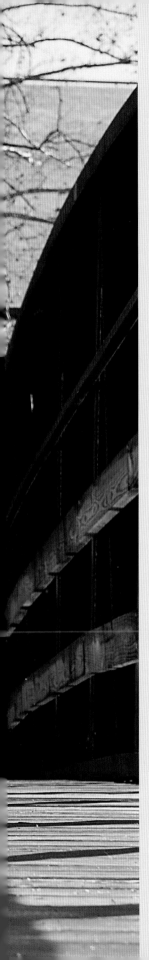

Chapter 1
Pump Up Your Heart with These Recipes

· ·

In the dozen or so times I've been asked to write magazine articles about heart-healthy foods, the editor has nearly always requested information on foods that lower cholesterol, making the assumption—as so many people do—that lowering cholesterol is the key to heart health.

It's not.

But lowering inflammation is. And the foods in these recipes do just that.

Let me explain.

Your heart is at the center of a vast network of blood vessels (veins, arteries, and capillaries) collectively called the vascular system. Because the heart and the blood vessels work so closely together, they are often collectively referred to as the cardiovascular system; another term for heart disease is cardiovascular disease.

When any of the major arteries in the body become damaged, blocked, or in some way dysfunctional, it means the heart has to work harder to pump blood through them—think of pumping water through a hose that's got a kink in it.

The major way that the vascular system becomes damaged is through chronic inflammation, which flies below the radar of pain but is ultimately at the "heart" of all cardiovascular disease. (See the Introduction.) Foods that tame the fires of inflammation are the key to a dietary program for heart health. The "real" heart-healthy foods are those that contain natural, powerful anti-inflammatory properties—apples, onions, salmon, berries, and dozens of others featured in this section. Take a look at the Heart-Friendly Veggie Parm, the Cobb Salad That Really Is Good for You, or the fabulous Longevity Lentil Loaf.

WHEN FAT IS YOUR FRIEND

One of the reasons that we feature cold-water fish such as salmon so prominently in this section is that they are a rich source of omega-3 fats. These fats—or more properly, fatty acids—are among the most anti-inflammatory compounds on the planet. In fact, that's why you'll see high-omega-3 foods in so many of the sections of this book. Inflammation, which can affect the brain, the joints, and virtually any other organ of the body, is a major player in every single degenerative disease.

Omega-3s are actually the building blocks of your body's anti-inflammatory factory. The body makes hormonelike substances called *prostaglandins* directly from fatty acids. Specifically, it makes the *inflammatory* prostaglandins from omega-6 fats (found in safflower, corn, soybean, sunflower, and other oils), and it makes *anti-inflammatory* prostaglandins from omega-3s. You need less of the former and more of the latter if you want to keep your heart (and body) healthy.

When I wrote *The 150 Healthiest Foods on Earth*, one of the criteria for inclusion of a food was that it contain natural anti-inflammatories. (That wasn't the only criteron, but it counted for a lot!) Fortunately, there are a ton of these compounds in the plant kingdom. Not to get too technical, but they're known as *phytochemicals* (phyto = plant), and they're grouped into many botanical classes, but the bottom line is that they act like plant versions of aspirin or ibuprofen. They calm the fires of inflammation, and that's the first step toward keeping your cardiovascular system in robust health.

Foods such as apples and onions, for example, are rich in a particularly potent anti-inflammatory called *quercetin*. (Check out the Hale and Hearty Apple Baked Beans—you're in for a treat!) And although more fruit and vegetable consumption in general is a great strategy for lowering the risk of heart disease and stroke (i.e., cardiovascular disease), the real superstars in the anti-inflammatory universe are green leafy veggies such as spinach and Swiss chard; members of the Brassica family such as cabbage, cauliflower, broccoli, and Brussels sprouts; and citrus fruits such as oranges and grapefruits. You'll

Highly processed foods are the handmaidens of diabetes and obesity, and both conditions strongly increase the odds of heart disease.

find many of them in the recipes that follow, for example the Low-Cal Heirloom Gazpacho or the Mahi Mahi with Macadamia Nut Crust and Peach Purée.

When it comes to keeping the heart healthy with food, you also have to consider what *not* to eat. Top of the list: highly processed foods. These foods are the handmaidens of diabetes and obesity, and both conditions strongly increase the odds of heart disease. Ditto with sugar. For that reason alone, you'll find minimum amounts of processed foods and sugar in the recipes that follow.

Earlier I mentioned that omega-6 fats are the "building blocks" of inflammatory compounds. You actually *need* some of these fats, and they're not all bad; but we eat too many of them (and not enough of the omega-3s). The recipes that follow attempt to minimize the use of vegetable oils (high in omega-6s) and balance them with more of the heart-healthy omega-9s (olive oil, macadamia nut oil) and the wonderful omega-3s (found in fish and flax).

Then there's our old nemesis cholesterol. While I have long been on record as believing that cholesterol is a vastly overrated health issue (especially compared to inflammation), I realize that many people are still deeply concerned about their cholesterol numbers. Not to worry. The foods that are known to help lower cholesterol will be found in abundance here: cold-water fish (again!), high-fiber fruits (apples), nuts, seeds, garlic, and onions. What a bonus that these foods all do "double duty" in healing and protecting the whole cardiovascular system!

NUTRIENTS YOU SHOULD KNOW

Two heart-healthy nutrients you may not have heard much about are arginine and taurine. Both are amino acids, and both play a huge role in heart health. The body uses arginine to make a phenomenal substance called *nitric oxide*. (Don't confuse this with nitrous oxide, the laughing gas of the dentist's office. It's very different!) The Nobel Prize in medicine was awarded in 1998 to the doctor who discovered the importance of nitric oxide to the health of the vascular system. It is a "signaling molecule" that regulates blood pressure and supports a healthy circulation. (Little trivia fact: Nitric oxide research ultimately led to the development of Viagra!) And arginine is the stuff out of which nitric oxide is born. That's why you'll find a ton of arginine-rich foods in this section, including nuts, seeds, eggs, fish, and crustaceans such as lobster and mussels.

Speaking of crustaceans, they're also a great source for that other nutrient you may not know about—taurine. Taurine is a natural diuretic and seems to help lower blood pressure. For many integrative nutrition–minded doctors, it's also a go-to nutrient for arrhythmia. When you're eating clams, shellfish, meat, or salmon, you're getting a nice healthy dose of the stuff.

One of the great nutrients for the heart is one you've definitely heard about, though you might not know why it's essential: potassium. Yup, the stuff found in bananas is actually something of a miracle nutrient for the heart. It's a member of a family of substances called *electrolytes* (charged ions, if you're up on your chemistry). Electrolytes conduct electricity in the body, and potassium plays a major role in the contraction of the heart. And you don't have to eat a banana to get it—it's found in all meats, some fish such as salmon (again!), and most fruits and vegetables. You'll see them all featured here.

Last but very far from least are the class of compounds known as antioxidants, also found in abundance in these recipes. Antioxidants fight damage to the heart and circulatory system in a different, but no less important, way than the anti-inflammatories. They help combat the cellular damage that occurs when you're exposed to toxins, pesticides, stress, and other bad actors. This damage takes place when rogue molecules called free radicals attack your cells (and DNA), which they do on a daily basis whether you want them to or not!

Antioxidants, such as vitamin A, zinc, selenium, vitamin C, and vitamin E, not to mention a veritable encyclopedia of those friendly phytochemicals I mentioned earlier, help stop those free radicals in their tracks. The foods in this section are loaded with them.

Enjoy!

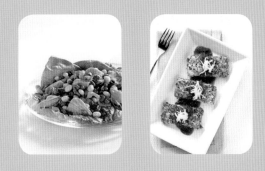

ENTRÉES

. . . .

Longevity Lemon Chicken with Kalamata Olives
Tasty Turmeric Turkey Burgers
Omega-Boost Salmon and Bean Salad
Protein-Packed Lake Trout Florentine
Mahi Mahi with Macadamia Nut Crust and Peach Purée
Unsaturated, Simple Shrimp Scampi
Heart-Friendly Veggie Parm
Longevity Lentil Loaf
Heartily Stuffed Acorn Squash
Hearty Split Pea–Sweet Potato Soup
Turkey, Wild Rice, and Cranberry Soup for the Heart and Soul

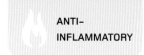

LONGEVITY LEMON CHICKEN WITH KALAMATA OLIVES

From Dr. Jonny: People who eat Mediterranean-style have significantly lower rates of just about everything you don't want, at least if you want to live long! This dish is a wonderful example of how to use Mediterranean principles in cooking. Olives and olive oil—the signature of a Mediterranean recipe—are loaded with polyphenols that protect the heart. Garlic lowers blood pressure and fights all sorts of microbes that can derail your health. The lemon, capers, and olives combine to make this a moist, tangy dish!

2 small lemons

1 whole chicken (about 4 pounds [1.8 kg]), giblets and excess fat removed, rinsed and patted completely dry

4 cloves garlic, minced

1 tablespoon (14 g) butter, softened

2 tablespoons (30 ml) olive oil

1 teaspoon oregano

1 teaspoon salt

½ teaspoon black pepper

2 red onions, skinned and quartered, divided

1 cup Kalamata olives, drained (100 g)

2 tablespoons (17.2 g) capers

1½ cups chicken broth (355 ml)

FROM CHEF JEANNETTE:

Various schools of thought differ about how best to roast a chicken. Some say roast at a high temperature for less time with frequent basting, others opt for the low temperature–longer-time-on-a-V-rack approach. My favorite no-fuss way to get perfect chicken every time with crispy skin and moist, tender meat is to use a clay pot. It's a no-brainer way to roast meats. Soak the terra cotta lid for about 10 minutes in cold water, replace it on the cooker, and place them on the lowest rack in a cold oven set to 425°F (220°C, gas mark 7). An hour to 90 minutes later, and voila! You have the perfect roast! If you have a clay cooker (I love my Schlemmer Topf!), use it to roast this dish for 75 minutes. You won't be disappointed!

Preheat oven to 325°F (170°C, or gas mark 3).

Lightly oil a shallow roasting pan with olive oil.

Zest one lemon and cut it into thin, half-moon slices.

Moving carefully so as not to puncture the skin, work your hand between the chicken skin and breasts as far as you can go, separating the skin from meat. Gently slide the lemon slices into the pockets you just created, dividing them evenly over the breasts.

Cut the remaining lemon into quarters and squeeze the juice into the breast pockets and cavity.

Place the squeezed lemon quarters and 1 prepared onion into the chicken cavity.

In a small bowl, mix together the zest, garlic, butter, olive oil, oregano, salt, and pepper. Using your hands, smear the mixture evenly over the skin of the entire chicken.

Place the prepared chicken into the prepared roasting pan, breast side up.

Surround the chicken with the remaining onion quarters, olives, and capers, and pour the broth gently into the bottom of the pan.

Bake for 75 to 90 minutes (depending on the size of the chicken, roughly 20 minutes per pound at this temperature) until the chicken thigh reads 180°F (82°C) on a meat thermometer.

Yield: 6 portions

Per Serving: 570 Calories; 42g Fat (66.6% calories from fat); 40g Protein; 7g Carbohydrate; 1g Dietary Fiber; 204mg Cholesterol; 963mg Sodium

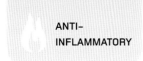
TASTY TURMERIC TURKEY BURGERS

From Dr. Jonny: This curried turkey burger is brimming with longevity ingredients such as yogurt and curry powder, which contains the superspice turmeric, a natural anti-inflammatory and anticancer compound, plus oats and eggs. Not a life-shortening trans fat in sight. The combination of spices, especially the ginger with the curry and mustard, will make you forget you ever heard the phrase "Do you want fries with that?"

High-heat cooking oil spray

1 pound (455 g) lean ground turkey

½ cup (40 g) quick-cooking oats

¼ cup (25 g) chopped scallions

1 tablespoon (15 g) Dijon mustard

1 clove garlic, minced

1 tablespoon (6 g) minced ginger

1 teaspoon (2g) curry powder

½ teaspoon cumin

½ teaspoon salt

½ teaspoon black pepper

1 egg, beaten

SAUCE

⅓ cup (77 g) plain yogurt (cow or soy)

¾ teaspoon curry powder

2 tablespoons (2 g) minced fresh cilantro

1 teaspoon fresh-squeezed lemon juice

1 teaspoon maple syrup, optional

Preheat grill or grill pan to medium heat.

In a large bowl, combine turkey, oats, scallions, mustard, garlic, ginger, curry, cumin, salt, pepper, and egg, and mix well, using your (clean!) hands if necessary. Divide mixture into 4 equal portions and form patties.

Coat a grill or grill pan with cooking oil spray and cook burgers until browned, 5 to 6 minutes per side. An instant meat thermometer should read 165°F (74°C).

While the burgers are cooking, whisk together the yogurt, curry powder, cilantro, lemon juice, and syrup, if using, in a small bowl.

Drizzle cooked burgers with sauce, to taste.

Yield: 4 burgers

Per Serving: 245 Calories; 11g Fat (39.6% calories from fat); 28g Protein; 10g Carbohydrate; 2g Dietary Fiber; 129mg Cholesterol; 424mg Sodium

FROM CHEF JEANNETTE:

These lean longevity burgers are great with lettuce and tomato on whole-wheat buns or whole-grain wraps. They're also good atop a fresh green salad if you want to avoid the starch altogether.

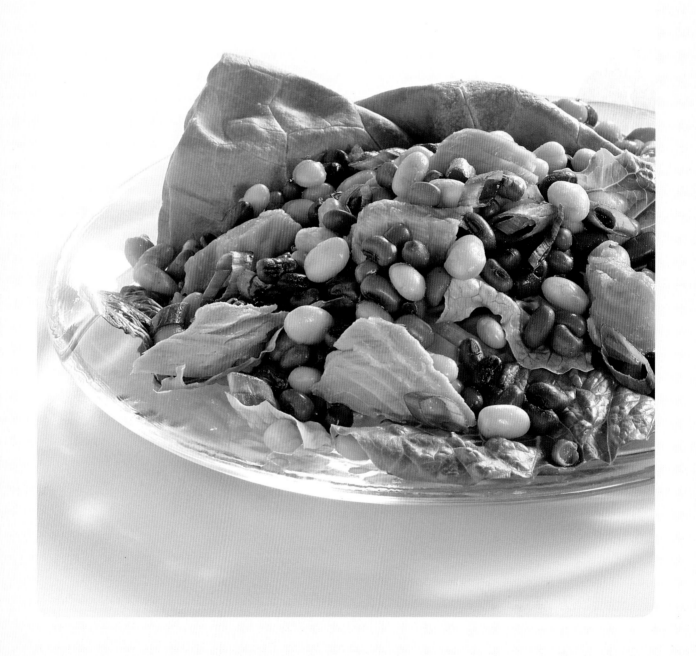

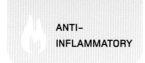

OMEGA-BOOST SALMON AND BEAN SALAD

From Dr. Jonny: Remember the saying "Beans, beans, good for the heart"? Well, it's true. And it's even truer when you combine beans with wild salmon. You get omega-3s from the fish—the best thing in the world for the heart and brain—and a ton of fiber from the beans. What could be bad? And if you're wondering what mirin is, it's a kind of rice wine used as an essential condiment in Japanese cuisine. (And it knocks out any fishy smell!) This light, no-cook dish has a nice Asian flair and is great for a summer evening dinner or a quick lunch anytime.

2 romaine hearts or 1 head Boston lettuce

2 teaspoons (10 ml) toasted sesame oil

1 tablespoon (15 ml) raw sesame oil

1 tablespoon (15 ml) mirin

1 tablespoon (15 ml) unseasoned rice vinegar

Juice of 1 lime (about 2 tablespoons [30ml])

1 teaspoon tamari

¼ teaspoon salt

1 can (7.5 ounces, or 214 g) wild Alaskan salmon
(we like Vital Choice), drained

1 can (15 ounces, or 400 g) navy beans, rinsed
and drained

1 cup (100 g) cooked adzuki beans, rinsed and drained if
using canned

¼ cup (25 g) diced scallions, bulbs removed

Wash the lettuce and separate the leaves. Arrange leaves into a bed in a salad bowl.

In a large bowl, whisk together sesame oils, mirin, rice vinegar, lime juice, tamari, and salt. Add salmon and break chunks apart into flakes with a fork. Add beans and scallions. Toss gently to combine well and spoon over lettuce bed.

Yield: 4 servings

Per Serving: 382 Calories; 5g Fat (10.9% calories from fat); 22g Protein; 64g Carbohydrate; 6g Dietary Fiber; 28mg Cholesterol; 821mg Sodium

FROM CHEF JEANNETTE:

Tuna salad is a favorite American lunch dish, but the heavy mayo typically used cancels out some of the longevity benefits of the fish. For a heart-healthy upgrade, try this version with salmon for the increased omega-3s and this lighter, more flavorful seed-oil dressing for a further boost of healthy fats. It makes a great wrap, too.

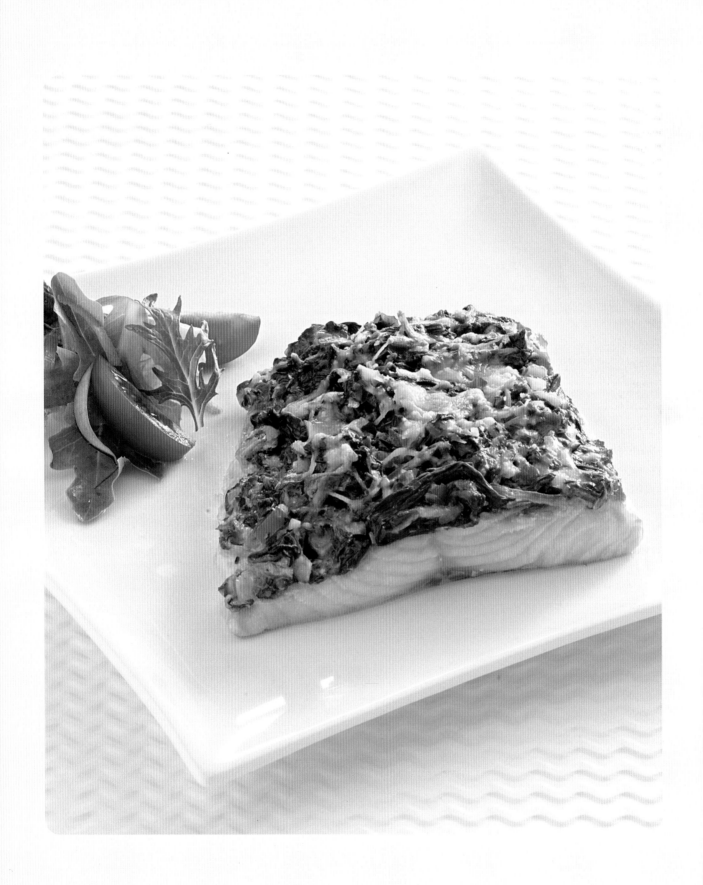

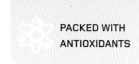
PROTEIN-PACKED LAKE TROUT FLORENTINE

From Dr. Jonny: By now, almost everyone knows that fish is great for the heart (and just about every other organ in the body as well). This recipe offers a healthy twist by replacing the classic butter and flour béchamel sauce with a high-protein tofu base. There's not a "bad" ingredient in the mix. The rich mix of antioxidants from the spinach helps fight oxidative damage (one of the Four Horsemen!) and nicely complements the protein from the fish and tofu. The mix of colors—yellow onions, red peppers, and green leafies—guarantees a panoply of phytonutrients that protect against inflammation (another of the Four Horsemen). Those colors, known as *anthocyanins*, protect the plant from free-radical damage, and they'll do the same for your heart. By the way, love that Parmesan cheese topping!

---

1 cup (235 ml) milk (cow's or unsweetened plain soy or almond milk)

⅓ cup (153 g) soft silken tofu, drained

½ teaspoon nutritional yeast*

2 teaspoons (10 ml) rice bran oil or olive oil

¼ cup (40 g) minced yellow onion

1 teaspoon dry sherry, optional

1½ tablespoons (14 g) minced red bell pepper

1 teaspoon fish bouillon (or use vegetable; we like organic Better than Bouillon)

½ teaspoon salt

¼ teaspoon fresh-ground black pepper

1 package (10 ounces, or 280 g) frozen spinach, thawed and drained well (squeezing against fine mesh sieve to remove excess liquid)

4 skinned lake trout fillets (6 ounces, or 170 g, each), rinsed and patted dry

2 tablespoons (10 g) fresh-grated Parmesan cheese

¼ cup (60 ml) dry white wine

Preheat the oven to 375°F (190°C, or gas mark 5).

In a food processor or blender, process milk, tofu, and yeast until very smooth and set aside.

Heat oil in medium sauté pan over medium heat. Add onion and sauté 2 minutes.

Add sherry, if using, and cook an additional 2 minutes. Add bell pepper and sauté about 2 minutes or until slightly softened. Add milk mixture, bouillon, salt, and pepper, and mix to combine. Remove from heat and stir in spinach.

Lightly oil a baking pan and lay out the fish fillets. Spoon the mixture evenly over all 4 fillets. Sprinkle Parmesan evenly over all and pour the wine into the baking pan.

Bake uncovered until the fish flakes and spinach centers are hot throughout, about 20 to 30 minutes.

Yield: 4 servings

Per Serving: 372 Calories; 18g Fat (44.0% calories from fat); 43g Protein; 8g Carbohydrate; 3g Dietary Fiber; 109mg Cholesterol; 494mg Sodium

*Nutritional yeast is available at your local health food store and many natural grocers. It is nutrient rich and imparts a depth of flavor similar to the umami of soy sauce and certain cheeses or mushrooms. It is frequently used with tofu and nondairy milks in many vegan recipes to provide a "cheesy" quality to the taste of the dish. If you can't find nutritional yeast, you can replace it with about six raw cashews, ground into a powder.

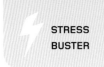
MAHI MAHI WITH MACADAMIA NUT CRUST AND PEACH PURÉE

From Dr. Jonny: You want heart health? We'll give you heart health—the power combo of the two healthiest fats on earth, omega-3s and omega-9s! Macadamia nuts are loaded with the latter and the fish have a nice dollop of the former. As for coconut oil, well, studies of the Trobriand Islanders in Papua New Guinea who eat the majority of their calories from coconut found that these folks had virtually no heart disease. The kudzu is a nice touch—it contains a number of useful compounds including some that are anti-inflammatory, antimicrobial, and possibly cancer-preventive. This dish has a rich, nutty flavor with a surprising burst of peaches. And who doesn't love peaches?

Cooking oil spray

1 tablespoon (15 ml) coconut or macadamia nut oil

4 skinless mahi mahi fillets (6 ounces, or 170 g each)

Sprinkle salt

Sprinkle fresh-ground black pepper

¾ cup (101 g) macadamia nuts, chopped fine

5 large, fresh, ripe peaches, peeled, pitted and sliced, (or one 10-ounce or 280-g bag frozen peaches, thawed)

1 tablespoon (15 ml) coconut oil

2 tablespoons (12 g) minced ginger

1 tablespoon (15 ml) wet sweetener (thawed frozen pineapple, orange, or apple juice concentrate; agave nectar; or rice syrup)

1 tablespoon (8 g) kudzu, optional for very juicy peaches

2 tablespoons (28 ml) water

Preheat the oven to 425°F (220°C, or gas mark 7).

Prepare a broiling pan with a small amount of spray in 4 places for each of the fish fillets.

In a large sauté pan, heat the coconut or macadamia oil over high heat. Rinse the fish pieces and pat dry. Season with salt and pepper and place the fish bottoms-down in the sauté pan. Sear the fish on 1 side until nicely browned, about 2 to 3 minutes.

Transfer the fish to the broiling pan, seared bottoms down. Evenly distribute the nuts over the tops of the fish pieces. Roast until fish is opaque, but still moist on the inside, checking frequently, about 8 to 10 minutes, depending on the thickness of the fillets. If the nuts become too brown before the fish is done, cover loosely with foil and reduce oven temperature to 375°F (190°C, or gas mark 5).

While the fish is cooking, prepare the sauce. Blend peaches in blender or food processor to purée consistency.

Heat the coconut oil in a medium sauté pan over medium heat. Add the ginger and sauté for about 2 minutes. Add peach purée and sweetener and bring to a low simmer. If the purée is runny, mix kudzu in water to dissolve and stir into simmering purée for about 30 seconds or until mixture thickens slightly. Remove from heat and drizzle lightly over roasted fish.

Yield: 4 servings

Per Serving: 429 Calories; 27g Fat (55.2% calories from fat); 34g Protein; 15g Carbohydrate; 4g Dietary Fiber; 124mg Cholesterol; 152mg Sodium

FROM CHEF JEANNETTE:

This recipe was originally conceived using delicious, fleshy Chilean sea bass. We have since learned, however, that the breed is being severely overfished and many of the fishermen are using equipment that ensnares seabirds. We switched it for the more eco-conscious mahi mahi, and it is just as delicious—and nutritious.

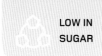

UNSATURATED, SIMPLE SHRIMP SCAMPI

From Dr. Jonny: I love scampi. It's light and delicious, but the traditional versions are swimming in oil and butter. (Not that there's anything wrong with that!) Here's a great alternative to the garden-variety scampi dishes, especially for those who are concerned about saturated fat. This easy, ultralight version is high on protein, low on saturated fat, and very high on taste! Garlic is one of the oldest medicinal foods on the planet, the cooked tomatoes add a ton of antioxidants, and the whole dish is just perfection as a summer evening meal. Tip: If you're interested in low-carbing it, see Chef Jeannette's hint about replacing all (or some) of the pasta with veggies. Pure genius!

1 pound (455 g) fresh, whole-wheat fettuccine, optional*

2 tablespoons (28 ml) olive oil

1 pound (455 g) large fresh shrimp, shelled and deveined

Pinch salt and 1 grind black pepper

3 large cloves garlic, minced

1 cup (180 g) diced fresh tomatoes, whatever is in season

1½ tablespoons (25 ml) fresh-squeezed lemon juice

½ teaspoon lemon zest

½ cup (120 ml) dry white wine

2 tablespoons (8 g) chopped fresh parsley

If using pasta, bring a large pot of salted water to a boil. Fresh whole-grain pasta will only take about 2 minutes to cook, so you will want to put it into the water just before the shrimp is ready so you can drain it and immediately add prepared scampi.

Heat olive oil in medium sauté pan over medium heat. Add shrimp, salt, and pepper, and sauté 1 to 2 minutes until they begin to turn pink, flipping them occasionally.

Add the garlic and sauté 30 seconds. Remove shrimp from pan and set aside. Add tomatoes and sauté 1 minute. Add lemon juice, zest, and white wine, and bring to a light simmer for a couple of minutes until the wine is reduced. Return shrimp to the pan and simmer until they are cooked through but still tender, just a minute or two.

Toss lightly with parsley and serve over hot pasta or with grilled veggies.

Yield: 4–6 servings

Per Serving: 393 Calories; 6g Fat (13.8% calories from fat); 23g Protein; 59g Carbohydrate; 4g Dietary Fiber; 115mg Cholesterol; 135mg Sodium

*You may leave out the pasta altogether if you'd prefer a low-carb dish. For the healthiest version, serve the scampi with grilled summer veggie shish kebab: Try 1-inch (2.5-cm) chunks of bell pepper, summer squash, sweet onion, zucchini, and mushrooms, lightly oiled and seasoned with salt and fresh-ground black pepper. Grill them over medium-high heat for 7 to 10 minutes for a grilled-but-still-hearty feel.

FROM CHEF JEANNETTE:

This is a quick-cooking dish—overcooking will result in rubbery shrimp, not the effect we're looking for in a fresh scampi! Prepare and measure all your ingredients before starting to cook to keep things moving right along.

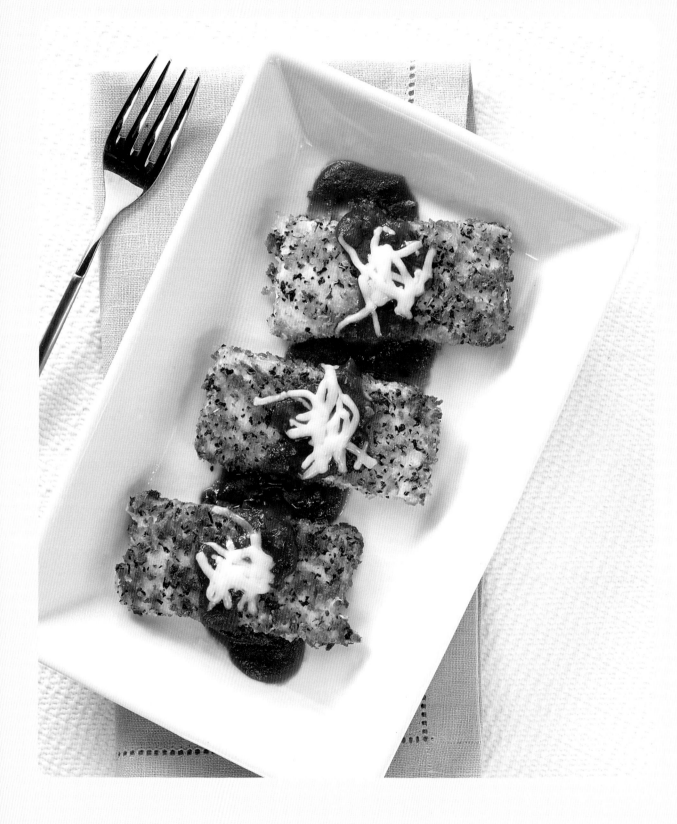

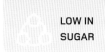
HEART-FRIENDLY VEGGIE PARM

From Dr. Jonny: Every time I go out with my beloved niece, she orders her favorite dish, "chicken parm" (apparently a favorite of teenagers everywhere). Actually, chicken parm crosses the generational barrier, as just about everyone loves it as a comfort food! This dish, however, is just so much better for you than the traditional version. You'll never miss the fat from the frying, and believe it or not, the texture is very close to chicken. Unlike chicken parm from the local take-out, there's not an ingredient in this mix that isn't good for the heart. Here's a test: Try serving it at home without telling anyone it's a "healthier" version of the old favorite and see whether anyone notices the difference. Bonus points—it'll pass muster with the growing population of vegetarian teens!

High-heat cooking oil spray

1 package (12.3 ounces, or 340 g) extra-firm tofu

SAUCE

1 can (14.5 ounces, or 413 g) puréed tomatoes

2 tablespoons (32 g) tomato paste

2 cloves garlic, minced

1 teaspoon dried oregano

¼ cup (10 g) chopped fresh basil (or 1 teaspoon dried)

½ teaspoon salt

¼ teaspoon red pepper flakes or fresh-ground black pepper

2 tablespoons (28 ml) red wine

TOFU

¾ cup (90 g) whole-wheat or whole-wheat panko bread crumbs

2 tablespoons (10 g) fresh-grated Parmesan cheese

½ teaspoon onion powder

½ teaspoon garlic powder

¾ teaspoon dried oregano

¾ teaspoon dried basil

1 egg, beaten

2 tablespoons (28 ml) olive oil

½ teaspoon salt

¾ teaspoon fresh-ground black pepper

¼ cup (25 g) fresh-grated Parmesan cheese

¼ cup (30 g) shredded mozzarella cheese

(continued on next page)

FROM CHEF JEANNETTE:

If you're running short on time, you can use a high-quality prepared sauce instead of making your own. You can serve this dish traditionally, over a small amount of whole-grain angel hair pasta, but for the best low-carb, low-cal, longevity version, try it over roasted and separated spaghetti squash. And don't forget a huge green salad!

Drain tofu and place between 2 plates. Place heavy cans on top plate and let sit for 20 minutes to 1 hour to remove excess water.

Preheat the oven to 375°F (190°C, or gas mark 5).

In the meantime, coat a 9 x 13-inch (23 x 33-cm) baking pan with cooking oil spray. Set aside.

For sauce: In a small saucepan over low heat, mix together puréed tomatoes, tomato paste, garlic, oregano, basil, salt, pepper, and red wine. Allow to warm as you prepare and cook the tofu.

For the tofu: In a small bowl mix together bread crumbs, cheese, onion powder, garlic powder, oregano, and basil. Pour bread crumb mixture into shallow dish with sides, such as a pie plate.

Place beaten egg in a shallow bowl or lipped plate.

Using a cheese slicer or sharp chef's knife, slice the tofu lengthwise very thinly, into 6 approximately ¼-inch (0.5-cm) slices.

Heat the 2 tablespoons of olive oil in large skillet over medium heat.

Pat each tofu slice gently with paper towel to remove any remaining moisture.

Season each slice with salt and pepper, dip into the egg, then press into the crumb mixture, coating all sides well.

In 2 batches, lightly fry the tofu in the hot skillet until evenly browned on both sides, about 3 minutes per side.

Make a thin layer of sauce on the bottom of the prepared baking pan. Lay the tofu out in a single layer on the sauce. Cover with remaining sauce and sprinkle cheeses over the top. Bake for 15 to 20 minutes until hot throughout and cheese is melted.

Yield: 4 servings

Per Serving: 349 Calories; 19g Fat (46.9% calories from fat); 20g Protein; 27g Carbohydrate; 3g Dietary Fiber; 67mg Cholesterol; 899mg Sodium

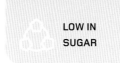

LONGEVITY LENTIL LOAF

From Dr. Jonny: My mother wasn't much of a cook, but she did make meat loaf. Unfortunately, she used factory-farmed meat, with its usual accompaniments—steroids, antibiotics, and hormones. This lentil loaf is a whole different ball game. The benefits of legumes and lentils are legion for the heart—more fiber, more nutrients, and none of the bad stuff! And lentils are surprisingly quick cooking. The oats provide more fiber, which may help lower cholesterol. The combo of lentils, olive oil, onion, and garlic make this a longevity dream!

LOAF

Cooking oil spray

1 tablespoon (15 ml) olive oil

1 large onion, diced fine

2 cloves garlic, minced

1 carrot, peeled and diced fine

1½ cups (288 g) dried lentils, rinsed*

4 cups (950 ml) vegetable stock plus 2 cups (475 ml) water

1 bay leaf

1 cup (80 g) rolled oats

¾ cup (4 ounces, or 113 g) crumbled feta cheese

2 tablespoons (28 ml) fresh-squeezed lemon juice

1 teaspoon lemon zest

2 tablespoons (12 g) minced fresh mint

1 teaspoon dried thyme

2 tablespoons chopped fresh parsley (8 g) or cilantro (2 g)

¾ teaspoon garlic powder

¾ teaspoon sea salt

⅛ teaspoon black pepper

1 large egg, beaten

SAUCE

3 red bell peppers, halved and seeded

1 tablespoon (15 ml) balsamic vinegar

½ teaspoon olive oil

¼ teaspoon each salt and cracked black pepper

* Cut the prep time by using canned cooked lentils (drained and rinsed) and a jar of prepared roasted red peppers. Sauté the onion and carrots for 10 to 12 minutes or until soft, adding the garlic in for the last minute. Stir in the lentils and sauté for a minute or two, stirring well to combine. Skip the pepper-roasting step and follow the rest of the directions.

Preheat oven to high broil.

Heat oil in a soup pot over medium heat. Add onion and sauté 5 minutes. Add garlic and sauté 1 minute. Add carrot and sauté 1 minute. Add lentils and cover all generously with stock and additional water, if necessary. Add bay leaf, increase heat, and bring to a boil. Lower heat to a simmer, cover, and cook for 25 to 35 minutes or until lentils are tender. Drain all and discard bay leaf.

While lentils are cooking, make the sauce. Lay the cut peppers face down on a broiling sheet. Broil for 10 to 15 minutes until they are charred all over. Remove from heat and place in a bowl, covering tightly with plastic wrap for about 10 minutes until they are cool enough to handle. Set the oven to 350°F (180°C, or gas mark 4).

Slip skins off with your hands and place peeled peppers, vinegar, olive oil, salt, and pepper into food processor or blender. Process until smooth, scraping down the sides if necessary. Set aside.

Spray a standard loaf pan with cooking oil and set aside. In a large mixing bowl, combine cooked lentil mixture, oats, cheese, lemon juice and zest, herbs, garlic powder, salt, and pepper and mix well to combine. Add egg and mix thoroughly to bind. Spoon mixture into prepared loaf pan to make a loaf shape and bake for 40 to 50 minutes until cooked through, covering lightly with foil for last 10 minutes if top becomes too brown. Pour sauce over individual portions and serve.

Yield: 4 to 6 generous servings (1 loaf)

Per Serving: 347 Calories; 10g Fat (24.3% calories from fat); 20g Protein; 48g Carbohydrate; 18g Dietary Fiber; 52mg Cholesterol; 1228mg Sodium

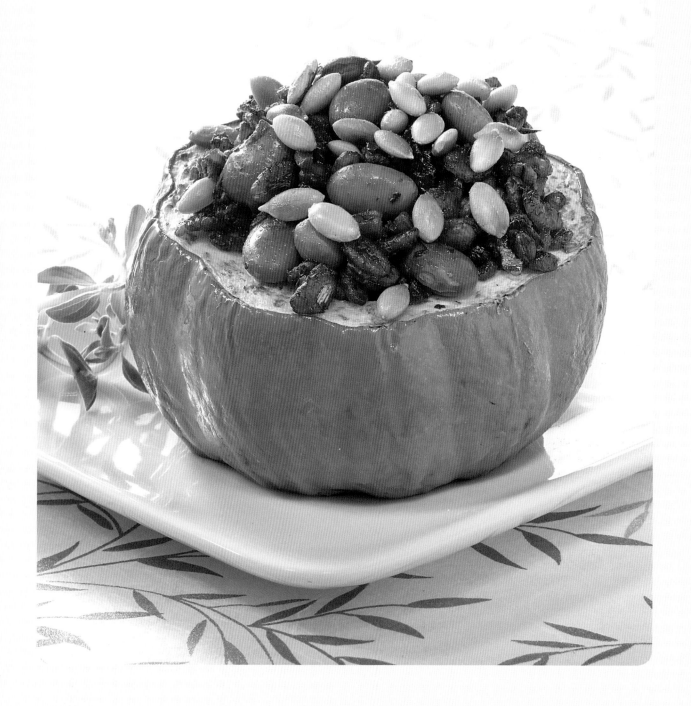

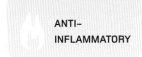

ANTI-
INFLAMMATORY

HEARTILY STUFFED ACORN SQUASH

From Dr. Jonny: Here's a heart-healthy, long-life recipe for squash, one of my favorite vegetables. Squash always reminds me of sweet potatoes—they share similar textures and colors, and both are terrific sources of immune-boosting vitamin A. Both barley and beans are high in fiber, especially a kind of soluble fiber called *beta-glucan*, which binds with cholesterol to help lower LDL, the "villainous" flavor of cholesterol your doctor is always nagging you about. Chef Jeannette added a light combo of Mexi-spices and delicious pumpkin seeds that make this dish a real treat.

High–heat cooking oil spray

⅓ cup (60 g) pearl barley (quick–cooking okay)

2 large acorn squash

1 tablespoon (15 ml) olive oil

1 small white onion, diced fine

1 clove garlic, minced

1 teaspoon dried oregano

½ teaspoon ground cumin

¼ teaspoon chili powder

1 cup (171 g) cooked pinto beans, drained and rinsed (if using canned)

1½ tablespoons (25 ml) tamari

¼ cup (35 g) pepitas (roasted pumpkin seeds)

Cook barley according to package directions, or use 1 cup (157 g) of precooked barley (regular pearl barley will cook in about 50 minutes, quick-cooking takes about 15 minutes).

Remove the stems and slice the squash in half, lengthwise. With a heavy spoon, scoop out all fibers and seeds.

Preheat the oven to 400°F (200°C, or gas mark 6). Lightly coat a baking pan with cooking oil spray or use a cooking rack, and place the acorn halves in/on it face up.

On the stovetop, heat the olive oil over medium in a large sauté pan. Add the onion and sauté for 4 minutes. Add garlic, oregano, cumin, and chili powder and sauté 3 to 4 more minutes until onions are soft and starting to caramelize. Stir in cooked barley, pinto beans, and

tamari, and gently stir to combine. Reduce heat to low and continue to cook for about 7 minutes until mixture is heated through and flavors have combined.

Spoon bean and barley mixture evenly into acorn halves, taking care not to let any drop into the pan (it will burn). Tightly cover the pan with aluminum foil and place in preheated oven.

Cook for 45 to 50 minutes until squash is soft when pierced with a fork.

Sprinkle pepitas evenly over 4 halves and serve.

Yield: 4 large servings

Per serving: 261 Calories; 6g Fat (18.8% calories from fat); 7g Protein; 49g Carbohydrate; 9g Dietary Fiber; 0mg Cholesterol; 294mg Sodium

FROM CHEF JEANNETTE:

This dish is both filling and satisfying. With its complement of high-fiber and high-protein ingredients, it makes an excellent vegetarian entrée. Pair it with a leafy green or a dark salad for a great fall or winter lunch or dinner. Reducing the overall meat content of your meals by replacing it with nutrient-dense vegetarian alternatives can extend your life by helping to protect your precious heart and veins.

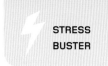

HEARTY SPLIT PEA–SWEET POTATO SOUP

From Dr. Jonny: You could just about live on this soup. (And I did for about two days!) Traditional split pea soup is made with ham, which I usually don't recommend because it's high in sodium and almost always from factory-farmed animals. This version is not only low in fat (if you care about that) but high in heart-friendly fiber and potassium—and that's something you don't often see in soup, especially soup that tastes this good. The mellow sweetness of the sweet potatoes compensates for the conventional saltiness of the ham—you'll never miss it. And split peas are a great vegetarian source of protein.

2 tablespoons (28 ml) olive oil

1 large Vidalia onion, diced

2 cloves garlic, crushed and chopped

4 medium carrots, sliced into thin rounds

1 large stalk celery, cut into thirds

1 large sweet potato, peeled and cut into
    ½-inch (1-cm) cubes

½ teaspoon dried thyme

1 pound (455 g) split peas, sorted, rinsed, and drained

8 cups (2 L) vegetable or chicken broth

¼ to ½ teaspoon red pepper flakes, to taste

1 package (10 ounces, or 280 g) frozen spinach, thawed
    but not drained

Salt, to taste, optional

2 tablespoons (28 ml) lemon juice or cooking sherry

Heat oil over medium heat in a large, heavy-bottom soup pot. Add onion, garlic, carrot, and celery, and sauté for about 5 minutes. Reduce heat to low and cook for 10 minutes, stirring often. Add sweet potato and thyme and sauté for about 2 minutes. Add split peas, broth, and red pepper flakes; increase heat to medium high, and bring to a boil. Reduce heat to medium low and cook, covered, for 1 hour. Remove the celery pieces, stir in the spinach and salt, if using, and cook, uncovered, for 10 to 20 minutes until soup reaches desired thickness. Stir in lemon juice (or sherry). Remove from heat and purée partially with immersion blender (or in a regular blender) to desired consistency.

SLOW-COOKER VARIATION

Combine all ingredients except spinach, salt, and lemon. Cover and cook on low for 7 to 8 hours or on high for 4 to 5 hours. Add spinach and salt for last 30 minutes of cook time. Stir in lemon juice just before serving.

Add additional water if soup is too thick.

Yield: about 8 cups

Per Serving: 443 Calories; 8g Fat (16.2% calories from fat); 22g Protein; 73g Carbohydrate; 21g Dietary Fiber; 3mg Cholesterol; 1772mg Sodium

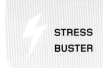
TURKEY, WILD RICE, AND CRANBERRY SOUP FOR THE HEART AND SOUL

From Dr. Jonny: Turkey is a healthy source of protein, but try to find one that is free range—it's easier than you might think because lots of organic turkey farms exist around the country. The longevity quotient of this satisfyingly rich soup is increased by the additions of the unexpected tart cranberries, loaded with cell-protecting plant chemicals called anthocyanins. What a great way to get cranberries into heavy rotation on your longevity diet!

2 tablespoons (60 ml) olive oil

3 large shallots, diced

2 medium carrots, peeled and cut into ½-inch (1.5 cm) rounds

4 cups (950 ml) chicken broth or turkey stock

1 teaspoon (5 ml) organic chicken Better than Bouillon

2 tablespoons (60 ml) marsala wine

½ teaspoon tarragon

¼ teaspoon thyme

1/3 cup (53 g) wild rice

8–10 ounces (225–280 g) turkey tenderloin or cutlets (or 1 large chicken breast)

½ teaspoon salt

½ teaspoon pepper

1 can red beans, drained and rinsed

1 cup (150 g) hominy, drained and rinsed (or 1 cup [150 g] frozen corn)

1 1/3 cup (48 g) dried cranberries

Put the turkey into the freezer (a 10-minute chill in the freezer will make it easier to dice).

In a large soup pot, heat the olive oil over medium heat. Add the shallots and sauté for 3 minutes. Add carrots, stir to combine, and sauté for another 3 minutes. Pour the broth over all and add the Better than Bouillon, wine, tarragon, and thyme. Increase heat to high and bring soup to a low boil. Add the wild rice. Lower heat and simmer, covered, for 30 minutes.

In the meantime, cut the turkey into ¾-inch (1.9 cm) cubes. Sprinkle with salt and pepper and toss to combine. Store in a covered bowl in the refrigerator.

After the soup has simmered for 30 minutes, add the turkey cubes and bring the soup back up to a steady simmer for 10 minutes. Add the beans, hominy, and cranberries, and cook for another 5–10 minutes or until turkey and rice are completely cooked.

Yield: 4 servings

Per Serving: 470 Calories; 14g Fat (27.4% calories from fat); 35g Protein; 50g Carbohydrate; 15g Dietary Fiber; 46mg Cholesterol; 1349mg Sodium

FROM CHEF JEANNETTE:

This recipe was inspired by members of the Wampanoag tribe I spoke with on a visit to Plimoth Plantation, in Plymouth, Massachusetts. The plantation is a living museum staffed, in part, by descendants of local Native American tribes. Wild turkey, cranberries, and roughly ground corn were seasonal staples of the fall in southern New England. When I asked about the eating habits of this indigenous tribe, I was told that food was available and cooking over the communal fires all day long. Both adults and children would eat when they felt hungry, and stop "when the hunger left them," not until they were stuffed to the brim!

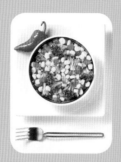

SIDE DISHES

· ·

Low-Cal Heirloom Gazpacho
Heart-Healthy Corn and Broccoli Fiesta
Hale and Hearty Apple Baked Beans
Nutted Quinoa Protein Pilaf with Caramelized Onions
Potassium Powerhouse:
Tzimmes with Sweet Potatoes, Figs, and Almonds

LOW-CAL HEIRLOOM GAZPACHO

From Dr. Jonny: So here's the deal: The only strategy that's been proven to extend life in absolutely every species ever studied has been calorie restriction. Which, as you might guess, is not the most popular eating plan around. But you don't have to be a fanatic to get the life-extending benefit of eating fewer calories. Just cutting back about 25 percent will do it for most people, and there's no better (or easier) way than to simply choose dishes that taste great but don't contain a ton of calories. Enter this dish, which is practically calorie free! (Okay, I exaggerate, but not by much.) Except for the little bit of heart-healthy olive oil, there's almost nothing in this recipe that tips the calorie scale past the double digits, and it's absolutely packed with nutrients for the heart. Flavorful and bright, this is best made in the deep summer when tomatoes are at their freshest.

2 tablespoons (28 ml) red wine vinegar

2 tablespoons (28 ml) olive oil

4 ripe heirloom tomatoes, diced

¾ cup (98 g) frozen corn, unthawed

½ cup (107 g) grated raw zucchini

1 green bell pepper, diced fine

1 English cucumber, peeled and diced

½ cup (50 g) diced scallions

2 cloves garlic, minced

1 to 2 teaspoons (3 to 6 g) minced jalapeño pepper, to taste (or 2 shots hot pepper sauce)

4 cups (950 ml) tomato-based vegetable juice (We like Knudsen's Very Veggie)

Juice of 1 lime

¼ cup (4 g) fresh cilantro, chopped

¼ cup (15 g) fresh parsley, chopped

Salt, to taste

Cracked pepper, to taste

Pinch Sucanat

In a small bowl, whisk together vinegar and olive oil.

In a large refrigerator storage container (preferably glass), mix together tomatoes, corn, zucchini, bell pepper, cucumber, scallions, garlic, and jalapeño. Pour the vinegar oil over the top, mix to combine, and refrigerate for 1 hour to overnight.

Pour the tomato and lime juices over the marinated vegetables and add herbs, mixing gently to combine. Season to taste using salt and pepper, adding tiny pinches of Sucanat as necessary to cut acidity. Chill in the refrigerator for at least 2 hours.

Serve ice cold.

Yield: about 4 servings

Per Serving: 191 Calories; 7g Fat (32.1% calories from fat); 5g Protein; 30g Carbohydrate; 6g Dietary Fiber; 0mg Cholesterol; 901mg Sodium

FROM CHEF JEANNETTE:

Want to make it a low-cal meal? Add 1 pound (455 g) of cooked medium shrimp when you combine the veggies and juices just before chilling.

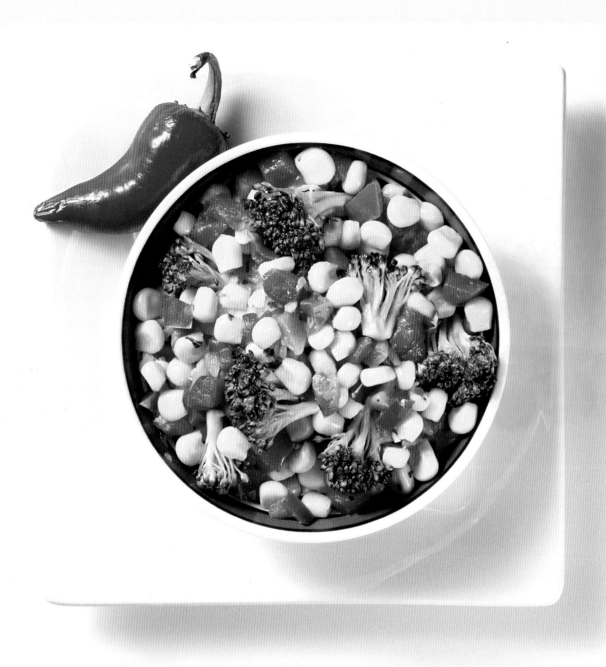
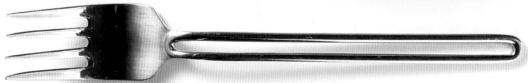

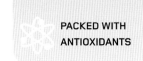
HEART-HEALTHY CORN AND BROCCOLI FIESTA

From Dr. Jonny: Vegetables (and fruits) are the best source of the mineral potassium, which helps regulate heartbeat. Many researchers believe that one of the reasons people who consume the most fruits and vegetables live the longest is because of their potassium intake. Potassium also helps lower blood pressure, particularly in people who have hypertension. Here's a flavor-rich dish with a southwestern flare. The chiles give it just the right amount of warmth. Corn was always one of my favorite veggies growing up (even though it's actually a grain), and this is a great way to eat it. A terrific variation on traditional Mexican fare.

1 tablespoon (14 g) butter

1 teaspoon olive oil

⅓ cup (80 ml) chicken or vegetable broth

1 clove garlic, finely minced

1 teaspoon dried basil

½ teaspoon salt

1 can (6 ounces, or 170 g) diced green chiles (mild), drained

¼ cup (37 g) finely diced red bell pepper

2 cups (260 g) frozen corn

1 large bunch broccoli, stemmed and cut into 1-inch (2.5-cm) florets (or one 10-ounce [280-g] package frozen broccoli florets)

In a large saucepan, melt butter over medium heat. Stir in olive oil, broth, garlic, basil, and salt. Add chiles, bell pepper, corn, and broccoli, and cover.

Reduce heat to medium low and cook, stirring occasionally, for about 10 minutes until broccoli reaches desired tenderness.

Yield: 4 servings

Per Serving: 165 Calories; 5g Fat (26.0% calories from fat); 7g Protein; 27g Carbohydrate; 7g Dietary Fiber; 8mg Cholesterol; 524mg Sodium

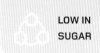
HALE AND HEARTY APPLE BAKED BEANS

From Dr. Jonny: I frequently have beans for breakfast. Call me crazy, I know. But the thing is, nothing keeps your blood sugar even like beans, and they satisfy for hours. (Sometimes I have them as a side dish with my eggs.) Beans are a powerful food to improve overall health and specifically to prevent heart disease, according to nutrition experts at Michigan State University, who reviewed 25 years of research involving beans and various health issues. And just for good measure, women in the famous Nurses' Health Study who ate four or more servings of legumes a week were 33 percent less likely to develop colorectal adenomas, a noncancerous tumor that can progress into colon cancer. The thing I love about this particular recipe is the tangy apple flavor, which you'd never expect in a bean dish; it makes it sweet and spicy at the same time. In addition to breakfast, this meal is really satisfying on a cold night!

1 teaspoon olive oil

1 small yellow onion, diced

2 cups (386 g) dried pinto beans, picked over, soaked overnight, and drained

½ cup (43 g) dried apple, pulsed in food processor to the size of large raisins

3 tablespoons (60 g) blackstrap molasses

2 tablespoons (30 g) Dijon mustard

½ to ¾ teaspoon cayenne or chipotle pepper

¼ teaspoon liquid smoke

1 teaspoon epazote*, optional, to help with bean digestibility

2 cups (475 ml) apple cider (also good with hard cider!)

3 cups (710 ml) low-sodium vegetable broth, plus extra if needed

½ teaspoon salt or to taste

In a large heavy-bottom pot, heat oil over medium burner and sauté onion for 4 minutes.

Add beans, apple, molasses, mustard, cayenne, liquid smoke, epazote (if using), cider, and broth, stirring to combine. Bring to a boil, reduce heat to maintain a low simmer, cover, and cook for 90 minutes to 2 hours or until beans are tender. After the first 45 minutes, stir and check liquid level every 30 minutes or so, adding more broth if necessary.

Add salt to taste at end of cooking time.

Yield: about 8 cups

Per Serving: 370 Calories; 1.7g Fat (5% calories from fat); 14.2g Protein; 57g Carbohydrate; 11g Dietary Fiber; 0mg Cholesterol; 781mg Sodium

FROM CHEF JEANNETTE:

Many people avoid beans because of their, ahem, digestibility issue. That's a mistake, though, if you want to live a long and fruitful life. (Most all of the people from the Blue Zones eat beans on a regular basis.) The sugars particular to beans are the primary gas culprits, but you can increase the digestibility of beans by cooking them until they are very tender and adding a few select spices or a bit of soaked and diced kombu, a dried sea vegetable.

* Epazote, a Mexican herb, is one of the best natural additions for helping the digestive system break down bean sugars. When cooking, use up to 2 teaspoons dried epazote or 6 fresh leaves per pound of beans. You'll find it in ethnic supermarkets or in the bulk herb bins of many natural food stores.

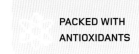
NUTTED QUINOA PROTEIN PILAF WITH CARAMELIZED ONIONS

From Dr. Jonny: Quinoa (pronounced keen-wah) is such a life-fortifying food that the ancient Incas considered it "food of the gods." Though it looks, tastes, and cooks like a grain, it's actually a seed—and higher in heart-friendly protein than any grain we know of. Add corn and beans and you've hit a trifecta of foods found among the longest-lived societies on Earth. The depth and sweet, nutty taste of this nontraditional pilaf will surprise and delight you.

1 teaspoon butter

1 tablespoon (15 ml) almond or macadamia nut oil

2 medium yellow onions, sliced thin

2 tablespoons (28 ml) white wine

½ teaspoon Sucanat

¼ teaspoon salt

1 cup (170 g) quinoa

1½ cups (355 ml) vegetable broth

½ cup (120 ml) apple cider

¼ cup (38 g) dried currants

½ cup (65 g) frozen corn kernels, thawed

1 cup (177 g) cooked white beans (great northern or cannellini work well), rinsed and drained if canned

¼ cup (35 g) toasted pepitas (pumpkin seeds)

¼ cup (36 g) toasted sunflower seeds (tamari-coated work well)

¼ cup (34 g) chopped toasted cashews

Salt, optional, to taste

DRESSING

3 tablespoons (45 ml) olive oil

1 teaspoon honey

1 tablespoon (15 ml) apple cider vinegar

1 teaspoon high-quality curry powder

Pinch salt

For pilaf: Heat the butter and oil in a medium sauté pan over medium-high heat. When butter starts to foam, add onions and white wine. Stir to combine and sauté for 4 to 5 minutes until onions begin to soften. Sprinkle Sucanat and salt over all, reduce heat to medium low, and cook for 15 to 20 minutes, stirring often, until lightly caramelized, adding a tablespoon or two (15 to 20 ml) of water if the onions get too dry.

For sauce: While onions cook, dry-toast the quinoa in a 2-quart saucepan over medium heat for 3 to 4 minutes, shaking the pan frequently to toast evenly and prevent browning. Add broth and cider to quinoa, increase temperature to high, and bring to a boil. Reduce heat and simmer, covered, for about 15 minutes until tails have "popped" and liquids are absorbed. Let it rest for 3 minutes, covered, then gently fluff grains with a fork and fold in caramelized onions, currants, corn, beans, seeds, nuts, and salt; cover for 3 minutes.

In a small bowl, whisk together oil, honey, vinegar, curry, and salt until well blended. Drizzle over quinoa mixture and mix gently to combine. Add salt to taste and serve at room temperature.

Yield: 4 to 6 servings

Per Serving: 424 Calories; 20g Fat (41.0% calories from fat); 11g Protein; 53g Carbohydrate; 7g Dietary Fiber; 2mg Cholesterol; 515mg Sodium

FROM CHEF JEANNETTE:

This versatile dish makes a great side to a lamb, fish, or chicken entrée, or on its own as a vegetarian entrée over a bed of cooked greens or salad.

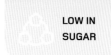
POTASSIUM POWERHOUSE: TZIMMES WITH SWEET POTATOES, FIGS, AND ALMONDS

From Dr. Jonny: This dish is a delight for the heart because it's absolutely loaded with potassium heavyweights such as sweet potatoes, carrots, and figs. Potassium helps keep your heart contracting regularly, and it also lowers blood pressure. (In fact, health professionals believe that one of the many important reasons that people who eat the most fruits and vegetables have the healthiest hearts has to do with the high potassium content of these foods.) Almonds add additional heart-healthy minerals, plus fiber and good fat, and the sweet potatoes add a nice dose of vitamin A. Traditionally served for the Jewish New Year celebration Rosh Hashanah, this is a lovely side dish for any holiday meal. After tasting the figs in combo with the sweet potatoes, you'll never want to go to back to nutritionally empty marshmallows often served with sweet potatoes!

High-heat cooking oil spray

4 medium sweet potatoes, peeled and cut into 1-inch (2.5-cm) chunks

4 medium carrots, peeled and cut into ½-inch (1-cm) slices

6 dried figs, chopped

1 tablespoon (14 g) butter, melted

1 tablespoon (15 ml) almond oil

1 tablespoon (15 ml) mirin

1 tablespoon (15 ml) maple syrup

1 teaspoon sweet white miso

¾ teaspoon ground cinnamon

½ teaspoon ground ginger

½ cup (55 g) sliced toasted almonds

Preheat the oven to 400°F (200°C, or gas mark 6).

Lightly coat a 9 x 13-inch (23 x 33-cm) baking pan with cooking oil spray and set aside.

Steam potatoes and carrots in a large steamer or stockpot fitted with a steamer basket for 15 minutes.

In a small bowl, cover figs with warm water and set aside to soak while preparing the dressing.

In another small bowl, whisk together melted butter, oil, mirin, syrup, miso, cinnamon, and ginger.

Spoon steamed potatoes and carrots into the prepared baking pan. Drain figs and spoon over veggies. Pour the dressing evenly over all and stir gently to mix.

Cover with foil and bake for 20 minutes or until all veggies are soft. Uncover, stir gently, sprinkle with almonds, and return to oven for 5 more minutes.

Yield: 6 servings

Per Serving: 264 Calories; 9g Fat (30.7% calories from fat); 4g Protein; 43g Carbohydrate; 8g Dietary Fiber; 5mg Cholesterol; 88mg Sodium

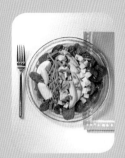

SALADS

· ·

Cobb Salad That Really Is Good for You
Potassium–Powered Roasted Sweets Salad

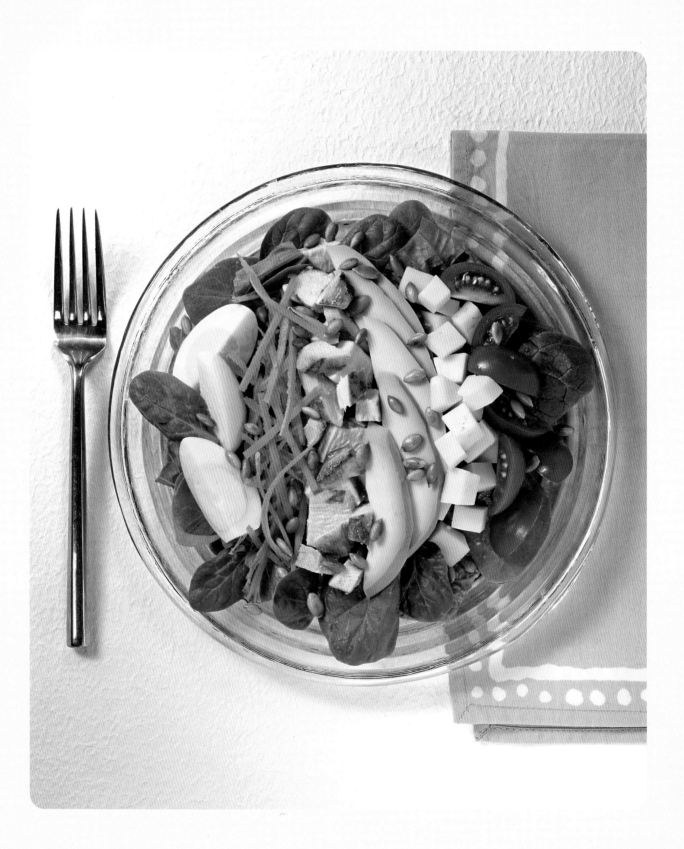

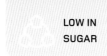

COBB SALAD THAT REALLY IS GOOD FOR YOU

From Dr. Jonny: Here's another example of how to make familiar foods into longevity dishes. Your "regular" Cobb salad is loaded with fatty, sugary ranch dressing and top-heavy on the meat and cheese, leaving little room for veggies. Chef Jeannette reversed the formula and made it taste better at the same time! When you're craving something salty and smoky, try this salad. The smoky flavor—from the Gouda and the dressing—has a tang and bite that will knock your socks off, and with its generous helpings of spinach, avocado, and tomatoes, it will extend your life in the bargain!

SALAD

6 cups (330 g) dark romaine lettuce, chopped

2 cups (60 g) baby spinach

½ cup (55 g) grated carrots

4 ounces (115 g) cooked chicken or turkey breast, cubed or thinly sliced (for a vegetarian option, substitute 6 ounces (170 g) unseasoned artichoke hearts, drained and quartered, about 2 to 3)

½ cup (60 g) smoked Gouda cheese, diced into small cubes

1 avocado, peeled, pitted, and sliced thin

2 cups (360 g) raw Campari tomatoes (4 to 6 depending on size), quartered

2 boiled eggs, quartered lengthwise

2 sliced, caramelized onions, optional (see page 49 for recipe for Caramelized Onions)

¼ cup (35 g) toasted pepitas (pumpkin seeds)

DRESSING

1 garlic clove, crushed

2 tablespoons (28 ml) balsamic vinegar

1 teaspoon horseradish mustard (or Dijon)

¾ teaspoon prepared horseradish

1 teaspoon tomato paste

1 teaspoon raw honey

¼ teaspoon salt

¼ teaspoon fresh-ground black pepper

2 drops liquid smoke

⅓ cup (80 ml) olive oil

For salad: Make a bed of romaine in a large salad bowl. Arrange the rest of the ingredients in separate sections around the salad bed, Cobb-style, or toss together gently to combine.

For dressing: Process all the ingredients except the oil in blender or all in a small bowl with immersion blender. Gradually add oil in a thin stream to emulsify. Dress salad to taste.

Yield: 4 servings

Per Serving: 493 Calories; 37g Fat (66% calories from fat); 20g Protein; 23g Carbohydrate; 8g Dietary Fiber; 148mg Cholesterol; 580mg Sodium

FROM CHEF JEANNETTE:

Neither Jonny nor I are fans of bacon. Nutritionally, most bacon is almost pure saturated fat, with harmful nitrates and sugars added to the mix. It's a life-shortener. But many people love bacon, and there's no denying that its smoky flavor adds a nice depth to certain dishes, including Cobb salad. So, I sometimes use a less-than-natural "fakin' bacon" product to capture that essence. I like Bac'Uns, a vegan Frontier product with a decent ingredient list and 3 grams of protein per serving. Try sprinkling a tablespoon (5 g) of Bac'Uns on this salad. For a more "natural" bacon texture, you can cook up a couple of slices of turkey bacon, similar in flavor but with almost no saturated fat—be sure to look for nitrate-free!

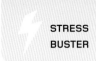
POTASSIUM-POWERED ROASTED SWEETS SALAD

From Dr. Jonny: I just love this recipe. It's a less calorie-dense way to eat a delicious vegetable that is typically covered in butter, maple syrup, and marshmallows. Yams are a staple of the bodybuilding community. They are also a fantastic source of potassium, which helps regulate heartbeat and is associated with lower blood pressure. This fabulous dish offers so much sweetness from the apples and raisins—and crunchiness from the nuts—that you'll never miss the gooey stuff. Pine nuts fit in beautifully both from a taste and a longevity point of view (remember, those who eat 5 ounces of any kind of nuts a week have significantly less heart disease). Hint: I'd recommend using Grade B maple syrup—it's richer in nutrients and cheaper than Grade A!

YAM

1 large yam or sweet potato, peeled and diced into ½-inch (1-cm) cubes

1 tablespoon (15 ml) unflavored vegetable oil

1 teaspoon maple syrup

½ teaspoon ground cinnamon

½ teaspoon ground cumin

½ teaspoon salt

SALAD

6 cups (330 g) hearty mixed seasonal salad greens

⅓ cup (37 g) grated carrots

1 crisp eating apple, cored and sliced thin, unpeeled (Honeycrisp, if you can find it)

1 cubed and roasted yam (see directions above)

¼ cup (35 g) raisins (black or golden)

¼ cup (35 g) toasted pine nuts

DRESSING

¼ cup (60 ml) apple cider

¼ cup (60 g) natural applesauce (no sugar added)

1 tablespoon (15 ml) apple cider vinegar

1 teaspoon raw honey

Preheat the oven to 400°F (200°C, or gas mark 6).

In a medium bowl, whisk together the oil, syrup, cinnamon, cumin, and salt. Add yam cubes and toss gently to coat. Lay cubes out in single layer on a baking sheet and cook for 15 to 20 minutes (until soft and lightly caramelized), turning once if browning too quickly. Sweet potatoes will take longer to soften than yams, up to 25 minutes.

Make a bed of greens in a large salad bowl and sprinkle carrots over the lettuce. Arrange apple slices over the lettuce bed and spoon yam over all. Top with raisins and sprinkle with pine nuts. Whisk dressing ingredients together and pour over arranged salad base, to taste.

FROM CHEF JEANNETTE:

If you're trying to reduce your daily calorie load but don't want to give up all the comfort foods, try this dish. The dressing uses no oil. It is simple and light tasting, but thick enough to coat the ingredients and add some body to the flavors, so the only fat you're eating is the small amount on the yam and the oils in the pine nuts.

This salad works well both warm and chilled. If you want to make it a meal, toss in a cup of cooked garbanzo or great northern beans to bump up the protein and fiber.

Yield: 4 servings

Per Serving: 250 Calories; 7g Fat (25.1% calories from fat); 5g Protein; 44g Carbohydrate; 8g Dietary Fiber; 0mg Cholesterol; 299mg Sodium

BREAKFASTS

· ·

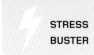
THE HEART-HEALTHIEST OATMEALS ON EARTH I

From Dr. Jonny: For a longevity combo, it's hard to beat oats, berries, and seeds, and this recipe has all three. Oats have fiber, berries are loaded with antioxidants that help fight one of the Four Horsemen of Aging (oxidative damage), and sesame seeds add a whopping 75 percent of the daily value for copper and almost half of the daily value for manganese. Bonus: The beta-glucan in oats helps lower cholesterol. I love this unusual combination of spices. This is one of my favorite breakfast recipes.

¾ cup (60 g) whole oat groats

¼ cup (46 g) whole-wheat or rye berries

4 cups (975 ml) water

½ cup (72 g) whole raw almonds

½ cup (72 g) raw sunflower seeds

¼ cup (32 g) sesame seeds (raw or toasted)

1 cinnamon stick, optional

¼ teaspoon ground cardamom, optional

¼ teaspoon ground nutmeg, optional

¾ cup (109 g) fresh or dried berries of your choice (try fresh blueberries or dried goji berries)

Combine the oats, wheat berries, water, almonds, sunflower and sesame seeds, cinnamon stick, cardamom, and nutmeg in a slow cooker. Cook on low for 8 hours.

Stir in the berries, let warm for 5 minutes, and serve.

Yield: 4 to 6 servings

Per Serving: 225 Calories; 16g Fat (58.5% calories from fat); 8g Protein; 17g Carbohydrate; 6g Dietary Fiber; 0mg Cholesterol; 9mg Sodium

FROM CHEF JEANNETTE:

If you like sweeter oatmeal, stir in half a mashed banana or ½ to ¾ cup (125 to 180 g) of unsweetened applesauce before serving. Oat groats also work as a savory dish: Simply omit the sweet spices when cooking and season to taste with a small amount of tamari sauce before serving. They're also great with chopped chives or scallion stirred in, even for breakfast! To add a little more calcium and some friendly intestinal flora, stir in a few tablespoons of plain yogurt to individual portions of either the sweet or savory version.

Slow-cooked whole oat groats are a major improvement over instant oatmeal. Most conventional oatmeal has a lot of added life-shortening sugar and sodium. The original groats

have been stripped and flattened as well, increasing their overall glycemic load. Using the whole groat is not only better for longevity, but also yields a creamier, more satisfying oatmeal that you can flavor yourself with ingredients that add to the nutrient punch rather than diminishing it. If you want an even bigger fiber boost, add ¼ cup (25 g) of wheat germ or ground flaxseed before serving.

If you have access to a large or natural grocer or co-op, look for the cheapest oat groats in the bulk section; the grains look a little like brown rice. If you can't find whole oat groats, you can use steel-cut oats (steel cut are just chopped groats), which are readily available at most supermarkets.

**STRESS
BUSTER**

THE HEART-HEALTHIEST OATMEALS ON EARTH II

From Dr. Jonny: One of the few pieces of conventional nutritional wisdom that I actually agree with is that oats are good for the heart. They contain a ton of fiber, they're low glycemic, and they contain important compounds such as beta-glucan. This tasty, fruity oatmeal dish is so easy to make because you can prepare it the night before and cook it the next morning. And it's not just a carb fest—it's loaded with protein from the whey protein powder. If you use the almond or hemp milk (which I recommend!) you can avoid any reactions to dairy, and there's not a drop of "bad" sugar in the mix to boot.

3 cups (240 g) whole rolled oats (not instant)

¼ cup (60 g) Sucanat, xylitol, or erythritol

¼ cup (25 g) ground flaxseed

⅓ cup (40 g) vanilla whey protein powder

2 teaspoons (5 g) ground cinnamon

½ teaspoon ground nutmeg

¼ teaspoon ground cardamom

½ teaspoon salt

2 teaspoons (9 g) baking powder

2 eggs

1 cup (235 ml) milk (can be cow's or unsweetened soy, almond, or hemp milk)

½ cup (125 g) applesauce

¼ cup (60 ml) maple syrup

2 tablespoons (28 ml) coconut or almond oil, melted

2 teaspoons (10 ml) vanilla extract

3 fresh peaches, unpeeled, pitted, and chopped, or 1 bag (10 ounces, or 280 g) frozen peaches, thawed

¾ cup (116 g) frozen blueberries*

Preheat the oven to 350°F (180°C, or gas mark 4). Lightly oil a 9-inch (23-cm) deep-dish pie plate.

In a large bowl, mix all dry ingredients together (oats through baking powder).

In a medium bowl, beat eggs into milk and mix in remaining wet ingredients (through vanilla extract).

Pour wet ingredients into dry and stir well to combine. Stir in fruit.

Bake in pie plate for 50 to 60 minutes or until cooked through (not jiggly) and just lightly browned on top.

Yield: about 6–8 servings

Per Serving: 306 Calories; 9g Fat (26.0% calories from fat); 12g Protein; 46g Carbohydrate; 5g Dietary Fiber; 62mg Cholesterol; 290mg Sodium

FROM CHEF JEANNETTE:

Nutritionally speaking, hemp milk is among the best of the alternate grain and seed "milks." It's made from pulverized hemp seeds and provides both omega-6 and omega-3 essential fatty acids in a balanced 3 to 1 ratio. It also contains a high concentration of essential amino acids, making it a great source of both healthy fats and protein. It's easier to digest than soy milk, and the micronutrients are easier to assimilate. Hemp seeds also present a much lower allergy risk than soy. The tradeoff for this great nutrient profile is a less "neutral" flavor. Hemp milk has a heavier consistency than soy, almond, or rice milk and a nuttier, somewhat earthy flavor. Right now it's mostly available only in natural food stores, but as it gains more prominence, we think you'll start to see it alongside the soy and almond milks in the supermarket.

* Using frozen blueberries rather then fresh will help them retain their shape over the long cooking time.

ANCIENT AMARANTH SWEET CEREAL

From Dr. Jonny: I'm not a huge fan of grains, especially the processed varieties that line our supermarket shelves and create all kinds of gluten-related problems for so many people. But before you give up on the idea of cereal for breakfast, consider this recipe, which uses one of the most ancient grains, amaranth. Actually amaranth, like quinoa, is a seed, but I won't tell if you won't. It looks like a grain, cooks like a grain, and tastes like a grain— only richer and sweeter. It's way higher in protein than most grains (9 grams per cup!), has a respectable 5 grams of fiber, and is high in potassium—a mineral with the critical job of helping your heart beat! The nuts offer a nice dose of heart-healthy fats, and the flaxseeds offer additional fiber. Tip: To me, this tastes fine without any additional sweetener, but man oh man, when you add a little raw honey or Grade B maple syrup, look out! You'll never lust after ordinary cereal again!

1 cup (193 g) amaranth

2 cups (475 ml) water

1 cup (235 ml) apple cider (or water)

1 Granny Smith apple, unpeeled, chopped

½ cup (55 g) grated carrot

½ teaspoon ground cinnamon

2 tablespoons (40 g) maple syrup or honey, optional

⅓ cup (37 g) chopped toasted pecans

2 tablespoons (13 g) ground flaxseed

In a large saucepan, mix together the amaranth, water, and cider. Bring to a boil and add the apple, carrot, and cinnamon. Reduce heat and simmer, covered, for about 25 to 30 minutes or until amaranth is tender and gelatinous. Stir in syrup or honey, if using, and pecans and flaxseed.

Yield: about 6 servings

Per Serving: 227 Calories; 7g Fat (26.9% calories from fat); 6g Protein; 37g Carbohydrate; 7g Dietary Fiber; 0mg Cholesterol; 14mg Sodium

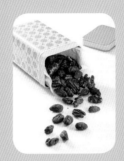

SNACKS and DESSERTS

. . . .

Chocolate Mixed Nuts for Heart Health
Heart–Healthy Hike 'n' Bike Trail Mix
Heavenly, Heart–Healthy Cinnamon Cocoa Brownie Pudding
Nutrient–Rich Date–Nut Rolls

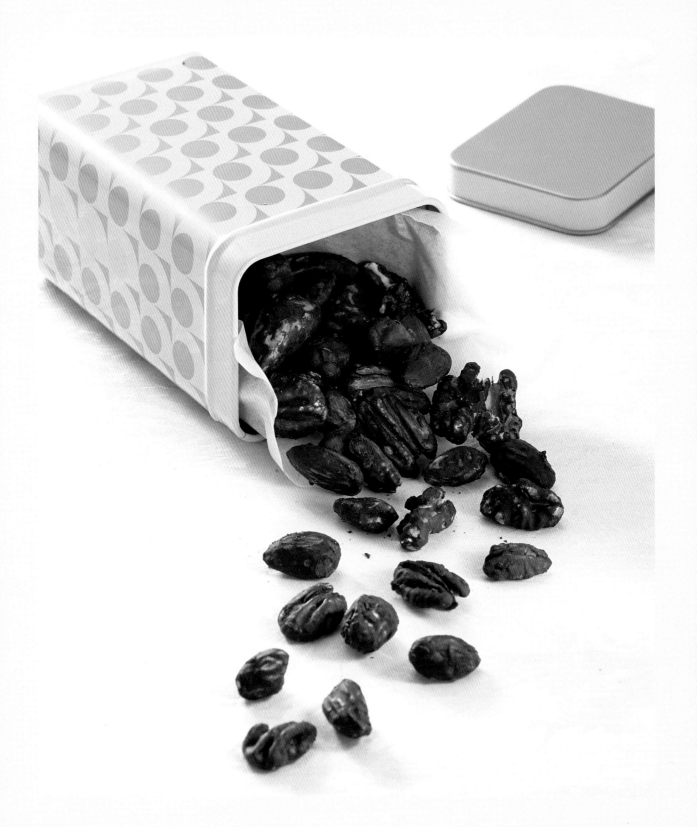

CHOCOLATE MIXED NUTS FOR HEART HEALTH

From Dr. Jonny: Nuts are a fabulous longevity food. In a major Harvard University study, women who ate more than 5 ounces of nuts a week had a 35 percent lower risk of heart disease than those who didn't. And I love this particular combo for heart health, which includes Brazil nuts, a fabulous source of the anticancer nutrient *selenium*. The aromatic recipe tastes chocolaty but with an exotic hint of spice! The Adventists, an American group of especially healthy and long-lived folks, would be proud: They attribute part of their exceptional longevity to daily doses of all different types of nuts.

---

1 large egg white

¼ cup (60 ml) pure maple syrup

¼ teaspoon vanilla

3 tablespoons (15 g) high-quality cocoa powder, sifted*
(try Ghirardelli)

½ teaspoon ground cinnamon

¼ teaspoon salt

⅛ teaspoon ground cloves

½ cup (67 g) unsalted Brazil nuts**

½ cup (72 g) unsalted almonds

½ cup (55 g) unsalted pecans

½ cups (50 g) unsalted walnuts

½ cup (67 g) unsalted hazelnuts

½ cup (62 g) unsalted pistachios

Preheat the oven to 325°F (170°C, or gas mark 3).

Line a large baking sheet with parchment paper.

In a large bowl, whip egg white by hand with whisk for 30 seconds until foamy.

Add syrup, vanilla, cocoa, cinnamon, salt, and cloves, and whisk together until smooth.

Stir in nuts until all are well coated.

Spoon nuts onto prepared baking sheet and spread out to a single layer. Bake for 10 minutes and stir nuts. Bake for 10 minutes more.

Allow nuts to cool thoroughly. They will harden as they cool.

Break apart and store in glass container in the refrigerator.

Yield: 3 cups (about 450g)

Per Serving: 179 Calories; 16.5g Fat (77% calories from fat); 5.3g Protein; 5.6g Carbohydrate; 2.8g Dietary Fiber; 0mg Cholesterol; 54mg Sodium

* If you don't have a sifter, simply flatten any lumps with a fork before adding to recipe.
** Raw or roasted nuts work equally well for all varieties in the recipe.

FROM CHEF JEANNETTE:

Typically, chocolate-covered nuts are packed with fat and sugar. This heart-healthy version has extra protein from the egg white and uses only a minimal amount of sweetener, but it will satisfy even a hardcore sweet tooth.

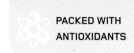
HEART-HEALTHY HIKE 'N' BIKE TRAIL MIX

From Dr. Jonny: Who doesn't love trail mix? No one I know! This version will not only delight your taste buds, but will make your heart sing as well. Another great—and sinfully delicious—way to get more heart-healthy nuts, fiber, and cocoa in your diet. Best of all, you don't need much of it to satisfy. It's crunchy, sweet, and unbelievably satisfying. Note: The grain-sweetened dark chocolate chips will make you forget all about the M&Ms in the store-bought version!

½ cup (72 g) almonds, raw or roasted

½ cup (67 g) hazelnuts, raw or roasted

½ cup (55 g) pecans, raw or roasted

1 cup (175 g) dark chocolate chips
   (we like grain-sweetened)

½ cup (62 g) dried cherries (or goji berries)

1 cup (63 g) unsweetened whole-grain "chex-style"
   cereal (e.g., oat, wheat, rice, etc.)

In a large bowl, gently mix all ingredients together. Store in a cool place in an airtight gallon-size zip-closure bag or Mason jars.

Yield: 4 cups (about 600 g)

Per Serving: 106 Calories; 4g Fat (31% calories from fat); 1.8g Protein; 18g Carbohydrate; 2.1g Dietary Fiber; 0mg Cholesterol; 106.4mg Sodium

FROM CHEF JEANNETTE:

Trail mix just begs to be customized to your tastes. It's so easy to make, and anything dry and bite-size can join your mix. All dried fruits can work, but we like the berries best for their life-enhancing antioxidant content. One of my favorite combos is a mix of nuts, dark chocolate chips, goji berries, and crystallized ginger. Goji berries contain eighteen amino acids and up to twenty-one trace minerals and are a rich source of carotenoids, fiber, and vitamin C.

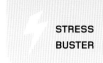
HEAVENLY, HEART-HEALTHY CINNAMON COCOA BROWNIE PUDDING

From Dr. Jonny: A chocolate brownie pudding for the heart? You're kidding, right? Nope. This sweet, crispy, creamy, deep chocolate decadence is meant for special occasions when you just need something to hit all those pleasure receptors but don't want to shorten your life with the heavy sugars and calories of conventional rich desserts. Dark cocoa is a heart-healthy food and one of the seven ingredients in the polymeal. Cocoa lowers blood pressure, almonds provide heart-healthy fat, and the whole-grain flour is a step above the nutritionally empty white version. Using xylitol, a natural sugar alcohol, as a sweetener instead of nasty old white sugar helps dampen what would otherwise be a humongous increase in blood

WET MIX

1 cup (120 g) whole-wheat pastry flour

½ cup (120 g) xylitol

2 tablespoons (10 g) high-quality natural cocoa powder (we like Ghirardelli)

2 teaspoons (9 g) baking powder

½ teaspoon ground cinnamon (Saigon, if you can find it)

¼ teaspoon salt

½ cup (120 ml) milk (cow's, soy, or almond)

2 tablespoons (28 ml) almond oil

1 teaspoon vanilla

⅔ cup (73 g) sliced toasted almonds (or ½ cup [60 g] walnuts or pecans [55 g])

DRY MIX

⅔ cup (150 g) xylitol

1 teaspoon ground cinnamon (Saigon)

¼ cup (20 g) high-quality natural cocoa powder

1½ cups (355 ml) boiling water

For wet mix: Preheat the oven to 350°F (180°C, or gas mark 4).

In a mixing bowl, whisk together flour, xylitol, cocoa, baking powder, cinnamon, and salt. Add milk, oil, and vanilla, and blend on low until just combined. Fold in almonds. Spoon into an ungreased 8 x 8-inch (20 x 20-cm) baking pan and spread to evenly cover the bottom; there will be only a thin layer of batter.

For dry mix: In a small bowl, whisk together ⅔ cup (150 g) xylitol, cinnamon, and ¼ cup (20 g) cocoa, and pour evenly over top of batter. Pour boiling water over all and do not mix.

Carefully place into oven and bake for 30 minutes or until brownie on top is cooked (test with a toothpick) and pudding below is bubbling.

Cool for at least 10 minutes before serving—pudding beneath is HOT!

Yield: 9 servings*

Per Serving: 212 Calories; 8g Fat (27.1% calories from fat); 5g Protein; 45g Carbohydrate; 4g Dietary Fiber; 2mg Cholesterol; 177mg Sodium

* Do not get carried away with this dessert and have multiple servings at once! It uses a lot of xylitol, which can cause some harmless, but potentially unpleasant gastric side effects when consumed in excessive quantities.

NUTRIENT-RICH DATE-NUT ROLLS

From Dr. Jonny: After all this time we're still fighting the battle to rescue nuts from their undeserved reputation as being fattening and bad for you. In case you missed the memo, they're anything but. Women in the Nurses' Health Study—that 30-year-and-counting respected study of more than 100,000 women done at Harvard—found that women who ate an ounce or so of nuts five times a week had a 35 percent lower risk of cardiovascular disease! Here's another super way to get nuts into your diet. Warning: These are very rich and not exactly low calorie. But they're absolutely loaded with nutrients. The only sweetener is natural dates ("nature's candy") complete with their fiber intact.

1 packed cup (150 g) pitted dates

¾ cup (109 g) almonds, raw or roasted

¾ cup (101 g) cashews, raw or roasted

½ cup (130 g) raw almond butter

¼ teaspoon ground cardamom

⅓ cup (40 g) toasted sesame seeds

Place the dates in a small bowl and cover with warm water for 10 to 15 minutes, until soft. Drain, reserving some of the water.

Add the almonds and cashews to a food processor and pulse about 5 times to break them up, then process steadily for 5 to 7 seconds or until they are very coarse crumbs (⅛ to ¼ inch, or 0.3 to 0.5 cm). Pour nuts into bowl and set aside.

Add the soaked dates and almond butter to a food processor and process until a "dough" is formed. You may have to scrape down the sides to get it to hold together. If your dates are very dry, you may need a tablespoon or so of the soaking water to help it form a dough, but don't overmoisten it. Sprinkle in the cardamom and nuts and process until well blended.

Pour the sesame seeds onto a shallow plate and press the dough into 1 ½-inch (4-cm) balls with your hands. Roll in the sesame seeds to coat to taste and store in the refrigerator, separating the layers with parchment to prevent sticking.

Yield: about 25 rolls

Per Serving: 92 Calories; 7g Fat (61.3% calories from fat); 2g Protein; 7g Carbohydrate; 1g Dietary Fiber; 0mg Cholesterol; 2mg Sodium

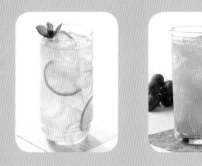

DRINKS

. . . .

Heart-Warming Spiced Cocoa
Spice of Life Mulled Wine
Sunny Iced Green Heart-Tea
Happy Heart Sparkling Red Grape Juice

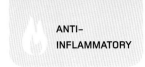

HEART-WARMING SPICED COCOA

From Dr. Jonny: So just about everyone knows by now that cocoa is great for the heart, but how to consume it without the added fat, sugar, and emulsifiers that come in most chocolate bars? Simple. Try this amazing spiced cocoa. Sure it has a drop of sweetener, but it's a great way to get cocoa into "heavy rotation" on your diet. I love this as a before-bed drink. This spiced-up version has cinnamon, which helps lower blood sugar. Best of all this is delicious hot or cold, and you can enjoy it all year round. I do!

SPICE MIX

4 teaspoons (9 g) ground cinnamon

1 teaspoon ground nutmeg

1 teaspoon ground mace

1 teaspoon ground cloves

½ teaspoon black pepper

In a small bowl, mix all spices together well.

Per Serving (excluding unknown items): 8 Calories; trace Fat (28.7% calories from fat); trace Protein; 2g Carbohydrate; 1g Dietary Fiber; 0mg Cholesterol; 1mg Sodium. Exchanges: 0 Grain(Starch); 0 Fat.

HOT CUP

1½ tablespoons (8 g) high-quality cocoa powder

1½ tablespoons (22 g) sweetener, or to taste (try xylitol, erythritol [Truvia], Sucanat, or brown rice syrup)

½ teaspoon Spice Mix (see above)

1 cup (235 ml) milk (cow's, unsweetened soy, almond, or rice)

Slice of fresh orange peel, optional

Combine all ingredients in a small saucepan over medium heat and whisk together until milk is steaming but not boiling. Garnish with orange peel, if using.

You can also blend cooled cocoa with ice cubes and half a frozen banana for a spiced smoothie in warm weather.

Per Serving (using 2% cow's milk): 56 Calories; 2g Fat (30.4% calories from fat); 2g Protein; 10g Carbohydrate; 1g Dietary Fiber; 8mg Cholesterol; 30mg Sodium.

NO-COOK "SPICY ICY"

2½ tablespoons (12 g) high-quality cocoa powder

2½ tablespoons (37 g) sweetener, or to taste (try xylitol, erythritol, Sucanat, or brown rice syrup)

¾ teaspoon Spice Mix (see above)

1 cup (235 ml) milk (cow's, unsweetened soy, almond, or rice)

Approximately 1½ cups ice cubes

In a blender, gently blend all ingredients together except ice until well incorporated.

Add ice and blend until it reaches a "slushy" consistency.

Yield: about 4 large mugs

Per Serving (using 2% cow's milk): 69 Calories; 3g Fat (25.3% calories from fat); 3g Protein; 14g Carbohydrate; 1g Dietary Fiber; 8mg Cholesterol; 31mg Sodium.

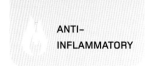

SPICE OF LIFE MULLED WINE

From Dr. Jonny: I know, I know—you were waiting for this one! Well, go ahead and indulge. The research is very clear that red wine is good for the heart. A study in the American Journal of Clinical Nutrition showed that moderate wine drinkers have lower mortality related to high blood pressure. And in 1992, Harvard researchers declared that moderate red wine consumption was one of "eight proven ways to reduce coronary heart disease risk." Red wine was one of the seven key ingredients in the polymeal. Bonus: Red wine contains reseveratrol, a flavonoid found to extend life in just about every species studied. The pungent and fruity combination of spice and citrus makes this warm and relaxing drink perfect for enjoying on a frosty night, or over the cold-weather holidays with friends.

1 bottle (750 ml) dry red wine (Cabernet Sauvignon, Shiraz, Merlot, etc.)*

Juice of 2 oranges

2 to 3 tablespoons (40 to 60 g) mild honey or agave nectar, to taste

6 thin ginger slices, peeled (about the size of quarters)

6 cinnamon sticks

2 teaspoons whole cloves

4 lightly crushed cardamom pods (or ¼ teaspoon powdered)

4 allspice berries (or ¼ teaspoon powdered)

¼ teaspoon ground nutmeg

4 unpeeled orange rounds (thin slices width-wise)

4 unpeeled lemon rounds (thin slices width-wise)

SLOW COOKER (best method)

Pour the wine, orange juice, and honey into a slow cooker and stir gently to combine. Add the spices (through nutmeg) and stir again. Float the fruit rounds on the top. Cover and heat on low for 3 to 4 hours or on high for 2 hours. Do not allow to boil. Stir gently to mix the honey and serve, straining the wine through a double-mesh sieve.

* Because you are mulling with a sweetener and strong spices, you can choose cheaper wine for this recipe. Hearty choices, such as those suggested above, work well.

STOVETOP

Pour the wine, juice, and honey into a large heavy-bottom pot over medium-low heat and stir gently to combine. Add the spices (through nutmeg) and stir again. Float the fruit rounds on the top. Partially cover and heat for 10 to 15 minutes until hot, but don't let it boil. Reduce heat to low and cook for another 10 to 15 minutes until very fragrant. Stir gently again to mix the honey and serve, straining wine through a double-mesh sieve.

Yield: about 4 large mugs

Per Serving: 57 Calories; 2g Fat (5.5% calories from fat); 4g Protein; 64g Carbohydrate; 17g Dietary Fiber; 0mg Cholesterol; 132mg Sodium

FROM CHEF JEANNETTE:

Using a slow cooker, with its airtight seal, will prevent evaporation and keep the nutrient content of the wine as intact as possible.

If you are a teetotaler, you can enjoy this recipe made with fresh-pressed apple cider instead of the wine—just omit the sweetener.

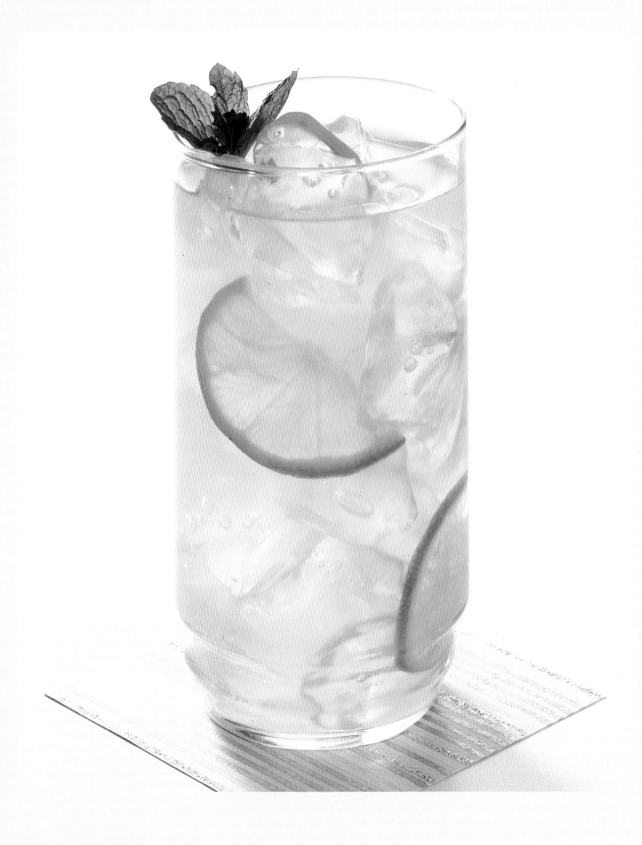

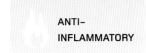
SUNNY ICED GREEN HEART-TEA

From Dr. Jonny: Every time I'm asked by a magazine editor to come up with "ten top tips" for living longer, I put this tip on the list: Drink green tea every day! It's loaded with catechins and phenols, which have been found to protect the heart and brain and extend life, not to mention help protect against cancer (a nice little "side effect" of this heart-healthy drink). Plus—drum roll, now—it tastes great! Lightly sweetened and bright with that hint of lime, it's incredibly refreshing on a hot summer afternoon!

CONCENTRATE

4 cups (950 ml) water

4 lemon green tea bags (we like Yogi Lemon Ginger Green Tea)

3 tablespoons (60 g) to ¼ cup (85 g) raw honey, to taste

3 to 4 teaspoons (15 to 20 ml) ginger juice*, to taste

Juice of 3 limes

Fresh mint leaves for garnish, optional

Bring the water to a boil and remove from the heat. Add tea bags and allow to steep for 10 minutes. Remove tea bags and stir in honey until completely dissolved, reheating tea slightly, if necessary. Add ginger juice and lime juice to tea.

FULL PITCHER

Pour hot concentrate into a glass pitcher.

Add 1½ to 2 trays of ice, stirring to combine as it melts.

Garnish with mint leaves, if desired.

* For ginger juice, you can buy it premade (we like The Ginger People brand), put the root through a juicer, or simply peel and grate a chunk of the root and squeeze the gratings with your hand to produce fresh juice.

INDIVIDUAL SERVINGS

Once cool, pour concentrate in a Mason jar and store in fridge.

To make tea, fill a glass with ice and top with cool (or hot) concentrate to taste.

Garnish with mint leaves, if desired.

Yield: 4 tall glasses

Per Serving: 8 Calories; trace Fat (1.1% calories from fat); trace Protein; 2g Carbohydrate; trace Dietary Fiber; 0mg Cholesterol; 1mg Sodium

FROM CHEF JEANNETTE:

After a swim at the beach in the blistering summer heat, a tall glass of iced tea hits the spot like nothing else. This citrusy green-tea version will beat any of those premade concoctions in bottles or cans for both taste and health benefits.

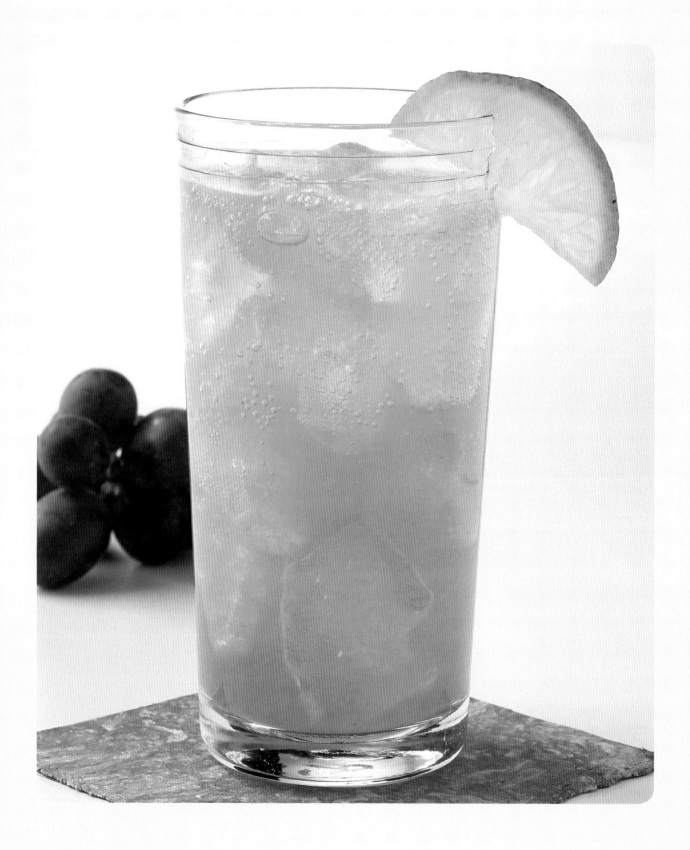

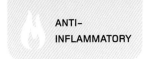

ANTI-
INFLAMMATORY

HAPPY HEART SPARKLING RED GRAPE JUICE

From Dr. Jonny: The skins of red (and dark) grapes are a virtual treasure trove of heart-healthy nutrients, including the life-extending polyphenol called resveratrol (the "secret ingredient" in red wine). The vitamin C in oranges and lemons helps protect your vascular system against aging oxidative damage (one of the Four Horsemen of Aging). And apples are a top source of *quercetin*, a member of the flavonoid family that happens to be one of the best anti-inflammatories in the plant kingdom. What a great nonalcoholic longevity alternative to champagne!

1½ pounds red seedless grapes (about 3½ cups, or 525 g), stemmed

2 apples, unpeeled, stemmed, and quartered

2 oranges, peeled and quartered

1 lemon, peeled and halved

1 cup (235 ml) cold seltzer, or to taste

Put the grapes through the juicer in small bunches, using apple and orange quarters to push them through. Finish with the lemon, mix gently, and combine with seltzer in a pitcher. Add ice to taste and serve.

Yield: 4 glasses

Per Serving: 127 Calories; 1g Fat (3.1% calories from fat); 2g Protein; 33g Carbohydrate; 5g Dietary Fiber; 0mg Cholesterol; 8mg Sodium

FROM CHEF JEANNETTE:

You can try switching out the oranges for 2 cups (250 g) of red raspberries when they're in season for an additional antioxidant/vitamin C blast. Feel free to spice or sweeten up this drink to your taste. Try adding juice of an inch (2.5 cm) of ginger, a quarter cup (6.5 g) of mint leaves, or float a tender rosemary sprig in your pitcher. For a sweeter drink, stir in honey or liquid stevia to taste before adding the seltzer.

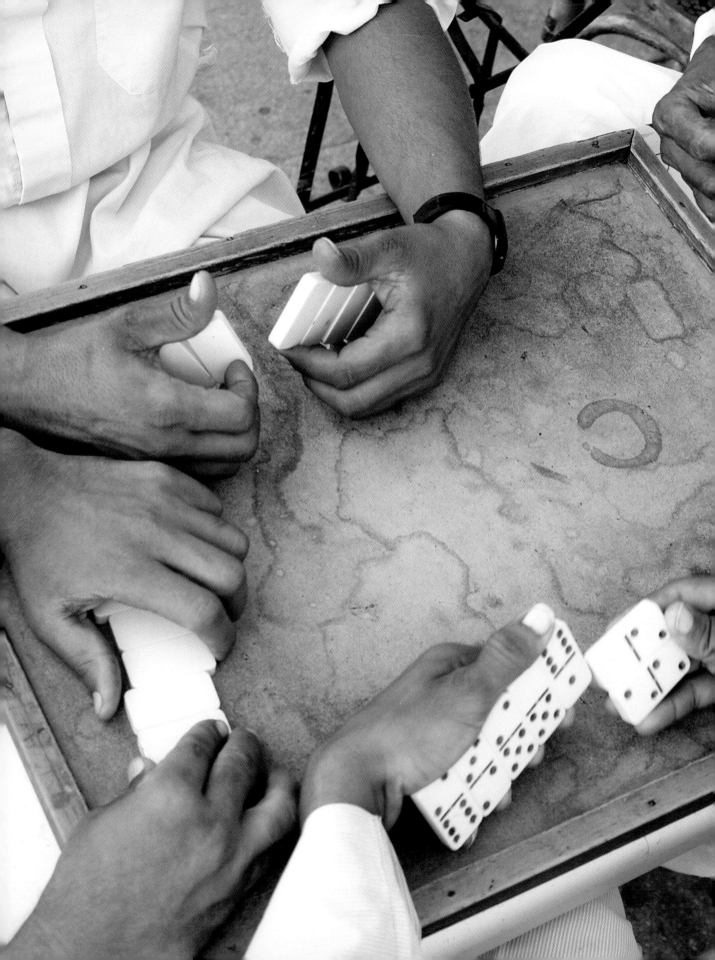

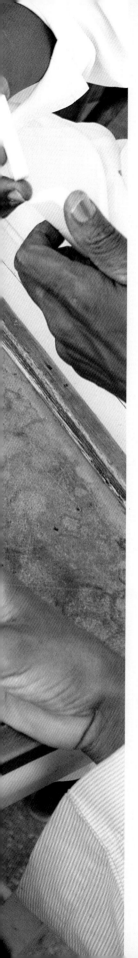

Chapter II
What to Eat to Keep Your Brain's Neurons Firing Past Ninety

· ·

ENTRÉES

Mega Omega Fettuccine Alfredo

A Movable, Mediterranean Feast of Striped Bass

Brain Wave: Orange-Poached Salmon with Teriyaki Glaze

Spinach-Stuffed Flounder with Tomato-Olive Tapenade

Shell Power: Mussels and White Beans Tuscany

Low-Cal Curried Halibut Stew

Protein-Powered Pan-Seared Tuna with Orange-Peppercorn Crust

Smart Shrimp Spring Rolls with Peanut Pesto

Pure and Simple Lamb Kebabs

Collard Roll-Ups with Black-Eyed Pea Hummus and Onion Chutney

Fiery Free-Radical-Fighting Mole Sauce

Wake-You-Up Spicy Shrimp with Thai Rice Noodles

Mellow, Miso-Marinated Pacific Cod

SIDE DISHES

Roasted Delicatas for Squashing Stress

Memorable, Mouthwatering Sweet Potato–Garbanzo Curry

Nutted and Nutritious Brown Rice Bonanza

Grilled Eggplant Sauté, Sardinian Style

Herbed Spaghetti Squash—Nature's Pasta

SALADS

Gift from the Gods Greek Salad

Mediterranean Dried-Herb Salad

BREAKFASTS AND SNACKS

Jonny's Brainy Breakfast Scramble

Mind-Full Middle Eastern Stewed Eggs

Salmon Frittata, Nova Scotian Centenarian Style

Brain Gain Tuna Spread

Rise and Brine Gravlax Canapés

Afternoon Pick-Me-Up Potassium Miso Soup

DESSERTS

Coconut Lemon Custard Tastes-like-Cheesecake

Sweet Bean Paste—Dessert That's Good for You

DRINKS

Anti-Inflammatory Virgin Bloody Mary

Dehydration Destroyers: Flavor Waters

Turn-Up-the-Volume Berry-Cherry Pom Juice Cocktail

Ever hear of type 3 diabetes?

Well, pull up a chair.

There's not a baby boomer alive who doesn't worry about losing her mental faculties as she ages to a disease such as Alzheimer's. And, plenty of us are also pretty scared of diabetes. According to the International Diabetes Foundation, the number of people suffering from it has increased from 30 million to 230 million just in the past two decades. Alzheimer's and diabetes.

Two diseases of aging, two diseases that strike fear in the hearts of anyone wanting to live long and well. Could they be related? We know there's a huge dietary component to diabetes; what about a diet connection to dementia?

This isn't the place to go into a deep discussion of the mechanisms of diabetes, but suffice it to say that it all revolves around an important hormone called *insulin*. When you have too much of it in your system, bad things happen. And new research is showing that insulin is a key player in the brain.

When your body makes too much insulin—a situation that is definitely related to diet—your brain decides to do the exact opposite. If you've got high levels of insulin in your body, there's a good chance your brain is running a deficit.

THE HIGHS AND LOWS OF INSULIN

Insulin deficit in the brain is the beginning of a really big problem, at least if you want to live a long life with your brain working at full capacity. Insulin is so important to the brain that one important researcher has coined the term type 3 diabetes to refer to the form of insulin deficiency linked to brain deterioration as well as the high sugar–high insulin conditions that are typical of diabetes.

Insulin actually controls an enzyme that makes *acetylcholine*, a major neurotransmitter that's involved in thinking and memory. (Note: The building blocks for acetylcholine are found in eggs, thank you very much!) Researchers have long known that a deficiency of acetyl-choline is one of the characteristics shared by dementia and Alzheimer's patients, which makes perfect sense. If you think of acetylcholine as a kind of fuel for the brain, low levels of insulin basically turn off the brain gas.

The best way to interrupt this cycle is to get rid of high levels of insulin in the body.

Let's work backward: What causes insulin to skyrocket in the body and sometimes get stuck there?

All together, class: Sugar does!

Sugar and processed carbs (which your body basically treats the same as sugar) cause your blood sugar to rise and your insulin levels to go up as well. But that insulin is supposed to keep your blood sugar in check. In diabetics, this system doesn't work well. There's too much sugar and too much insulin, and health havoc results. We now know that one of the bad consequences is that deficit of insulin in the brain we talked about. Remember, high levels in the body, low levels upstairs.

So, conclusion number one: Use your diet to normalize insulin levels in the body!

PROTECT YOUR BRAIN WITH THE RIGHT FOODS

The recipes in this section are designed to normalize insulin levels.

That's why you'll find recipes filled with foods that are known as "low glycemic"—they don't raise blood sugar (or insulin) all that high or all that quickly. The recipes are also filled with the greatest brain-protecting foods on Earth. For example, cold-water fish such as wild salmon, mackerel, and tuna all have a large repository of anti-inflammatory omega-3s, long known to protect cell membranes in the brain from damage that can impair your functioning and slow you down. (No wonder grandma said fish was brain food!)

You'll also find eggs—no surprise because they contribute the building blocks for that "brain gas" acetyl-choline, the stuff that keeps you sharp and helps you think and remember.

Those who followed the Mediterranean diet the most consistently had an unbelievable 48 percent lower risk of developing Alzheimer's than those who didn't, researchers found. Now that's a brain-protecting diet!

What you *won't* find is sugar. Or, at least you'll find as little of it as possible and only when it is absolutely necessary to make a recipe taste a certain way. Sugar has gotten a bad rap among those concerned with longevity, and the bad rap is 100 percent justified. Research from Columbia University Medical Center implicates high blood sugar levels in memory lapses. Researchers now think that even for those who are perfectly healthy with nary a hint of diabetes, controlling blood sugar just might be the key to preserving memory!

But we didn't choose the foods in these delicious recipes only because they're low sugar, or, as they say, low glycemic. These foods also pack a powerful nutritional wallop—as well as being pretty darn delicious. Blueberries, for example, are the ultimate memory food and have been shown in research to make rats smarter! (Nope, I'm not making this up. Blueberry-eating rats had better memory and better performance on a variety of maze tests than non-blueberry-eating rodents. That's because the berries contain polyphenols, compounds that actually help brain cells communicate better with one another.)

Best of all, these tasty dishes fit nicely with a dietary strategy named after a part of the world where they traditionally have much lower rates of heart disease than we do in America—the Mediterranean. But, you say, we all know the Mediterranean diet is protective of the heart.

What has it got to do with the brain?

Actually, more than we thought. Researchers have found that patients who adhere most closely to a Mediterranean-type diet—one loaded with vegetables, fruit, legumes, fish, and olive oil, all the foods in this section—had an almost 30 percent lower risk of developing mild cognitive impairment (compared with those who followed the Mediterranean diet the least). And, those who followed the Mediterranean diet the most consistently had an unbelievable 48 percent lower risk of developing Alzheimer's.

Now that's a brain-protecting diet!

Last, you'll find the foods in this section just loaded with antioxidants. You may recall from *The Most Effective Ways to Live Longer* that oxidative damage is one of the Four Horsemen of Aging. Oxidation damages your cells and your DNA and nowhere more dramatically than in the brain. Foods and spices such as the ones used for the recipes in this section—most especially the vegetables and fruits—are packed with antioxidants such as vitamin C to help stave off the aging effects of free radicals on your brain cells.

And none of this would probably matter if the food didn't taste so amazingly good.

It does.

Enjoy!

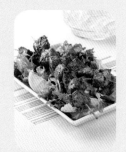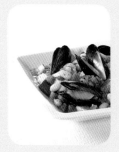

ENTRÉES

. . . .

Mega Omega Fettuccine Alfredo

A Movable, Mediterranean Feast of Striped Bass

Brain Wave: Orange-Poached Salmon with Teriyaki Glaze

Spinach-Stuffed Flounder with Tomato-Olive Tapenade

Shell Power: Mussels and White Beans Tuscany

Low-Cal Curried Halibut Stew

Protein-Powered Pan-Seared Tuna with Orange-Peppercorn Crust

Smart Shrimp Spring Rolls with Peanut Pesto

Pure and Simple Lamb Kebabs

Collard Roll-Ups with Black-Eyed Pea Hummus and Onion Chutney

Fiery Free-Radical-Fighting Mole Sauce

Wake-You-Up Spicy Shrimp with Thai Rice Noodles

Mellow, Miso-Marinated Pacific Cod

MEGA OMEGA FETTUCCINE ALFREDO

From Dr. Jonny: Wild salmon is one of the richest sources of omega-3s, arguably one of the five top nutrients for brain health. Omega-3s are fatty acids that get incorporated into the cell membrane, making the membrane fluid and making it easier for information to get in and out of the cells. This may be one reason why fish is considered "brain food." Another is that 60 percent of your brain is fat, most of it DHA, one of the two important fatty acids found in wild salmon. Whatever the reasons, omega-3s are good for the brain and good for longevity. The broccoli, shallots, and olive oil—not to mention the wild salmon—in this dish turn ordinary pasta into a luscious and creamy longevity feast.

1 pound (455 g) dried, whole-grain fettuccine

2 tablespoons (28 ml) olive oil

4 medium shallots, diced

2 cups (142 g) bite-size broccoli florets

½ cup (120 ml) dry white wine

1 cup (460 g) silken tofu

¾ cup (175 ml) milk (cow's, unsweetened soy, or almond milk)

½ teaspoon salt

½ teaspoon tarragon

½ teaspoon ground nutmeg

½ teaspoon white pepper

1 cup (100 g) finely grated Parmesan cheese, divided

1 can (7.5 ounces, or 214 g) boneless, skinless, wild Alaskan salmon, drained (or 1 pound [455 g] cooked, shelled shrimp)

¼ cup (25 g) ground flaxseed

¼ cup (15 g) chopped fresh parsley, optional

Bring a large pot of water to a boil. Cook pasta until al dente according to package directions. Drain in colander, reserving ¼ cup (60 ml) of the cooking liquid.

Heat oil in a large, ovenproof skillet over medium-high heat. Add shallots and sauté 3 minutes. Add broccoli florets and sauté for 2 minutes. Add the wine and cook until evaporated, 4 to 5 minutes.

Meanwhile, combine silken tofu and milk in food processor or blender and process for 20 seconds or until smooth and creamy. Pour tofu-milk mixture over vegetables in pan. Stir in salt, tarragon, nutmeg, pepper, and ¾ cup (75 g) of the Parmesan until well combined. Fold in salmon, reduce heat to medium low, and cook gently for about 7 minutes until heated through.

Return pasta and reserved cooking liquid to its cooking pot over medium heat.

Gently stir in tofu mixture and flaxseed to combine. Sprinkle remaining ¼ cup (25 g) Parmesan over the top, garnish with parsley, if using, and serve immediately.

Yield: 6 servings

Per Serving: 468 Calories; 15g Fat (29.5% calories from fat); 27g Protein; 53g Carbohydrate; 4g Dietary Fiber; 30mg Cholesterol; 453mg Sodium

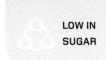

A MOVABLE, MEDITERRANEAN FEAST OF STRIPED BASS

From Dr. Jonny: Can the Mediterranean diet slow down brain aging? Maybe even help prevent Alzheimer's? A study in the journal *Archives of Neurology* investigated the effect of eating in a Mediterranean style on something called MCI—mild cognitive impairment. Mild cognitive impairment is defined by the Alzheimer's Association as "a condition in which a person has problems with memory, language, or another mental function severe enough to be noticeable to other people and to show up on tests, but not serious enough to interfere with daily life." While not everyone who is diagnosed with MCI goes on to develop Alzheimer's, those with MCI definitely have an increased risk for doing so. So, what did the research in the *Archives of Neurology* show? Those who adhered more closely to a Mediterranean diet lessened their risk of developing MCI. I'd say that makes the Mediterranean diet a pretty good protective treatment for the brain, wouldn't you? Researchers certainly think so. Anyway, this piquant bass dish is very much in the tradition of Mediterranean eating—fish, garlic, olives, olive oil—what's not to like? Best of all, you'll remember where you put your car keys!

3 cloves garlic, chopped

1 can (13.75 ounces, or 390 g) artichoke hearts, drained

½ cup (50 g) pitted Kalamata olives

1 tablespoon (15 ml) olive oil

Juice of 1 lemon

1 teaspoon lemon zest

1 teaspoon dried oregano

¼ cup (15 g) parsley

½ teaspoon cracked black pepper

2 teaspoons (3 g) capers

½ cup (75 g) crumbled feta cheese

1 can (14.5 ounces, or 413 g) diced tomatoes, drained

1½ pounds (710 g) striped bass fillets, skinless and deboned

Salt and black pepper, to taste

Preheat the oven to 400°F (200°C, or gas mark 6).

In a food processor, combine the garlic, artichoke hearts, olives, olive oil, lemon juice, zest, oregano, parsley, and pepper. Pulse several times, scraping down the sides as necessary, until you have a chunky blend. Stir in the capers, feta, and tomatoes.

Rinse fish and pat dry. Lightly salt and pepper to taste and place in small roasting pan. Spoon vegetable mix evenly over the top of the fish. Cook uncovered for 35 to 40 minutes or until fish is cooked through.

Yield: 4 servings

Per Serving: 395 Calories; 18g Fat (39.9% calories from fat); 41g Protein; 20g Carbohydrate; 7g Dietary Fiber; 137mg Cholesterol; 649mg Sodium

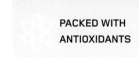

BRAIN WAVE: ORANGE-POACHED SALMON WITH TERIYAKI GLAZE

From Dr. Jonny: There's probably no better brain food in the world than wild salmon. Why? Because it's loaded with omega-3 fats. We've long known that these "wellness molecules" protect brain cells by acting as natural anti-inflammatory agents, as well as helping to keep the cell membranes nice and fluid so that information (such as feel-good neurotransmitters) can flow easily in and out. And, wild salmon contains a powerful antioxidant called astaxanthin, which gives wild salmon its natural red color. All in all, this is a restaurant meal made for dining in. The moist, rich glaze base makes it especially elegant. Serve with candlelight and fine red wine!

4 cups (950 ml) no-sodium vegetable broth or water

2 cups (475 ml) orange juice

Juice of 1 lemon

¼ cup (60 ml) apple cider vinegar

2 tablespoons (28 ml) mirin

2 teaspoons (10 ml) soy sauce

4 skinless fillets (6 ounces, or 170 g each) salmon, rinsed

TERIYAKI GLAZE

½ cup (120 ml) low-sodium tamari

½ cup (120 ml) orange juice

Zest of 1 orange

1 tablespoon (15 g) Sucanat

1 tablespoon (20 g) honey

1½ tablespoons (9 g) minced fresh ginger

1 tablespoon (8 g) toasted sesame seeds

In a sauté pan or skillet, add the broth, juices, vinegar, mirin, and soy sauce and bring to a boil over high heat. Simmer, uncovered, for 5 minutes. Gently place the salmon pieces into the simmering liquid, taking care that they are fully covered. (If not covered, add more broth or water.) Cover and simmer over low heat for 7 minutes.* Remove pan from heat and allow fish to sit in hot water until cooked through (translucent), 3 to 5 minutes.

While the salmon is poaching, prepare the glaze. In a medium saucepan over high heat, whisk together the tamari, orange juice, zest, Sucanat, honey, and ginger, and bring to a boil. Reduce heat and simmer, uncovered, for about 15 minutes or until reduced and slightly thickened.

Pour a small amount of the teriyaki glaze onto each of 4 plates and place the fish in the center. Sprinkle sesame seeds over all and serve.

Yield: 4 servings

Per Serving: 359 Calories; 7g Fat (18.5% calories from fat); 40g Protein; 32g Carbohydrate; 1g Dietary Fiber; 88mg Cholesterol; 1762mg Sodium

* If your fillets are very thick, you may need to keep them over a simmer for a couple of minutes longer. If they are ¾ inch (2 cm) or less, 7 minutes should be sufficient. Watch them closely to see that they don't overcook.

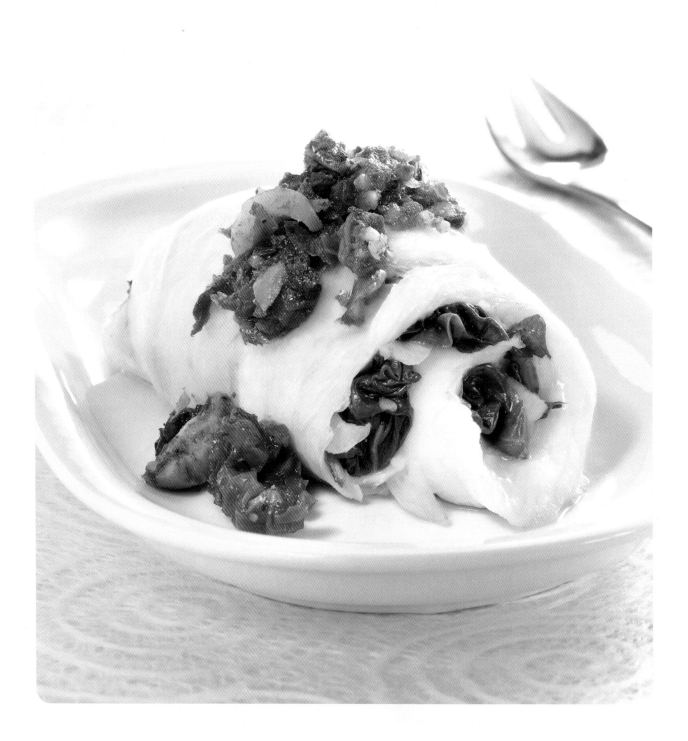

SPINACH-STUFFED FLOUNDER WITH TOMATO-OLIVE TAPENADE

From Dr. Jonny: A ton of research has demonstrated the association of a Mediterranean diet with lower rates of heart disease, but recent research has shown the effects of Mediterranean-style eating on brain health. One major study showed that the more people adhered to Mediterranean principles, the lower their risk for Alzheimer's, and another showed the same relationship to mild cognitive impairment. No one is 100 percent sure why this is so. It may be that the Mediterranean diet reduces inflammation in the brain, a likely possibility because that's precisely what omega-3 fats in fish do, but the rich array of antioxidants in the vegetables and the phenols in olives and olive oil could certainly be part of the reason as well. No matter. The verdict is in: The more you can adhere to basic traditions of a Mediterranean diet, the more you protect your brain and its ability to function optimally. How nice to know you can do it with food that tastes this good!

FLOUNDER

Olive oil cooking spray

4 flounder fillets (6 ounces, or 170 g each)

Salt and black pepper, to taste

1 tablespoon plus two teaspoons (25 ml) olive oil

4 shallots, diced

1 clove garlic, minced

12 ounces (340 g) baby spinach (about 4 packed cups)

¼ teaspoon cracked black pepper

½ lemon

TAPENADE

¼ cup (25 g) cured green olives, pitted

½ cup (55 g) oil-packed sun-dried tomato halves, drained

½ teaspoon dried oregano

1 tablespoon (15 ml) olive oil

1 tablespoon (15 ml) balsamic vinegar

2 teaspoons (3 g) capers

Preheat the oven to 350°F (180°C, or gas mark 4).

Coat a small baking dish (8 x 8 inch, or 20 x 20 cm) with olive oil cooking spray and set aside.

Rinse fillets and pat dry. Lightly salt and pepper. Lay them out on a work surface and prepare spinach.

In a large sauté pan, heat 1 tablespoon (15 ml) olive oil over medium heat. Add shallot and sauté for about 3 minutes until soft. Add garlic, spinach, and cracked pepper, cover, and cook until spinach is wilted, about 2 to 3 minutes. Remove from heat.

Spoon spinach evenly over 4 fillets and roll them up, placing them (seam side down) in prepared baking pan. Drizzle the remaining 2 teaspoons (10 ml) olive oil and squeeze lemon over all. Bake for 20 minutes or until fish is cooked through.

For tapenade: While fish is cooking, combine olives, tomatoes, oregano, olive oil, and vinegar in food processor. Pulse several times and then process briefly until a smooth paste is formed. Stir in capers, and spoon over hot, cooked flounder fillets to taste.

Yield: 4 servings

Per Serving: 186 Calories; 13g Fat (57.0% calories from fat); 12g Protein; 10g Carbohydrate; 3g Dietary Fiber; 20mg Cholesterol; 207mg Sodium

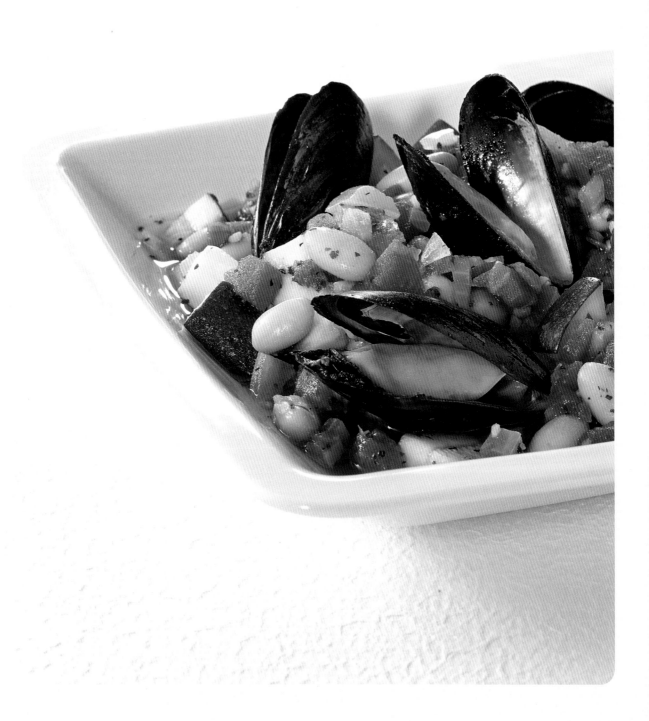

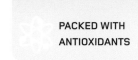

SHELL POWER: MUSSELS AND WHITE BEANS TUSCANY

From Dr. Jonny: Most people know that the brain needs glucose (sugar) to function, but not enough people appreciate how important protein is for optimal brain function. After all, brain chemicals known as *neurotransmitters*, which help you think and remember, are themselves proteins, built from the amino acids found in protein foods such as mussels. One study found that brain protein synthesis (that's tech talk for the assembly of important brain chemicals) was affected by the quality of dietary protein. In other words, you need good-quality dietary protein for your brain to function at its best, and mussels are a great, low-calorie source. Mussels are also high in zinc, a mineral that plays an important role in the transfer of information between brain cells and is found in high amounts in a section of the brain called the hippocampus. Mussels go especially nicely with high-fiber beans, a dietary staple in every long-lived society in the Blue Zones. And hey, they're color coordinated to boot!

1 tablespoon (15 ml) olive oil

1 large red onion, chopped

4 cloves garlic, crushed and chopped

1 cup (235 ml) dry white wine

2 pounds (900 g) mussels (about 40), scrubbed

1 can (14.5 ounces, or 413 g) diced tomatoes, undrained

1 cup (235 ml) vegetable broth

1 teaspoon white wine vinegar

1 can (14.5 ounces, or 413 g) cannellini beans, drained and rinsed

1 medium zucchini, halved lengthwise and sliced thick (½-inch, or 1-cm slices)

1 teaspoon dried basil

½ teaspoon dried oregano

1 bay leaf

Salt, to taste

Cracked black pepper, to taste

⅓ cup (20 g) chopped fresh parsley

In a large soup or stockpot heat the oil over medium heat. Add the onion and sauté 5 to 6 minutes until soft. Add the garlic and sauté 1 minute. Add wine, stirring to combine, and bring to a simmer. Add mussels, cover, and steam until just opened, about 4 to 5 minutes.* Remove mussels and set aside in a large bowl.

Add tomatoes (with juice), broth, vinegar, beans, zucchini, basil, oregano, bay leaf, salt, and pepper and bring to a low simmer, cooking for 10 to 15 minutes or until zucchini is tender. Stir in parsley, add mussels, and cook, covered, for about a minute until the mussels are just reheated.

Remove the bay leaf and serve immediately.

Yield: about 6 servings

Per Serving: 461 Calories; 7g Fat (14.5% calories from fat); 36g Protein; 58g Carbohydrate; 13g Dietary Fiber; 43mg Cholesterol; 721mg Sodium

* Discard any mussels that do not open with the others. If you wish, you may shell the mussels and add them to the stew cleaned, just before serving. This makes less mess and work for your eaters, but the presentation is not as special.

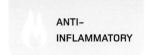

ANTI-
INFLAMMATORY

LOW-CAL CURRIED HALIBUT STEW

From Dr. Jonny: How can something that tastes this delicious be good for your brain? First, there's wild halibut, an extremely low-calorie fish filled with protein and about ½ gram of omega-3s, not to mention B_{12}. Then there's turmeric, known for its anti-inflammatory properties. Finally, there's a virtual alphabet of brain-supporting nutrients from the onions, tomatoes, and peppers. The dish is sweet and spicy—feel free to "dial down" the heat by reducing the amount of curry, ginger, or red pepper flakes.

1 fresh pineapple, peeled, cored, and cut into rings or 1 can (14 ounces, or 400 g) pineapple chunks, drained*

½ teaspoon sweet paprika

1½ tablespoons (25 ml) coconut oil

1 large yellow onion, chopped

1 tablespoon (6.3 g) curry powder

1 teaspoon coriander

¾ teaspoon ground cumin

¾ teaspoon turmeric

¼ to ½ teaspoon red pepper flakes, to taste

2 tablespoons (12 g) minced fresh ginger

1 garlic clove, minced

2 large bell peppers, any color, seeded and chopped

4 cups (475 ml) vegetable broth

1 can (14.5 ounces, or 413 g) fire roasted or regular diced tomatoes (do not drain)

½ teaspoon salt

¼ teaspoon black pepper

1 pound (455 g) wild halibut, skinned, deboned, and cut into 2-inch (5-cm) pieces

1 tablespoon (15 ml) fresh-squeezed lime juice

¼ cup (4 g) chopped fresh cilantro

Preheat your grill to medium.

Lay the pineapple rings out in a single layer on a platter and sprinkle them lightly with paprika. Grill the pineapple rings for about 2 minutes per side until lightly caramelized. Remove from heat, stack, and cut the rings into 6 to 8 pieces each.

Heat the oil over medium heat in a large, heavy-bottom soup pan. Add the onion and cook until softened, about 5 minutes. Add the curry, coriander, cumin, turmeric, pepper flakes, ginger, and garlic, and sauté for 1 minute, stirring constantly. Add the peppers and sauté for about 30 seconds, stirring to coat and prevent sticking. Pour in broth and tomatoes, scraping the bottom to loosen any spices. Increase the heat and bring to a boil. Stir in the salt and black pepper, reduce heat, cover, and simmer until the peppers are tender, about 10 minutes.

Add the fish and continue to simmer for about 5 minutes until it is cooked through, but still tender. Stir in the lime juice and cilantro and serve.

Yield: 6 servings

Per Serving: 234 Calories; 8g Fat (29.0% calories from fat); 20g Protein; 23g Carbohydrate; 4g Dietary Fiber; 25mg Cholesterol; 773mg Sodium

FROM CHEF JEANNETTE:

Fresh pineapple doesn't ripen after picking, so try to choose a ripe one: The leaves should be green and look fresh, the "eyes" on the skin plump. It should be firm and give off a strong sweet smell of pineapple. Remove the crown from the pineapple, slice it in half the long way, and then quarter it. You can then cut out the core and cut off the rind. These quarters can be cut up into chunks and grilled shish-kebab style.

* If using canned pineapple, skip the grilling step and add it to the stew when you add the tomatoes. To avoid the unnecessary added sugars, always look for fruit canned in water or its own juice instead of "syrup."

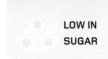

PROTEIN-POWERED PAN-SEARED TUNA WITH ORANGE-PEPPERCORN CRUST

From Dr. Jonny: One of my go-to dishes at restaurants is seared tuna. I just love it. While not as high in brain-boosting omega-3 fatty acids as wild salmon, it's still got plenty of them. And it's a fabulous source of protein, delivering a hearty dose of amino acids to the brain. Preventing strokes is certainly on my list of must-do things for protecting the brain, and data from the famed Nurses' Health Study showed that women who ate fish such as tuna two to four times per week had a 27 percent reduced risk of stroke compared to women who ate fish only once a month. More frequent fish eating—five times per week—reduced the risk of certain types of strokes by an incredible 52 percent. And it's not just women who are protected; research published in the July 2004 issue of the medical journal *Stroke* showed that eating fish is protective against stroke in men as well. Taste-wise, this dish can't be beat—the spicy, aromatic rub brings out the very best in the tuna. You'll love this recipe. I do!

Juice of 1 orange

2 tablespoons (28 ml) mirin, optional

4 tuna steaks (6 ounces, or 170 g each; we like Vital Choice tuna medallions)

½ teaspoon black peppercorns

2 teaspoons (3.5 g) pink peppercorns

1 teaspoon coriander seeds

½ teaspoon fennel seeds

½ teaspoon salt

¼ teaspoon Sucanat

2 teaspoons (3.5 g) orange zest

1½ teaspoons plus 1½ tablespoons (25 ml) neutral-flavored high-heat oil (rice bran, if you have it)

In a small bowl, whisk together the orange juice and mirin, if using.

Rinse the tuna and pat dry. Place in a shallow glass dish and pour juice mixture over all. Set aside while preparing other ingredients.

In a small dry skillet over medium heat, toast peppercorns, coriander, and fennel until very fragrant, 3 to 5 minutes (do not scorch the fennel). Grind mix to the consistency of cracked black pepper in a spice grinder.

In a small bowl, mix together the ground spices, salt, Sucanat, and zest.

Drain the tuna steaks and pat dry. Drizzle about 1½ teaspoons of the rice bran oil onto the steaks and lightly oil their surfaces. Rub the spice mixture lightly and evenly all over the steaks.

Heat the remaining rice bran oil in a large, heavy skillet over high heat. Add the tuna steaks and sear for 1 minute. Reduce the heat to medium and gently flip the steaks over. Sear the other side for 1 minute for medium rare (if desired, reduce heat and cook longer for more doneness).

Yield: 4 servings

Per Serving: 329 Calories; 14g Fat (40.1% calories from fat); 40g Protein; 8g Carbohydrate; 2g Dietary Fiber; 65mg Cholesterol; 376mg Sodium

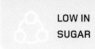

SMART SHRIMP SPRING ROLLS WITH PEANUT PESTO

From Dr. Jonny: Okay, boys and girls, which do you think your brain would rather have: Chinese fried egg rolls dripping in grease or these light and fresh-tasting shrimp spring rolls? No contest, right? Shrimp are absolutely loaded with the important amino acids your body needs to string together to make brain chemicals, known as neurotransmitters, that are needed for thought, memory, cognition, attention, and good mood. And while you've undoubtedly heard that red wine confers longevity benefits by providing an important antioxidant known as *resveratrol*, what you might not know is that peanuts are also a good source of this anti-aging nutrient. Finally, there's basil, one of the most versatile spices around and also one that has generated a fair amount of research. Studies have shown that compounds in basil oil have potent antioxidant, anticancer, antiviral, and antimicrobial properties. Betcha can't say that about fried Chinese egg rolls!

SHRIMP

2 tablespoons (28 ml) fresh-squeezed lime juice

2 tablespoons (28 ml) unseasoned rice vinegar

1 tablespoon (15 ml) tamari

12 cooked large shrimp, peeled, deveined, and cold

PEANUT PESTO

²/₃ cup (97 g) roasted peanuts

2 tablespoons (28 ml) peanut oil

2 tablespoons (28 ml) light coconut milk

1 tablespoon (15 ml) Thai fish sauce

1 tablespoon (15 g) Sucanat

Juice of 2 limes

½ teaspoon cayenne pepper

¹/₃ cup (5 g) packed fresh cilantro

¼ cup (10 g) packed fresh Thai basil (or can use regular)

WRAPS

12 spring roll wraps (8 ½-inch or 21-cm rice sheets)*

²/₃ cup (33 g) mung bean sprouts

2 carrots, peeled and grated

1+ cups (70+ g) shredded white, Napa, or green cabbage (to fill out your rolls to desired size)

¼ cup (25 g) chopped scallions (greens only)

3 tablespoons (7.5 g) chopped fresh Thai basil (or can use regular)**

3 tablespoons (3 g) chopped fresh cilantro

3 tablespoons (18 g) chopped fresh mint

FROM CHEF JEANNETTE:

Because this dish is nearly all raw vegetables, it's not very filling, though the pesto—with its healthy fat—does give it a bit more staying power than the traditional dipping sauce for Thai spring rolls. If you're serving it as the centerpiece of a main meal, you might consider making an additional 4 to 8 rolls, or using more shrimp.

This pesto sauce can also be used with the shrimp and Thai rice noodles to make a light pasta dish.

---

* The first time I bought these, I got them from an Asian market. The problem was, there were no directions in English, so I had to go through some trial and error to figure out how to prepare them! You can also soak several of them in cold water for the couple of minutes it takes to make the rolls, or dip them individually into warm water for 10 seconds and remove.

** For a pretty presentation, lay whole basil leaves on the rice wrap at the bottom of your pile of shrimp and veggies. When rolling them, the leaves will show through the wraps.

In a medium bowl, whisk together the juice, vinegar, and tamari. Slice the shrimp in half lengthwise and add to the bowl, tossing gently to coat. Allow to marinate for 15 minutes in the fridge while you prep the peanut pesto.

For peanut pesto: Combine the peanuts, peanut oil, coconut milk, fish sauce, Sucanat, lime juice, cayenne, cilantro, and basil in a food processor and process until mostly smooth, scraping down the sides as necessary, about 20 to 30 seconds. Set aside.

For wraps: Drain shrimp well and place the wraps in a large bowl or pot of cold water.

In another large bowl, mix together the sprouts, carrot, cabbage, scallions, basil, cilantro, and mint.

Remove 1 wrapper and lay it flat on your work surface. Lay 2 halves of one shrimp across the lower third of the wrapper. Lay ¼ to ⅓ cup (60 to 70 ml) of filling over the shrimp. Fold the sides in over the filling and fold the bottom up over the filling, rolling tightly, away from you, until sealed. Lay on a platter, seam side down.

Serve the spring rolls with small bowls of the peanut pesto for dipping, or spoon it over the individual rolls.

Yield: 4 servings

Per Serving: 156 Calories; 10g Fat (32.9% calories from fat); 9g Protein; 35g Carbohydrate; 1g Dietary Fiber; 27mg Cholesterol; 146mg Sodium

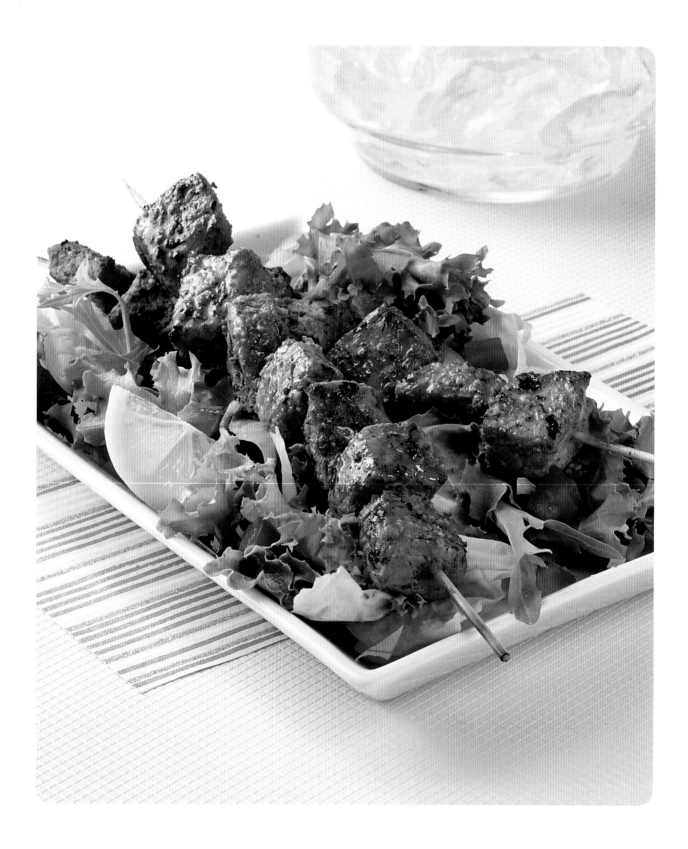

PURE AND SIMPLE LAMB KEBABS

From Dr. Jonny: By now you probably know that my all-time favorite brain nutrient is omega-3 fatty acids. Why? Because they get incorporated into the cell membranes of the nerve cells in the brain, allowing information to flow freely in and out of the cell. They also lower inflammation and improve mood, not to mention all the things they do for the heart. (But that's a separate topic!) So, why am I telling you this? Because lamb has more omega-3s than most meats (with the possible exception of grass-fed beef). That's because it's almost always grass-fed (animals that are grass-fed by definition have greater amounts of omega-3s in their meat). In addition, lamb almost never has all those brain-deadening "extras" you'll find in factory-farmed meat (that is, steroids, antibiotics, and hormones). The almonds provide magnesium, which protects the brain. It improves the neurologic outcomes of infants and adults who have had oxygen deprivation to their brain. (Some studies have shown that a higher daily magnesium intake may help prevent strokes.) The flavorful marinade makes the lamb juicy and succulent, but plan ahead; you'll need to marinate overnight for best results!

¼ cup (36 g) blanched skinless almonds

8 cloves garlic, crushed

2 medium yellow onions, coarsely chopped

⅓ cup (77 g) plain yogurt

Juice of 1 lemon

1 bunch cilantro (or ¼ cup [15 g] fresh parsley)

½ teaspoon turmeric

½ teaspoon ground cumin

½ teaspoon salt

½ teaspoon cracked black pepper

1½ pounds (710 g) lean lamb, cut into 1-inch (2.5-cm) cubes

Grind the almonds into a powder in the food processor. Add the garlic and pulse a few times to chop. Add the onions, yogurt, lemon juice, cilantro, turmeric, cumin, salt, and pepper and process until it forms a pasty purée, scraping down the sides as necessary.*

Spread the lamb cubes out in a glass storage dish and spoon marinade over all, mixing to coat all sides. Marinate meat from 3 hours to overnight, turning pieces over occasionally.

Preheat grill to medium low. Place the meat loosely on 4 metal skewers, removing as much of the marinade as possible. Grill until desired doneness, about 6 to 9 minutes, turning occasionally.

Yield: 4 servings

Per Serving: 466 Calories; 35g Fat (67.3% calories from fat); 27g Protein; 12g Carbohydrate; 2g Dietary Fiber; 101mg Cholesterol; 361mg Sodium

* Processing all that onion so finely releases a lot of tear gas. You can prepare for that by running a fan near where you're working so you don't get it in the face when you lift off the top. I know it's an odd remedy, but I also find it helpful to stick my head in the freezer when I get a face-full.

FROM CHEF JEANNETTE:

Middle Eastern shish kebabs are typically pulled off the skewers and rolled into naan or pita bread. To make a low-carb longevity version, serve it over a bed of crisp salad greens with lots of fresh chopped heirloom tomatoes and a drizzle of olive oil with lemon wedges for squeezing.

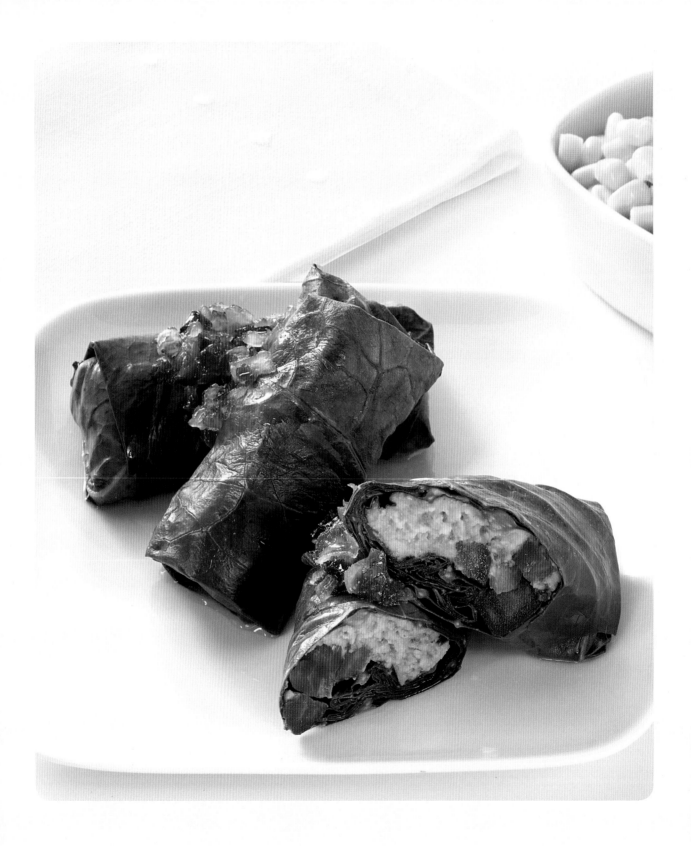

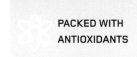

COLLARD ROLL-UPS WITH BLACK-EYED PEA HUMMUS AND ONION CHUTNEY

From Dr. Jonny: Black-eyed peas (the food, not the groovy hip-hop group) are loaded with folic acid, which has an interesting relationship to brain health. Research published in the prestigious medical journal *The Lancet* studied the effect of folic acid supplements on cognitive function and found that three-year folic acid supplementation improved performance on tests that measured information-processing speed and memory—areas that are known to decline with age. "Folic acid is often deficient in the elderly population," says Barbara Levine, R.D., Ph.D., of the Weill Cornell Medical College. "While many people think loss of cognition naturally occurs in the elderly, this may in part be a deficiency in folic acid." Folic acid also lowers a nasty little compound in the body called *homocysteine*, which has been linked to both heart disease and strokes. These collard roll-ups with black-eyed pea hummus are a nice little twist on southern "soul food" that'll feed your brain as well as satisfy your appetite!

ONION CHUTNEY

2 tablespoons (28 ml) olive oil

2 red or yellow onions, diced fine (about 2 cups, or 320 g)

1 teaspoon coriander

½ teaspoon ground ginger

½ teaspoon red pepper flakes

¼ teaspoon cracked black pepper

½ teaspoon salt

½ cup (120 ml) apple cider vinegar

¼ cup (60 g) Sucanat

12 to 14 good-size collard leaves (about 2 small bunches, or 1 large)

HUMMUS

2 cans (15 ounces, or 425 g, each) black-eyed peas, drained and rinsed (we like Eden Organics)

4 tablespoons (60 ml) apple cider vinegar

2 cloves garlic, crushed and chopped

2 teaspoons (10 ml) maple syrup

1 teaspoon ground cumin

1 teaspoon coriander

3 drops liquid smoke, optional

½ teaspoon salt

¾ teaspoon chipotle or cayenne pepper, or to taste

3 tablespoons (45 ml) high-lignan flaxseed oil (such as Barlean's) or olive oil

Chopped and seeded tomatoes, optional

MAKE THE CHUTNEY

Heat the oil in a medium saucepan. Add the onions and sauté for 5 minutes or until they begin to soften. Stir in the coriander, ginger, peppers, and salt and sauté for 2 minutes. Add the vinegar and Sucanat and bring to a boil. Reduce the heat, cover, and simmer for about 5 minutes. Uncover and continue simmering until the liquid is nearly gone and the onions are creamy, about 15 minutes. Set aside to cool.

COOK THE COLLARDS

While the chutney is cooking, bring a large pot of salted water to a boil. Lay the collards down and slice away the stems with a sharp knife from 3 to 4 inches (7.5 to 10 cm) into the bottom of the leaves. You should be

(continued on page 92)

left with oval leaves with narrow Vs cut out where the stems came out. Gently place the leaves into the boiling water and cook for 5 minutes.

Without tearing the leaves, drain them carefully in a colander, letting them cool while you make the hummus.

MAKE THE HUMMUS

Purée all the hummus ingredients from black-eyed peas to flaxseed oil in a food processor until well incorporated but still slightly chunky, scraping down the sides as necessary.

ASSEMBLE THE ROLL-UPS

Lay a collard leaf in front of you, uncut side down. (So the V will be at the top of the leaf.) Spoon a few tablespoons of hummus and chopped tomato, if using, onto the bottom of the leaf and roll the bottom edge up to cover it. Roll the sides in over the bottom fold and roll it, gently but tightly, away from you, from the bottom up.

Lay it on your serving platter, seam side down. Spoon cooled chutney over the rolls and serve.

Yield: 4 servings

Per Serving: 457 Calories; 19g Fat (44.0% calories from fat); 24g Protein; 30g Carbohydrate; 6g Dietary Fiber; trace Cholesterol; 1286mg Sodium

FIERY FREE-RADICAL-FIGHTING MOLE SAUCE

From Dr. Jonny: Hot peppers are a terrific way to spice up dishes. They're absolutely loaded with antioxidants such as vitamins C and A, which help prevent cell damage and diseases of aging. They also reduce inflammation, one of the dreaded Four Horsemen of Aging. The unsweetened cocoa powder adds heart-healthy magnesium and gives it a unique taste, spicy with a tinge of chocolate. What could be better?

2 teaspoons (10 ml) olive oil

½ sweet onion, diced fine

1 clove garlic, minced

1 tablespoon (5 g) unsweetened cocoa powder

1 teaspoon chili powder

1 teaspoon ground cumin

¼ teaspoon ground cinnamon

1 can (14 ounces, or 400 g) fire-roasted tomatoes, undrained

½ to 2 chipotle peppers in adobo sauce, diced* (use more or less depending on the heat level you like)

1 can (4 ounces, or 115 g) diced green chile peppers

¼ cup (35 g) raisins

* Most large grocery stores carry chipotles in adobo sauce in 6- or 8-ounce (128- or 225-g) cans in the Mexican food section. (See above for the health benefits of hot peppers.) They are very spicy; a little goes a long way. Try blending the remaining contents of the can in a blender or food processor to make a smoky, hot sauce that will keep for several weeks in your refrigerator. Use it to spice up beans, eggs, or salad dressings. You can also make a double batch of the whole sauce recipe and freeze some for later use.

Heat the oil in a medium saucepan over medium heat, and cook the onion until tender, 6 to 7 minutes. Add the garlic and sauté 1 minute. Add the cocoa powder, chili powder, cumin, and cinnamon, mixing to coat the onions and garlic. Stir in the tomatoes, chipotle, green chiles, and raisins. Bring to a boil, reduce heat to low, cover, and simmer for 10 minutes. Cool slightly and blend in a blender or food processor until smooth.

Pour over cooked chicken and serve over brown rice or in a sprouted corn tortilla with shredded lettuce, chopped fresh tomatoes, and avocado slices.

Yield: about 2 ¼ cups (535 ml)

Per Serving: 83 Calories; 2.3g Fat (24% calories from fat); 3.5g Protein; 15.5g Carbohydrate; 2.3g Dietary Fiber; 0mg Cholesterol; 494mg Sodium

FROM CHEF JEANNETTE:

Chipotles are among the hot peppers that contain the precious and healing substance known as capsaicin. Capsaicin is a very powerful antimicrobial and anti-inflammatory agent. Also, many cultures that feature these types of peppers as a regular part of their diet tend to suffer fewer strokes than those with "cooler" diets. Most of the capsaicin is in the spicy seeds and ribs, so include those in your dishes for the most potent nutritional "punch."

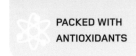

WAKE-YOU-UP SPICY SHRIMP WITH THAI RICE NOODLES

From Dr. Jonny: Did you ever notice that eating protein in the daytime tends to keep you more alert through the afternoon? I made that discovery years ago when, after eating a tuna sandwich and a glass of milk, I was suddenly more energetic and alert and stayed that way for hours. That's because most neurotransmitters—those chemicals in the brain responsible for alertness, memory, and cognition—are made from amino acids that come from—guess where?—protein! Like in shrimp! This terrific recipe provides a low-calorie (and low-fat if you care) source of protein. The rice noodles are light and digestible, which means you won't feel heavy and foggy after eating this sweet and spicy hot dish. Bonus: Rice noodles are gluten free, which is a great "pasta" option for many people.

½ pound (8 ounces, or 225 g) stir-fry rice noodles, linguine style, or soba noodles

2 tablespoons (28 ml) peanut oil

3 cloves garlic

3 tablespoons (18 g) minced ginger

1½ pounds (680 g) fresh medium shrimp, shelled and deveined*

⅓ cup (33 g) sliced scallions

2 tablespoons (28 ml) sake (or sherry)

3 tablespoons (45 ml) tamari

¼ teaspoon salt

2 tablespoons (32 g) tomato paste

2 tablespoons (28 ml) hoisin sauce

1 teaspoon red pepper flakes, or to taste

2 teaspoons kudzu + ½ cup (120 ml) vegetable broth or water

Prepare rice noodles al dente according to package directions.

While noodles are soaking, heat oil in large skillet over medium heat. Add garlic and ginger and sauté 30 seconds. Add shrimp, sprinkle with scallions, and sauté, stirring frequently, until shrimp turn pink (just cooked through), about a minute or two. Remove shrimp from pan and set aside. Add the sake, tamari, salt, tomato paste, hoisin sauce, and red pepper flakes, mix well, and bring to a simmer for about a minute.

In a small bowl, mix the kudzu into the vegetable broth until dissolved and add to simmering sauce, stirring until well incorporated and sauce thickens, 1 to 2 minutes.

Stir in shrimp and serve over warm rice noodles.

Yield: about 4 servings

Per Serving: 569 Calories; 12g Fat (18.5% calories from fat); 56g Protein; 59g Carbohydrate; 3g Dietary Fiber; 343mg Cholesterol; 1493mg Sodium

* For an easy, superspeedy version of this dish, use thawed, precooked shrimp and add them to the sauce just after it's thickened.

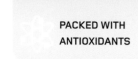

MELLOW, MISO-MARINATED PACIFIC COD

From Dr. Jonny: So a little background on this recipe. "Listen," I said one day to Chef Jeannette, "what are we going to do for people who say they just don't like fish and can't eat it? After all, there's just no substitute for the high-quality protein found in fish, which contains amino acids that your brain absolutely craves." This recipe was her answer. Sweet miso is a wonderful treatment for fish, absolutely perfect for mellowing the already mild taste of cod. And if you use real, traditional fermented miso, you'll also get a nice dose of probiotics. You probably already know from reading this book how helpful probiotics can be for the immune system, but what you might not know is that they can also benefit brain function. Preliminary research indicating the interrelationship between the nervous systems of the "gut" and the brain could mean cognitive benefits when probiotics are consumed. "The brain is not beyond the reach of probiotics," said Jia Zhao, Ph.D. And hey, this dish just might make you a fish lover.

⅓ cup (80 ml) sake (or sherry)

⅓ cup (80 ml) mirin

¼ cup (60 ml) sesame oil (or other unflavored, high-heat oil)

2 tablespoons (28 ml) tamari

½ cup (125 g) sweet white miso (or mellow white)

2 tablespoons (30 g) Sucanat

2 tablespoons (12 g) minced fresh ginger

4 pieces (6 ounces, or 170 g each) Pacific cod, skinless

Black sesame seeds, optional for garnish

In a small bowl, mix together the sake, mirin, sesame oil, tamari, miso, Sucanat, and ginger until well combined.

Place the fish in a shallow glass dish (or gallon-size zip-closure bag) and coat with marinade all over. Marinate covered (or sealed) in the fridge 4 hours to overnight.

Preheat the grill to medium high.* Scrape or wipe the marinade off the fish and grill for 10 to 12 minutes, turning at 6 minutes, or until fish is cooked through. Sprinkle with black sesame seeds to garnish, if using.

Yield: 4 servings

Per Serving: 441 Calories; 17g Fat (36.9% calories from fat); 36g Protein; 29g Carbohydrate; 2g Dietary Fiber; 63mg Cholesterol; 2287mg Sodium

* For another healthy cooking method, broil this fish in your oven for about the same length of time. Watch closely so it doesn't char. The longer you give this one to marinate (up to overnight), the richer the flavor will be.

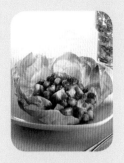

SIDE DISHES

· ·

Roasted Delicatas for Squashing Stress
Memorable, Mouthwatering Sweet Potato–Garbanzo Curry
Nutted and Nutritious Brown Rice Bonanza
Grilled Eggplant Sauté, Sardinian Style
Herbed Spaghetti Squash—Nature's Pasta

ROASTED DELICATAS FOR SQUASHING STRESS

From Dr. Jonny: Anyone who has ever seen a Popeye cartoon knows that spinach builds big biceps! (Okay, maybe not exactly, but it does provide vitamin K for your bones.) What you might not know is that largely because of its rich array of antioxidants, spinach helps protect the brain from one of the Four Horsemen of Aging—oxidative stress—which in turn reduces many of the effects of age-related decline in mental function. And a study in the medical journal *Neurology* suggested that three servings of green leafy, yellow, and cruciferous vegetables a day could slow the decline of mental performance by a whopping 40 percent. Use of the entire squash in the recipe below provides an assortment of nutrients including those found in the seeds, and roasting the whole squash pieces adds a nutty, sweet depth to the simple spinach. Enjoy!

2 small delicata squashes, or 1 large*

2 tablespoons (30 g) tahini

1 tablespoon (15 ml), plus 2 teaspoons (10 ml) Bragg Liquid Aminos (or tamari), divided

2 tablespoons (28 ml) water

¼ teaspoon garlic powder

1 ½ tablespoons (25 ml) coconut oil (we like Barlean's)

2 tablespoons (16 g) grated ginger

1 large bunch fresh spinach, chopped

¼ teaspoon crushed red pepper flakes, or to taste

1 tablespoon (8 g) toasted sesame seeds

* Nutrient-rich delicata squash, also called carnival squash or sweet potato squash, is a good source of potassium, iron, and vitamins A and C. It is a pale yellow, oblong squash, usually 5 to 8 inches (13 to 20 cm) long and 3 to 4 inches (7.5 to 10 cm) wide, with thin green stripes running along its length. They are in season in the fall, and you can usually find them in your regular grocery store. Another simple way to roast delicatas is to slice in half lengthwise, scoop out the seeds, and cook face down on a baking sheet in a 375°F (190°C, or gas mark 5) oven until soft, about 25 to 30 minutes. You can scoop the cooked flesh right out of the skin. You can also prepare this recipe with other greens, such as collards, but add a little extra liquid and steaming time (a few tablespoons of water and extra 5 minutes covered) so they are tender enough.

Preheat the oven to 375°F (190°C, or gas mark 5).

Cut off the ends of the squashes and slice widthwise into thin circular rounds (about ¼ inch or 0.5 cm each), leaving veins and seeds intact.

In a large bowl, whisk together the tahini, 1 tablespoon (15 ml) liquid aminos or tamari, water, and garlic powder. Add the squash slices and toss gently to coat.

Cover a large baking sheet with parchment paper and lay the slices out in a single layer. Roast for 15 minutes, turn the slices over, and roast for 10 to 15 minutes more or until tender.

In the meantime, prepare the spinach about 5 minutes before the end of the squash cook time. Melt the coconut oil in a large sauté pan over medium heat. Add the ginger and sauté for 2 minutes or until starting to brown. Add the spinach, pepper flakes, and remaining 2 teaspoons (10 ml) liquid aminos or tamari, and toss to coat. Sauté for 2 to 3 minutes or until wilted. Add sesame seeds and toss to combine. Remove from heat.

Lay roasted squash over sautéed spinach and serve.

Yield: about 4 servings

Per Serving: 127 Calories; 11g Fat (73.7% calories from fat); 2g Protein; 6g Carbohydrate; 2g Dietary Fiber; 0mg Cholesterol; 120mg Sodium

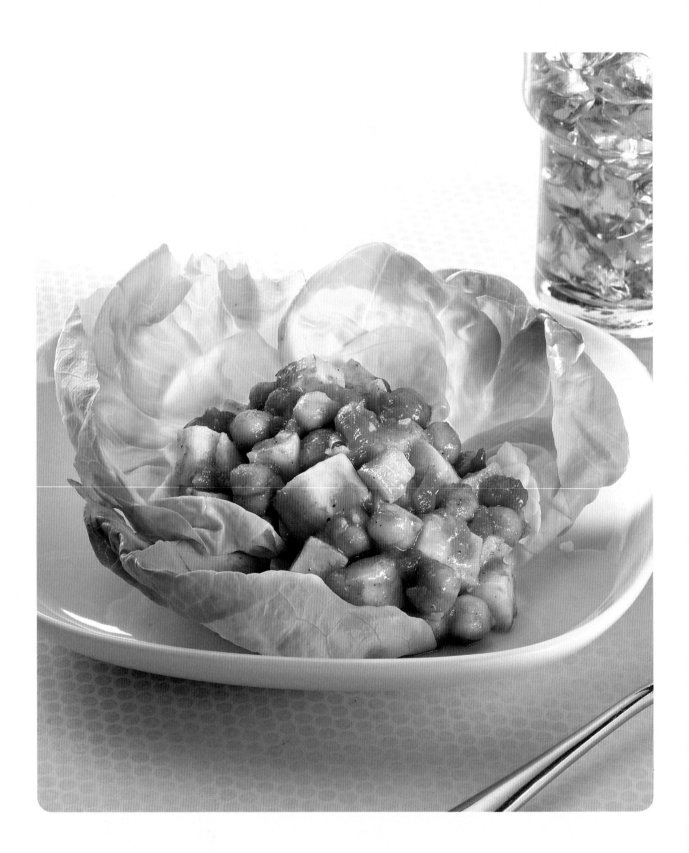

MEMORABLE, MOUTHWATERING SWEET POTATO–GARBANZO CURRY

From Dr. Jonny: No one knows for sure how to prevent Alzheimer's, dementia, and memory loss, but one thing that's becoming increasingly clear is that inflammation, one of the Four Horsemen of Aging, plays a huge part in the deterioration of the brain. And one of the most anti-inflammatory spices on Earth is turmeric. A superfood if there ever was one, turmeric is the spice that makes curry yellow; you'll get a nice dose of it in this dish. The stewed tomatoes are rich in antioxidants, which also help protect brain cells from the damaging effects of free radicals. This warming curry comes together easily and is great as a hearty side dish with a small amount of lamb, beef, or white fish. Or you can use it by itself as a nice vegetarian entrée.

1 can (14 ounces, or 400 g) stewed tomatoes, undrained, divided

2 tablespoons (28 ml) coconut oil (or olive oil)

1 yellow onion, diced fine

2 cloves garlic, minced

1 tablespoon (6 g) minced ginger

2 small sweet potatoes, peeled and cut into ½-inch (1-cm) cubes

½ teaspoon salt

½ teaspoon cracked black pepper

1 teaspoon ground coriander

½ teaspoon turmeric

½ teaspoon ground cumin

¼ teaspoon ground cloves

¼ teaspoon ground cinnamon

½ teaspoon dried shredded coconut (unsweetened), optional

1 can (14.5 ounces, or 413 g) garbanzo beans, drained and rinsed

¼ cup (65 g) tomato paste

¾ cup (175 ml) vegetable broth or water, plus more if necessary, to simmer potatoes

Pulse tomatoes a few times in food processor to chop and set aside.

Heat the oil in large sauté pan or Dutch oven over medium heat. Add the onion and sauté 3 to 5 minutes until translucent. Add garlic and ginger and sauté 1 minute. Add potatoes and ½ cup (200 g) of the stewed tomatoes and sauté for 5 to 10 minutes until potatoes have started to brown and tomato is somewhat dry. Add all spices and coconut and stir to combine. Pour in beans, remaining stewed tomatoes, tomato paste, and vegetable broth. Increase temperature and bring to a boil.

Reduce heat and simmer, covered, until potatoes are tender (about 10 to 15 minutes).

Yield: 6 servings

Per Serving: 397 Calories; 9g Fat (20.7% calories from fat); 16g Protein; 65g Carbohydrate; 15g Dietary Fiber; trace Cholesterol; 505mg Sodium

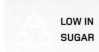
NUTTED AND NUTRITIOUS BROWN RICE BONANZA

From Dr. Jonny: Look at the diets of the areas around the globe known as the Blue Zones and several commonalities emerge: fish, whole grains, lots of vegetables, nuts, and berries. These foods protect organs such as the brain in dozens of ways, partly by providing nutrients necessary for brain function but also by providing antioxidants and anti-inflammatory properties to protect delicate brain tissue and nerve cells. This dish includes the Blue Zone mainstays and a dash of anchovies, which, by the way, are an underappreciated source of omega-3s. Hot and spicy, this dish simply sizzles with flavor. Portioned as a side dish, it's a great accompaniment to stews, soups, or marinated meats.

2½ tablespoons (40 ml) coconut oil, divided

1 large yellow onion, diced fine

¾ teaspoon red pepper flakes, or to taste

2 cloves garlic, minced

1 teaspoon anchovy paste

¼ cup (34 g) macadamia nuts, ground finely (can crush well or use the food processor)

⅓ cup (32 g) dried coconut

¾ teaspoon coriander

½ teaspoon salt

½ cup (67 g) toasted cashews

2½ cups (410 g) cooked brown basmati rice

½ cup (8 g) cilantro, chopped

In large skillet or Dutch oven, heat 1½ tablespoons oil over medium heat. Add the onion and pepper flakes and sauté 3 to 5 minutes until translucent. Add the garlic and anchovy paste and sauté 1 minute. Add the nuts and coconut and sauté 1 to 2 minutes or until just browned. Add coriander, salt, and cashews and sauté 1 minute. Add remaining tablespoon of oil and mix well. Gently fold in rice, stirring well to combine and warm, about 5 minutes. Stir in cilantro just before serving.

Yield: 4 to 6 servings

Per Serving: 268 Calories; 18g Fat (57.4% calories from fat); 5g Protein; 25g Carbohydrate; 2g Dietary Fiber; 0mg Cholesterol; 197mg Sodium

LOW IN
SUGAR

GRILLED EGGPLANT SAUTÉ, SARDINIAN STYLE

From Dr. Jonny: Ever wonder where eggplant gets its unusual color? I didn't think so—that question isn't usually number one on everybody's must-know list. But in case you're curious, it comes from a chemical called *nasunin*, properties of which are particularly useful for brain health. In animal studies, nasunin has been found to protect the fat in the membranes of brain cells, and though that may not seem like the sexiest assignment, it's critically important for brain function. If the membranes are protected from damage, they can do their job letting information in (and out) of the cell, making for better thinking, cognition, and mood. Nasunin is also a powerful antioxidant. And eggplant is a regular part of the diet of those stars of the Blue Zones, the folks in Sardinia. Want to really do it Sardinian-style? Serve this delectable dish with a salad of fresh anchovies (omega-3s!) and sun-dried tomatoes soaked in olive oil. Wow!

1 medium eggplant, sliced (½ inch or 1 cm thick)

3 tablespoons (45 ml) olive oil, divided

1 teaspoon fresh-squeezed lemon juice, optional

Salt and black pepper, to taste

3 cloves garlic

2 red bell peppers, seeded and diced

4 plum tomatoes, diced

½ teaspoon salt

½ teaspoon cracked black pepper

1 teaspoon red wine vinegar

Pinch Sucanat

¼ cup (28 g) oil-packed sun-dried tomatoes, drained and chopped

⅓ cup (13 g) chopped fresh basil

¼ cup (25 g) grated Pecorino cheese

In a large bowl, gently toss the eggplant with 1 table-spoon (15 ml) olive oil, lemon juice, salt, and pepper to taste, until evenly coated. Grill over medium heat for 3 to 4 minutes per side or until desired doneness, and set aside.

In a large sauté pan, heat the remaining 2 tablespoons (28 ml) of olive oil over medium heat. Add the garlic and sauté for 1 minute. Add the bell peppers, fresh tomatoes, salt, and pepper, and sauté until soft, about 5 to 6 minutes. Stir in the vinegar, Sucanat, and sun-dried tomatoes and sauté another minute. Add grilled eggplant slices and basil, top with the cheese, and serve.

Yield: 4 servings

Per Serving: 194 Calories; 13g Fat (58.4% calories from fat); 5g Protein; 17g Carbohydrate; 5g Dietary Fiber; 7mg Cholesterol; 371mg Sodium

FROM CHEF JEANNETTE:

Alternatively, roast the peppers when you roast the eggplant, or sauté the eggplant with the peppers (it will take about 10 to 15 minutes for the eggplant to soften in the skillet with the peppers). See page 39 for directions for roasting bell peppers. Substitute diced fresh mozzarella for the Pecorino cheese for a milder flavor.

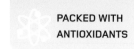

HERBED SPAGHETTI SQUASH—NATURE'S PASTA

From Dr. Jonny: Sometimes you protect an organ, such as the brain, by what you *don't* do to it—that is, feed it soda, sugar, or highly processed carbs such as spaghetti. Repeatedly overloading your body with high-glycemic (and high-calorie!) foods such as pasta can ultimately screw up the body's ability to respond to insulin. Researchers are now finding a direct link between too much insulin in the blood and not enough in the brain (they are calling it type 3 diabetes, and it's linked to Alzheimer's). Here's a way to eat something that tastes as good as pasta and won't do a single bad thing to your brain. Spaghetti squash—so named because it is stringy like its namesake—can easily replace the regular kind. With only 42 calories per cup, it's the lowest-calorie winter squash, making it a near-perfect choice for longevity. But its natural flavor is a little bland. Enter this terrific recipe, imbued with the crunch of pecan and delicious flavors from the hint of butter and light blend of fresh herbs. You'll love this savory dish.

---

1 medium spaghetti squash*

1 tablespoon (15 ml) olive oil

1 tablespoon (14 g) butter

1 large Vidalia onion, diced

3 cloves garlic, minced

½ teaspoon salt, or to taste

½ teaspoon cracked black pepper

½ teaspoon dried oregano

1 tablespoon (15 ml) balsamic vinegar

¼ cup (10 g) fresh basil, chopped

¼ cup (15 g) fresh parsley, chopped

⅓ cup (37 g) toasted pecans, coarsely chopped, optional

Preheat the oven to 375°F (190°C, or gas mark 5).

Pierce squash in 4 places with a sharp knife and place whole in a roasting pan.**

Bake for about 1 hour until soft when pressed. Allow squash to cool for at least 30 minutes and carefully cut open lengthwise. (Wear oven mitts to prevent burns— it's very hot inside the cooked squash.) Scoop out the seeds, pull the strands out, and separate them by dragging a large fork lengthwise through each half and placing into a bowl until you're left with 2 empty rinds.

Set squash strands aside and heat the oil and butter over medium in a large sauté pan. When foam subsides, add the onion and sauté for 5 minutes. Add the garlic and sauté for 1 minute. Add squash strands to the pan and stir gently to combine. Add salt, pepper, and oregano and sprinkle vinegar over all, stirring gently to combine. Remove from heat, stir in fresh herbs, sprinkle pecans over all, if using, and serve.

Yield: 4 to 6 servings, depending on the size of your squash

Per Serving: 89 Calories; 8g Fat (79.0% calories from fat); 1g Protein; 4g Carbohydrate; 1g Dietary Fiber; 5mg Cholesterol; 199mg Sodium

FROM CHEF JEANNETTE:

Add some heat with a sprinkle of red pepper flakes or try it topped with a little feta or freshly shaved Parmesan cheese and a green salad to make it a light vegetarian meal.

* Look for a squash that's more yellow in color than pale white—the deeper color indicates better ripeness.

** It takes a long time to roast the whole squash. A faster method is to cut it in half lengthwise (raw) and scoop the seeds out with a heavy spoon. Bake it face down for 30 to 45 minutes at the same temperature.

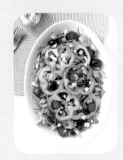

SALADS

. . . .

Gift from the Gods Greek Salad

Mediterranean Dried-Herb Salad

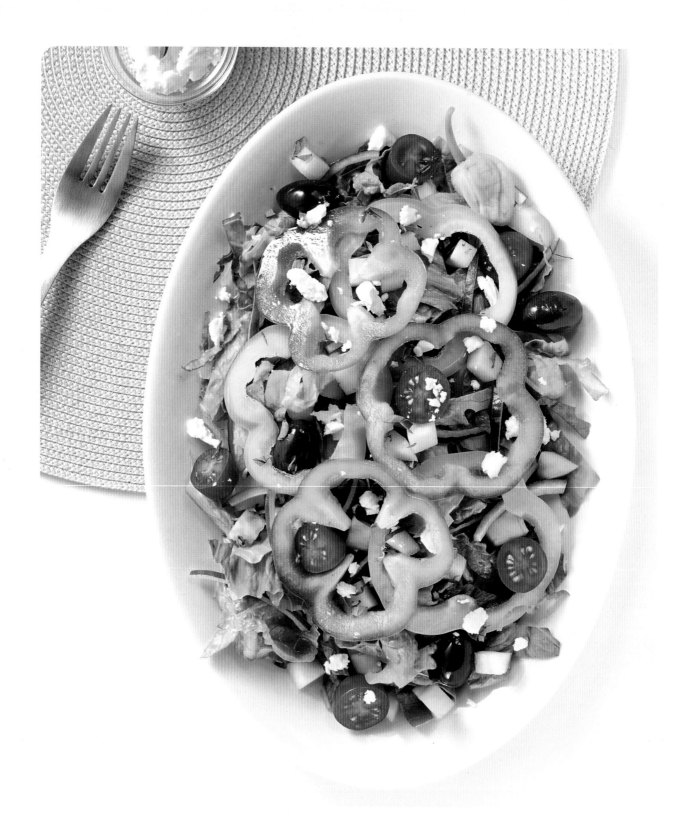

GIFT FROM THE GODS GREEK SALAD

From Dr. Jonny: Let's talk for a minute about the Mediterranean diet. At least two major studies, including a 2006 study from Columbia University, show that those who adhere most closely to the principles of Mediterranean eating have significantly lower risk of mental decline and Alzheimer's—40 percent lower in the Columbia study! And this Greek salad is a perfect example of Mediterranean eating. It also has an interesting twist that makes it even more brain protective: flaxseed oil. Rich in protective lignans, flaxseed oil adds some nifty anti-inflammatory omega-3s to the monounsaturated fats in the olive oil. This salad tastes ultrafresh and zippy.

DRESSING

3 tablespoons (45 ml) olive oil

2 tablespoons (28 ml) high-lignan flaxseed oil
(such as Barlean's)

Juice of 1 lemon

2 teaspoons red wine vinegar

2 cloves garlic, minced

1 teaspoon dried oregano

½ teaspoon dried basil

Pinch of salt

Grind or two of black pepper

SALAD BASE

6 cups (330 g) romaine lettuce, chopped into bite-size
pieces (about 1 large head or 2 hearts)

1 small red onion, halved and sliced thinly

1 small green bell pepper, seeded, ends removed, and
sliced into thin rings

1 small yellow bell pepper, seeded, ends removed, and
sliced into thin rings

1 medium cucumber, peeled and chopped

1 cup (150 g) grape tomatoes

6 small, pickled pepperoncini, whole

1 cup (100 g) Kalamata olives

²/₃ cup (100 g) crumbled feta cheese

In a small bowl whisk together all the dressing ingredients (or use an immersion blender).

In a large salad bowl, lay a base of the lettuce and arrange onions and pepper rings on the top. Sprinkle cucumber and tomatoes over peppers and arrange pepperoncini evenly around salad. Top with olives and crumble cheese over all.

Dress to taste.

Yield: about 4 servings

Per Serving: 356 Calories; 30g Fat (72.3% calories from fat); 7g Protein; 19g Carbohydrate; 4g Dietary Fiber; 22mg Cholesterol; 860mg Sodium

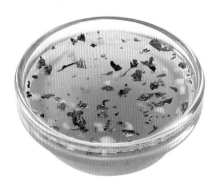

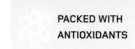
MEDITERRANEAN DRIED-HERB SALAD

From Dr. Jonny: Here's an interesting coincidence: On the very day I was writing this introduction, a new study came out showing that sticking to a Mediterranean diet may help prevent dementia. The Mediterranean diet, which has previously been shown to reduce heart disease, seems to lower the risk of having small areas of dead tissue in the brain that are linked to thinking problems. These areas are known as brain infarcts, and they're deeply involved in vascular dementia, the most common form of dementia next to Alzheimer's disease. Need I say more? This salad comes straight out of the Mediterranean diet playbook—rich in olives and olive oil, green vegetables, and tomatoes, it's fast and easy to assemble and will reward you with simple, bright flavors. The bitter bite of the greens is cut by the sharpness of the lemon and aids wonderfully in digestion.

1 medium head chicory, cored and torn into bite-size pieces

2 cups (60 g) baby spinach

1 cup (100 g) pitted Greek olives, halved

2 large heirloom tomatoes, chopped

½ cup (70 g) pine nuts

1 teaspoon dried oregano

¾ teaspoon garlic powder

½ teaspoon onion powder

¼ teaspoon dried marjoram

¼ teaspoon dried thyme

Pinch salt

Cracked black pepper, to taste

1 lemon

3 tablespoons (45 ml) olive oil

1 clove garlic, finely minced

In a large salad bowl, toss together greens, olives, tomatoes, and pine nuts. Evenly sprinkle herbs and spices to taste over all, using the given measurements as a guide only.

Roll the lemon hard under the heel of your hand to help release the liquid from the pulp. Slice in half and squeeze over the salad, removing the seeds and discarding.

In a small bowl, whisk together the olive oil and garlic and pour evenly over the salad. Toss to combine, correct seasonings, and serve.

Yield: 4 servings

Per Serving: 271 Calories; 24g Fat (75.6% calories from fat); 6g Protein; 12g Carbohydrate; 4g Dietary Fiber; 0mg Cholesterol; 227mg Sodium

FROM CHEF JEANNETTE:

To make it an ultrafast longevity meal with clean protein and omega-3 fatty acids, just add a drained can of chunk light or skipjack tuna, or anchovies, to taste.

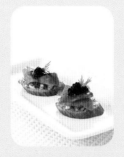

BREAKFASTS and SNACKS

Jonny's Brainy Breakfast Scramble
Mind–Full Middle Eastern Stewed Eggs
Salmon Frittata, Nova Scotian Centenarian Style
Brain Gain Tuna Spread
Rise and Brine Gravlax Canapés
Afternoon Pick–Me–Up Potassium Miso Soup

JONNY'S BRAINY BREAKFAST SCRAMBLE

From Dr. Jonny: I admit, I'm not the greatest cook in the world, which is why I coauthor these books with Chef Jeannette. But I have one special recipe I make really well, and I call it my Brainy Breakfast Scramble. The unique blend of ingredients, which I admit I originally chose for taste and ease of preparation, turn out to be a compendium of nutrients for brain health. And while most people don't immediately think of eggs as brain food, the truth is that they are just that, and here's why: Eggs (especially the yolks) are one of the best sources in the world of *choline*, a nutrient in the B-vitamin family that the body uses to make an important brain chemical called acetylcholine. *Acetylcholine* is a neurotransmitter that's vitally important in thinking, memory, and cognition; by giving the body exactly what it needs to produce more acetycholine, eggs deserve a place on the short list of brain foods. The apples are very high in an anti-inflammatory flavonoid called *quercetin*, which can calm the inflammatory fires in the brain (and body) that rob us of vital energy and life. This omelet tastes great and comes together so easily even a bachelor like me can whip it up in no time. Bonus points if you can get free-range, omega-3 eggs!

1 tablespoon (15 ml) coconut oil

2 teaspoons (9 g) butter

2 apples, unpeeled, cored, and cut into bite-size pieces

4 cups (120 g) baby spinach

4 eggs, lightly beaten

½ teaspoon turmeric

½ teaspoon lemon pepper, or to taste

¼ teaspoon salt, or to taste

Melt the oil and butter in a large skillet over medium heat. Add the apples and cook, stirring occasionally, until they brown lightly or turn translucent, about 4 to 6 minutes. Add the spinach and cook for 1 to 2 minutes until it begins to wilt. Pour the eggs over all and stir to mix well. Sprinkle in the turmeric, pepper, and salt, mix well, and continue to cook until the eggs reach desired doneness.

Yield: 2 large or 4 small servings

Per Serving: 169 Calories; 11g Fat (55.0% calories from fat); 7g Protein; 12g Carbohydrate; 3g Dietary Fiber; 217mg Cholesterol; 289mg Sodium

MIND-FULL MIDDLE EASTERN STEWED EGGS

From Dr. Jonny: If you've read any of my writing over the past decade you know that one of my pet dietary peeves is egg-white omelets. I think they're ludicrous. The yolks are what make eggs "brain food." They contain *choline*, the building block of one of the most important chemicals in the brain, acetylcholine, a neurotransmitter that is essential for thinking, memory, and cognition in general. This recipe breaks away from the standard American omelets and makes for a new (and quite delicious) presentation that's great hot or cold, good for breakfast or a snack. With their unusual Middle Eastern combo of spices, these eggs are sure to break up a humdrum breakfast habit!

1 can (14.5 ounces, or 413 g) whole stewed tomatoes, undrained

1 tablespoon (15 ml) olive oil

1 yellow or sweet onion, diced

1 clove garlic, minced

¼ cup (25 g) diced scallions

½ teaspoon ground cinnamon

¼ teaspoon allspice

Pinch turmeric

Pinch ground cumin

Tiny pinch ground clove

Tiny pinch ground nutmeg

½ teaspoon salt

¼ teaspoon cracked black pepper

Dash hot pepper sauce, or to taste

8 eggs, boiled, peeled, and halved lengthwise

Pulse the stewed tomatoes and juices a couple of times in a food processor or briefly blend in a blender until the tomatoes are chopped and set aside.

Heat the oil in a 12-inch (30-cm) skillet over medium heat. Add the onion and cook for 5 minutes. Add the garlic and scallions and cook 1 minute. Add the spices (through black pepper) and cook for 30 seconds, stirring constantly. Add the diced tomatoes and hot sauce, stir to combine, and cook for 3 minutes. Carefully add the egg halves, with the yolks facing up, gently spooning the tomato mixture over the tops of the eggs. Reduce the heat to medium low and simmer the eggs in the tomatoes, frequently spooning sauce over the tops, for 7 to 9 minutes, reducing the heat if the sauce gets too sputtery.

Yield: 4 servings

Per Serving: 223 Calories; 14g Fat (54.7% calories from fat); 14g Protein; 11g Carbohydrate; 2g Dietary Fiber; 424mg Cholesterol; 439mg Sodium

FROM CHEF JEANNETTE:

Our choice for eggs is always organic and cage free, preferably from a local farmer with chickens you can see running around. Some hens are fed omega-3-enhanced feed, and the omegas are available in the eggs. This is another great way to increase those essential fatty acids in your diet for brain health. These eggs are great served over a bed of almost any steamed green.

To boil the eggs, lay them in a single layer in a large soup pot and cover with cold water. Place pot over high heat, cover, and cook for 15 minutes, reducing heat to medium high and only partially covering once boiling. Pour the water off and allow them to cool, or place them in cool water to speed the process.

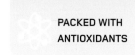

SALMON FRITTATA, NOVA SCOTIAN CENTENARIAN STYLE

From Dr. Jonny: There are an awful lot of centenarians in Nova Scotia, and I can't help wondering if it has to do with all the fish they eat. (Nova Scotia salmon, anyone?) Smoked salmon is rich in brain-protecting omega-3 fats as well as performance-enhancing vitamin D, and eggs are one of the best sources of choline, a B-vitamin relative the body uses to make neurotransmitters that help you think better! There's also choline in the cottage cheese, making this tasty frittata dish a real memory booster. And don't forget the panoply of nutrients in spinach. According to psychologist Barbara Shukitt-Hale, Ph.D., a daily dose of spinach extract fed to lab rats "prevented some loss of long-term memory and learning ability normally experienced by the 15-month-old rats." Spinach was also the most potent extract in protecting different types of nerve cells against the effects of aging.

Cooking oil spray

1 medium leek, roots and tough stalk removed

7 large eggs

1 cup (225 g) cottage cheese

1 tablespoon (4 g) fresh chopped dill or 1 teaspoon dried

½ teaspoon salt, or to taste

½ teaspoon cracked black pepper

2 shots hot pepper sauce, or to taste

1 tablespoon (8.6 g) capers, or to taste

1 tablespoon (15 ml) olive oil

2 cloves garlic, minced

2 cups (60 g) baby spinach

1 can (5.5 ounces, or 157 g) smoked sockeye salmon, drained and broken up (we like Vital Choice)

Preheat the oven to 350°F (180°C, or gas mark 4). Spray or butter a 9-inch (23-cm) deep-dish pie plate.

Cut the prepared leek in half lengthwise and then chop into 1-inch (2.5-cm) segments. Immerse pieces in clean sink or large bowl of water and separate to clean completely, removing all grit. Drain, rinse, and set aside.

In a large bowl, beat eggs with about 2 tablespoons (28 ml) water. Whisk in the cottage cheese, dill, salt, pepper, and hot pepper sauce. Stir in capers and set aside.

Heat the oil in a skillet over medium heat. Add leeks and sauté until soft, about 4 to 5 minutes.

Add garlic and sauté 1 minute. Stir in spinach and cook until just wilted, about 1 minute. Spoon leek-spinach mixture evenly into prepared pie plate. Stir salmon gently into eggs and pour mixture over leek-spinach mixture in pie plate. Bake for 20 to 25 minutes or until firm.

FROM CHEF JEANNETTE:

If your skillet is large enough, you can make your frittata right in the pan. Simply pour the egg mixture over the greens and cook uncovered over medium-low heat for 15 to 20 minutes, without stirring, or until eggs are set.

Yield: 4 servings

Per Serving: 280 Calories; 15g Fat (49.5% calories from fat); 27g Protein; 8g Carbohydrate; 1g Dietary Fiber; 385mg Cholesterol; 1333mg Sodium

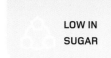

BRAIN GAIN TUNA SPREAD

From Dr. Jonny: To tell you the truth, I don't think I ever tried Neûfchatel till Chef Jeannette whipped up this rich-tasting little spread. And don't you love the recipe name? Tuna is a fabulous source of protein. It also contains *tyrosine*, an amino acid that our bodies use to build the neurotransmitter that brightens your day and gives you mental energy—dopamine. This spread has a pleasingly piquant flavo, and is great with veggie sticks or spread on whole-grain crackers. Tip: Try ordering canned tuna from Vital Choice, my favorite source for pristine, uncontaminated, and delicious fish both frozen and canned. I have a link to them on my website under "healthy foods." You may never go back to supermarket tuna again!

8 ounces (225 g) Neûfchatel or soy cream cheese

1 teaspoon lemon zest

1 tablespoon (15 ml) fresh-squeezed lemon juice

2 shots hot pepper sauce, or to taste

¼ cup (25 g) chopped scallions

1 to 2 tablespoons (4 to 8 g) chopped fresh parsley, to taste

2 cans (5 ounces, or 140 g each) water-packed tuna, drained*

⅓ cup (33 g) chopped Kalamata or niçoise olives

1 tablespoon (8.6 g) capers

* Choose skipjack or chunk light tuna for lowest ocean contaminants. Use one can for a lighter fish flavor, two for more omega punch. You can substitute canned salmon for more omega-3s.

In a food processor blend Neûfchatel, zest, lemon juice, pepper sauce, scallions, parsley, and tuna until well blended, scraping down the sides as necessary.

Using a stiff spatula or wooden spoon, stir in the olives and capers until mixed.

Serve at room temperature or chill in the refrigerator for 1 to 2 hours before serving.

Yield: about 8 servings

Per Serving: 169 Calories; 8g Fat (43.9% calories from fat); 10g Protein; 13g Carbohydrate; 2g Dietary Fiber; 11mg Cholesterol; 522mg Sodium

FROM CHEF JEANNETTE:

You can also cook this to make it a hot dish. Cover a mini loaf pan with high-heat cooking oil spray. Line with wax or parchment paper and spray with oil. Spoon the spread over the paper into the mold, trimming the edges so no paper is exposed. If you don't have a mini loaf pan, you can try it in individual lined and sprayed muffin tins. Bake at 400°F (200°C, or gas mark 6) for about 10 minutes, or until just browning and slightly puffed.

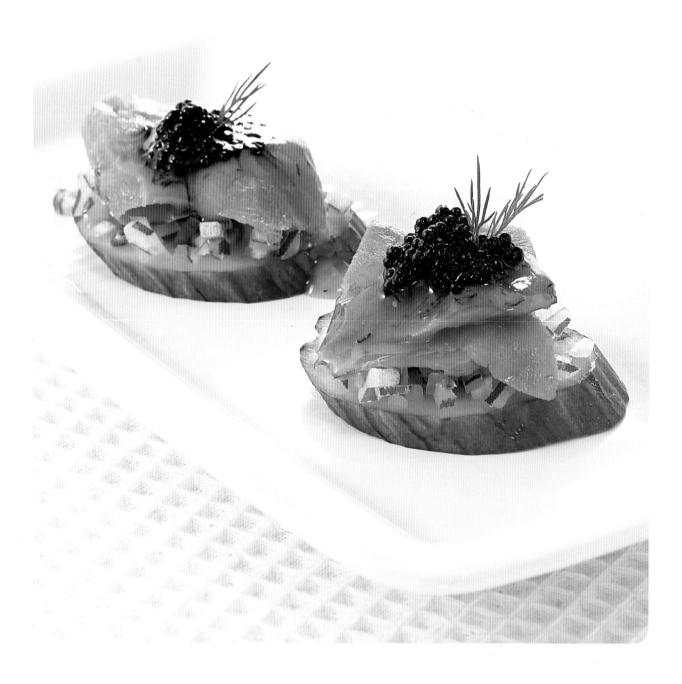

RISE AND BRINE GRAVLAX CANAPÉS

From Dr. Jonny: Your brain is about 60 percent fat by weight, and a great portion of that fat is in the form of a particular fatty acid called DHA (docosahexaenoic acid). And guess where DHA is found? In cold-water fish such as wild salmon. This omega-3 fatty acid is one of two found in fish (the other is EPA, or eicosapentaenoic acid). Both of these valuable omega-3s are needed for optimal brain health. They can improve mood, lower inflammation, and generally improve communication between the brain cells (neurons), making it easier for them to "talk" to each other (and improving memory, thinking, and cognition in the process).

GRAVLAX

4 tablespoons (60 g) Sucanat

4 tablespoons (72 g) sea salt

1 tablespoon (6.4 g) fresh-ground black pepper

1.5 to 2 pounds (710 to 900 g) highest-quality fresh wild salmon fillets, scaled and deboned, skin intact

1 large bunch dill

2 tablespoons (28 ml) Grand Marnier, optional

CANAPÉS

1½ tablespoons (22 g) Dijon mustard

1½ tablespoons (30 g) raw honey

1 teaspoon chopped dill, or to taste

¼ teaspoon black pepper, or to taste

1 large English cucumber, peeled and sliced into ¼-inch (0.5-cm) discs

1 red onion, sliced paper thin or diced fine

1 bunch fresh dill, snipped into small sprigs for garnish

1 ounce (28 g) black caviar or olive tapenade, optional, for garnish

For the gravlax: Three days prior to serving, sterilize a shallow glass or ceramic dish in the dishwasher.

In a small bowl, mix the Sucanat, salt, and pepper together. Evenly coat the fish with the mixture and place into the prepared dish, skin side down. Cover with dill and pour the Grand Marnier, if using, over all. Cover the fish with plastic wrap and lay a clean, heavy skillet carefully right on top of it (over the plastic). Add a couple of heavy cans to the skillet to weight it evenly (this helps the fish to release its juices, preparing the brine). Set the dish carefully in the refrigerator and leave it undisturbed for 3 days.

Prepare the canapés: In a small bowl, mix together the mustard, honey, dill, and pepper.

Slice prepared salmon into 1-inch (2.5-cm) squares, ¼ inch (0.5 cm) thick.

Assemble canapés on a large platter with a cucumber as the base, onion on the cucumber, salmon slice on the onion, topped with a bit of the mustard sauce, a sprig of dill, and a bit of the caviar or tapenade, if using.

Yield: approximately 24 canapés

Per Serving: 65 Calories; 2g Fat (22.9% calories from fat); 8g Protein; 4g Carbohydrate; trace Dietary Fiber; 26mg Cholesterol; 1183mg Sodium

FROM CHEF JEANNETTE:

The concept for this recipe comes from my (mostly) Norwegian friend and colleague, Judy Hestnes, R.D. and professional chef. Gravlax is a cured fish dish popular in several Scandinavian countries. Curing the salmon in the salt and sugar will cause it to create its own brine, but it means you will need to start preparations three days before you wish to serve it. But it's well worth it!

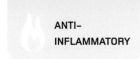

AFTERNOON PICK-ME-UP POTASSIUM MISO SOUP

From Dr. Jonny: Alkalizing and calming to the system, this ultralight, brothy soup will help calm your frazzled nerves when you really need a vacation but it isn't convenient to just fly off to Jamaica. And calming your nerves is central to reducing inflammatory stress hormones that can play havoc with brain health. In addition to being a comfort food, this soup is loaded with potassium, an alkaline mineral that's involved in the cellular pumps that regulate the transport of water and nutrients into the cell walls (including cells in the brain). Potassium deficiencies can cause the cells to fill with water and swell up. There's speculation that potassium deficiency may be partly responsible for chronic headaches. In any case, the combination of nutrients in this "snack" soup will give your brain a nice little boost. It's a great remedy for that annoying brain and nervous system crash that hits so many of us come 3 p.m.!

4 carrots, unpeeled, grated, and divided in half

2 potatoes, unpeeled and sliced thick

1 large yellow onion, unpeeled and quartered

½ head green cabbage, chopped

2 heads broccoli, chopped

3 stalks celery, chopped

½ cup (30 g) chopped parsley

1 piece kombu (2 inches, or 5 cm)

4 tablespoons (64 g) barley miso paste, or to taste

¾ cup (75 g) sliced scallions

1 cup (460 g) firm tofu, cut into ½-inch (1-cm) cubes

½ sheet nori, sliced or snipped into thin ribbons, optional

In a stockpot (or large soup pot), add half the grated carrots, all the potatoes, onion, cabbage, broccoli, celery, parsley, and kombu, and cover generously with cold water (about 10 cups, or 2.5 L). Bring soup to boil over high heat. Reduce heat, cover, and simmer for 30 minutes. Strain veggies out using a colander or double-mesh strainer and return 8 cups (2 L) of broth to the pot (removed from heat), storing any remaining broth in the fridge to sip as a tea. Discard steeped veggies. Stir in miso paste until dissolved. Gently add second half of grated carrots, scallions, tofu, and nori and stir gently to combine.

Rest soup for 2 minutes before serving.

Yield: 4 servings

Per Serving: 363 Calories; 9g Fat (19.0% calories from fat); 27g Protein; 57g Carbohydrate; 21g Dietary Fiber; 0mg Cholesterol; 847mg Sodium

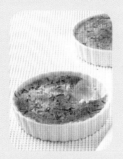

DESSERTS

· ·

Coconut Lemon Custard Tastes-like-Cheesecake
Sweet Bean Paste—Dessert That's Good for You

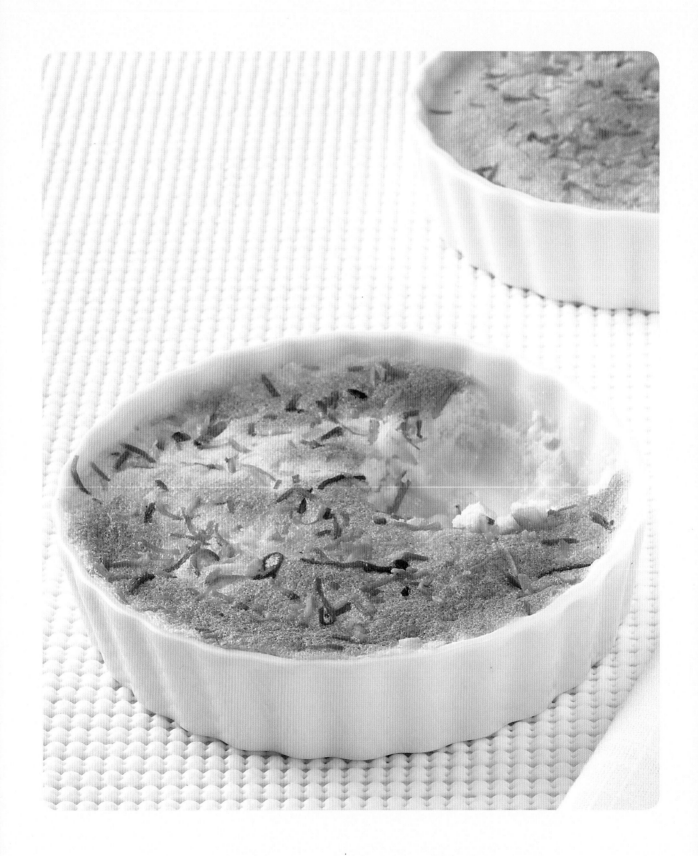

COCONUT LEMON CUSTARD TASTES-LIKE-CHEESECAKE

From Dr. Jonny: You probably already know that fish is "brain food." But did you also know that eggs are, too? Here's why: There's a chemical in your brain called *acetylcholine*. This chemical is classed as a neurotransmitter, *neuro* meaning "brain" and *transmitter* meaning, well, "transmission." That means it relays, or amplifies, signals (information) from one brain cell (neuron) to the next, and in the case of this particular neurotransmitter, it has great importance to thinking, cognition, and memory. Acetylcholine also plays an important role in sustaining attention. And guess what the body uses to make acetylcholine? Choline! A member of the B-vitamin family, choline is vital for the manufacturing of acetylcholine. And guess where choline is found? You got it: eggs. Particularly the yolks. So you can enjoy this creamy, coconutty custard knowing it's delivering important nutrients that allow your brain to function at peak potential.

1 cup (235 ml) soy milk

1 cup (235 ml) cow's milk

4 tablespoons (60 ml) coconut oil, plus extra for oiling pan

Juice and zest of 1 lemon

1¼ cups (300 g) xylitol, divided

⅔ cup (83 g) unbleached wheat flour

Pinch salt

4 egg yolks, beaten

4 egg whites

¼ cup (21 g) dried unsweetened coconut

2 tablespoons (12 g) toasted dried unsweetened coconut

Preheat the oven to 350°F (180°C, or gas mark 4).

Oil a 7 x 11-inch (18 x 28-cm) glass baking pan with coconut oil. Set the prepared pan into a roasting pan and fill the roasting pan with water to halfway up the side of the baking pan. Set aside.

In a medium pan over medium heat, combine the milks and coconut oil. Cook, whisking frequently, until the coconut oil is fully melted and well incorporated into the milk but before the milk boils, about 4 to 5 minutes. Remove from the heat and set aside.

In a medium bowl, mix together the lemon juice and zest and 1 cup (240 g) of xylitol. Add the flour, salt, and beaten yolks and whisk or beat them together until well incorporated.

Whisk the milk and oil mixture into the flour and yolk mixture. Set aside.

Beat the egg whites with a mixer until foamy. Continue to beat on medium high, gradually adding the remaining ¼ cup (60 g) xylitol until the mixture stiffens and just becomes glossy, but before it makes heavy peaks.

Gently whisk about half the egg white mixture into the batter until well incorporated. Gently fold in remaining egg white mixture one cup at a time—don't overmix it!

Sprinkle ¼ cup (21 g) dried coconut evenly over the bottom of the prepared pan and pour the batter over the top. Sprinkle the toasted coconut evenly over the top and gently place the pans in the oven. Cook for 30 to 35 minutes or until starting to brown lightly and top springs back when lightly pressed.

Yield: 9 servings

Per Serving: 232 Calories; 10g Fat (30.3% calories from fat); 6g Protein; 44g Carbohydrate; 2g Dietary Fiber; 98mg Cholesterol; 73mg Sodium

FROM CHEF JEANNETTE:

For this treat, I needed to use a small amount of white flour—the only time in the book—because egg whites are so light and fussy they wouldn't support the weight of whole-wheat pastry flour.

SWEET BEAN PASTE—DESSERT THAT'S GOOD FOR YOU

From Dr. Jonny: The Japanese have the right idea—desserts should be nutritious foods, and this sweet bean paste is a perfect example. Adzuki beans are very healthy. High in fiber, relatively low in calories, and when sweetened with honey, immensely satisfying at the end of a meal—or anytime at all.

**1 can (14.5 ounces or 413 g) adzuki beans,
drained and rinsed**

⅓ cup (155 g) honey

¼ teaspoon salt

Process the beans in a food processor, scraping down the sides frequently, for about a minute off and on or until mashed into a paste. Add the honey and salt and continue to process until it forms a very smooth paste. In a heavy medium saucepan, cook bean mixture at medium low for about 20 minutes, stirring occasionally. At 20 minutes or when it starts simmering, watch it more closely, stirring frequently over 10 to 15 minutes until it forms a thick paste. Store in the fridge.

Yield: about 1½ cups (375 g)

Per Serving: 36 Calories; .02g Fat (0% calories from fat); 1.3g Protein; 8g Carbohydrate; 1.3g Dietary Fiber; 0mg Cholesterol; 66mg Sodium

RED BEAN GEL CANDIES

2 tablespoons (7 g) agar flakes

2 cups (475 ml) water

⅓ cup (115 g) honey

½ cup (125 g) red bean paste

FROM CHEF JEANNETTE:

Red bean paste is actually one of my all-time faves—and nutritious to boot! These dessert ideas are very classically Japanese. If they don't appeal to you, try using it in other ways. I love sweet bean paste spread lightly on dry cookies, stuffed into chewy rice mochi, or topping my vanilla Rice Dream! With its earthy sweet quality, it is deeply satisfying.

Heat the agar flakes and water in a large saucepan over medium-high heat until it reaches a boil, stirring occasionally. Reduce heat to medium and simmer for 5 to 7 minutes or until flakes have dissolved completely. Add the honey and simmer for 5 minutes more.

In a small bowl, mix bean paste and ½ cup (170 g) of the agar-honey mixture until well incorporated (immersion blender works well for this). Add another ¼ cup (85 g) of the agar-honey liquid and blend well. Pour the bean mixture into the saucepan and whisk (or blend) to incorporate. Cook for 3 minutes until fully incorporated.

Pour into an 8 x 8-inch (20 x 20-cm) baking pan (glass, if you have it) and refrigerate for 1 to 2 hours until fully set and chilled. Slice into bars to serve.

Yield: 16 bars

Per Serving: 60 Calories; trace Fat (0.6% calories from fat); 2g Protein; 14g Carbohydrate; 1g Dietary Fiber; 0mg Cholesterol; 13mg Sodium

RED BEAN RICE BALLS

Process 1½ cups (245 g) cooked sweet brown rice with 1 to 2 tablespoons (20 to 40 g) honey and a touch of salt until it starts to form a dough, adding a little water if necessary. With wet hands, pinch off enough rice to roll a 1-inch (2.5-cm) ball and flatten it into a patty.

Pinch off enough bean paste to make a ½-inch (1-cm) ball and place it into the center of the rice patty. Pinch the ends of the rice up to cover the paste and roll the ball in toasted sesame seeds. Store in the fridge.

Yield: 22 to 24 rice balls

Per Serving: 38.5 Calories; trace Fat (0% calories from fat); 1.2g Protein; 8.9g Carbohydrate; 1g Dietary Fiber; 0mg Cholesterol; 72.9mg Sodium

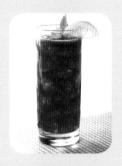

DRINKS

· · · · · · · · · · · · · · · · · · · ·

Anti-Inflammatory Virgin Bloody Mary
Dehydration Destroyers: Flavor Waters
Turn-Up-the-Volume Berry-Cherry Pom Juice Cocktail

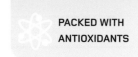
ANTI-INFLAMMATORY VIRGIN BLOODY MARY

From Dr. Jonny: Here's a real pick-me-up substitute for the usual vodka-laced ("bring-me-down") version of this popular cocktail. I won't say that you'll never miss the alcohol, but I will tell you that this version will do a heck of a lot more for your brain and your longevity than the "get soused on the airplane" version! Antioxidants from the tomato and the spices help calm oxidative damage, one of the Four Horsemen of brain aging. And compounds in celery with the unpronounceable names of luteolin and diosmin appear to block inflammation that causes the brains of Alzheimer's patients to start shrinking and dying.

6 large ripe heirloom tomatoes, quartered

Juice from 2 lemons

2 tablespoons (30 g) prepared horseradish, or to taste

½ teaspoon Sucanat

2½ teaspoons Worcestershire sauce (organic, please, to avoid high-fructose corn syrup!)

1 teaspoon tamari

¾ teaspoon fresh-ground black pepper

2 to 4 dashes hot sauce, or to taste

1 tablespoon (4 g) minced fresh parsley

4 stalks celery

In a blender, add all ingredients except celery and process until smooth, scraping down the sides as necessary. Chill well and serve over ice with a trimmed celery stalk.

Yield: 4 servings

Per Serving: 74 Calories; 1g Fat (9.5% calories from fat); 2g Protein; 17g Carbohydrate; 3g Dietary Fiber; 0mg Cholesterol; 135mg Sodium

DEHYDRATION DESTROYERS: FLAVOR WATERS

From Dr. Jonny: Several years ago, I was on a panel for the LA Times Festival of Health and Fitness along with a number of notable health practitioners. One doctor on the panel told the audience that he gave every patient who came to see him the same prescription on the first visit: Double the amount of water you're drinking and come back next week. "Virtually three-fourths of their symptoms disappear," the doctor said. Everyone else on the panel nodded vigorously. Your brain is about 78 percent water. Even a minor amount of dehydration can impair performance, memory, and thinking, not to mention longevity. These great flavored waters make it easier to get your eight-plus glasses a day. They're slightly alkalizing and way higher quality than the store-bought flavored variety. Crisp, refreshing, noncaloric, with a bunch of trace nutrients. What's not to like?

HOT SUMMER'S DAY–ADE

1 lime, peeled*

1 medium cucumber, peeled

3 liters pure spring water

Per Serving: 10 Calories; trace Fat (2.3% calories from fat); trace Protein; 6g Carbohydrate; trace Dietary Fiber; 0mg Cholesterol; 1mg Sodium

HINT OF MINT–ADE

1 large crisp "eating" apple, peeled

⅓ cup (30 g) mint leaves

3 liters pure spring water

Per Serving Serving (excluding unknown items): 16 Calories; trace Fat (4.3% calories from fat); trace Protein; 4g Carbohydrate; 1g Dietary Fiber; 0mg Cholesterol; 2mg Sodium

CITRUS SNAP–ADE

1 lemon or orange, peeled*

¼ cup (25 g) peeled and grated ginger

3 liters pure spring water

Per Serving: 25 Calories; trace Fat (9.1% calories from fat); 1g Protein; 6g Carbohydrate; 1g Dietary Fiber; 0mg Cholesterol; 1mg Sodium

* It's easiest to use a knife to peel lemons and limes. Just cut away the skins and white pith, which is bitter, with a paring knife in long strips.

To prepare any of these flavored waters, cut peeled fruit or vegetables into ½-inch (1-cm) segments: lemons, limes, and cucumbers can be cut in half lengthwise and then sliced into ½-inch (1-cm) half-moons; apples can be cored, sliced, and slices halved or quartered; oranges can be split into segments and the segments halved or quartered. Place the ingredients into your water jug, give it a shake, and chill for 12 to 24 hours in the refrigerator.

After soaking and chilling, strain out all veggie and fruit pieces through a double-mesh strainer into a large bowl. You may have to swirl the water around a bit to get everything out of the bottle. Using a funnel, carefully pour the flavor water back into your jug and enjoy. Keep refrigerated.

Yield: 3 liters

FROM CHEF JEANNETTE:

It's best to choose organic produce for your waters because you don't want to be filling them with pesticides and fungicides.

Once you have the concept, don't be afraid to experiment with your favorite ingredients/flavors. My favorite waters have a bunch of different things in them at once. I've added garden cilantro or basil to these combos for an offbeat taste. It works well with fresh berries, too!

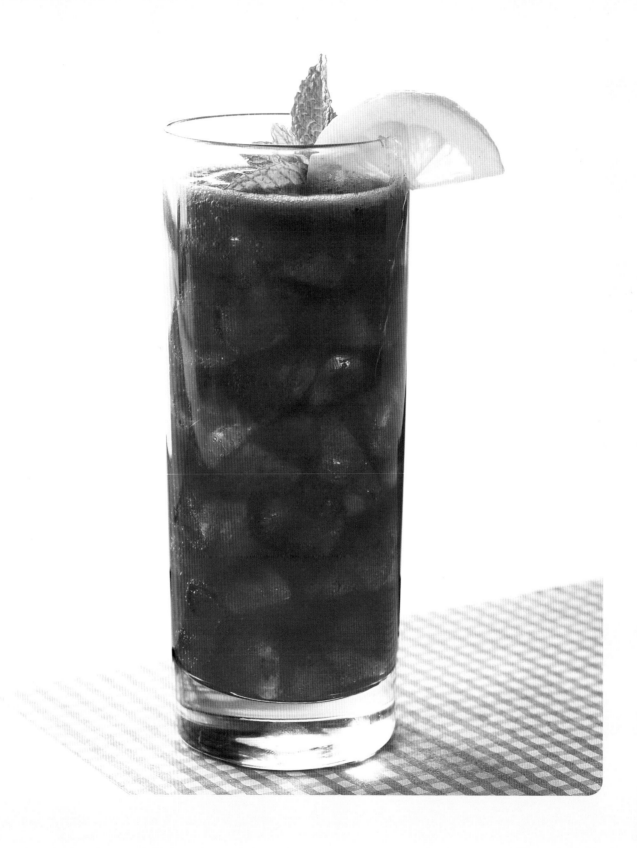

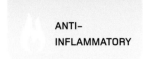

TURN-UP-THE-VOLUME BERRY-CHERRY POM JUICE COCKTAIL

From Dr. Jonny: When Jim Josephs, Ph.D., runs animal experiments at the Laboratory of Neuroscience at the U.S. Department of Agriculture's Human Nutrition Research Center on Aging, he has a little thing called the Rat Olympics. He tests the rats for things such as memory and motor function, strength, and coordination. Around middle age the rats start to decline. Then Josephs feeds them blueberries, and they begin to behave like young studs. Blueberries, you see, actually help nerve cells in the brain talk to each other. Special compounds in the blueberries called *polyphenols* actually turn up the volume on the phone lines these cells use to communicate with one another, resulting in better brain function: better memory, better motor coordination, better everything. But blueberries aren't the only brain food in this nice little cocktail. Pomegranate juice, black cherry juice, and strawberries are filled with antioxidants and anti-inflammatory properties that help protect brain tissue as well. I love this drink as a nonalcoholic alternative at cocktail hour, and no one will even know you're not drinking the hard stuff.

½ cup (120 ml) unsweetened black cherry juice

½ cup (120 ml) unsweetened pomegranate juice

1 cup (235 ml) water or sparkling water

2 cups (290 g) fresh blueberries

2 cups (290 g) fresh strawberries

Ice, to taste

Mint leaves or lemon wedges, optional for garnish

In a small pitcher, mix together black cherry juice, pomegranate juice, and water. Juice blueberries and strawberries and add liquids to pitcher. Stir gently to combine, pour over ice, and garnish with mint leaves or lemon wedges, if using. If you don't wish to ice the juice, add more water or seltzer to thin, as desired.

Yield: 4 glasses

Per Serving: 99 Calories; 1g Fat (4.5% calories from fat); 1g Protein; 24g Carbohydrate; 3g Dietary Fiber; 0mg Cholesterol; 12mg Sodium

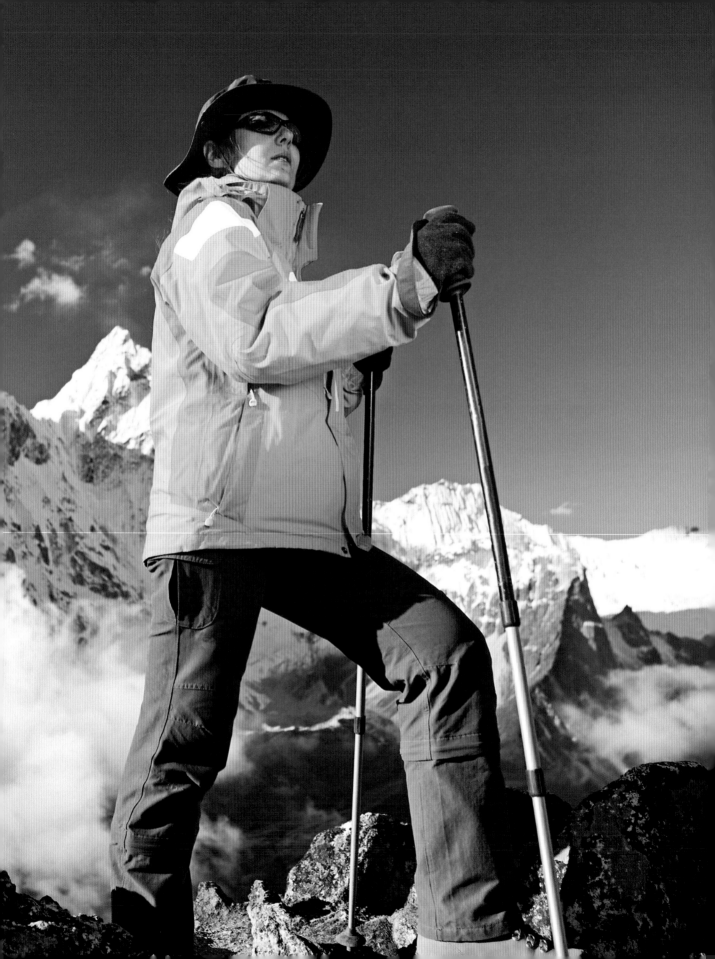

Chapter III

Help Your Muscles, Bones, and Tendons Stay Fit, Firm, and Flexible with This Fare

. . . .

ENTRÉES

Nutrient Blast Orange Black–Bean Soup

Anti-Aging Apple-Pumpkin Ginger Soup

An Ocean of Nutrition: Grilled Lobster and Mango with Coconut Cream

Fresh Caesar Salad with Mustard-Grilled Shrimp

Blood Orange–Scallop Salad with Feta and Macadamia

Protein Blast Asian Grilled Chicken

Bone-Building Bell Peppers Stuffed with Seafood Quinoa

Strengthening Mustard-Hoisin Lettuce Wraps

Better Butternut Flax Mac and Cheese

Leaner, Better Turkey-Basil Meat Loaf

Tangy Antioxidant Creole Seafood Stew

SIDE DISHES

A Sea of Nutrients: Cold Marinated Shrimp Salad

Vitamin Overload Stir-Fried Chard

Bone Up on Baked Okra

Krispy Kale: A Vitamin K Extravaganza

Not Your Average Green Beans

SALADS

Bone-Building Mandarin-Broccoli Salad

Fabulous Fruit-and-Veg Vitamin C Salad

BREAKFASTS AND SNACKS

Better Bones Muffins

Potassium-Powered Raw Muesli

Sweet and Savory Magnesium-Calcium Combo Snacks

Bone-sational Mexi-Tofu Dip

Easy Edamame Hummus

DESSERTS

Not Your Mother's Pumpkin Pie

Gingered Mango and Green Tea Freeze

DRINKS

Creamy Green Smoothie

Day-at-the-Park Dreamsicle Shake

Carrot-Orange Juice for Strong Bones

Antioxidant Almond Nog

I f I ask you right now to think about what being really old looks like, what's the picture that immediately comes to mind?

Chances are you think of someone frail. Someone not very strong, not very mobile, not able to move around very easily, and maybe not even able to walk independently, certainly not at full stature. (There's a reason we have clichés like "little old lady.")

That frailty and brittleness you probably conjured up comes—at least partially—from having muscles that atrophy over the years and bones that are far from rock solid and strong.

And here's a surprising fact for you: Most people who go into assisted living don't go there because they can no longer remember things or because they have heart disease. They go there because they're no longer able to perform everyday tasks for themselves! (Makes sense—*assisted* living, right?) And that lack of ability comes from weak bones and weak muscles. After all, if you can't open a jar, get out of a chair, walk the stairs, or pick up the groceries, you're gonna need a bit of help.

So, the best thing to do, in my humble opinion, is not let those bones and muscles get so weak in the first place.

Fortunately, it's not all that hard to keep them strong.

IT'S NOT JUST THE CALCIUM

Since this isn't a book on lifestyle, I won't talk about the obvious connection between strong muscles, strong bones, and exercise. (I covered most of that in *The Most Effective Ways to Live Longer* as well as *The Most Effective Natural Cures on Earth*.) But there is a huge connection between strong bones and diet.

You can eat in such a way as to protect your bones and muscles. (And you get a double layer of protection from that way of eating if you combine it with daily exercise, which I hope you'll do!)

When it comes to nutrients for strong bones, everyone thinks about eating (or taking) calcium, but believe me, it's about much more than calcium. You need vitamin K, the newest superstar of the bone nutrients, and one that's in plentiful supply in dishes such as Krispy Kale. You also need magnesium, found in virtually all the vegetables in this section, and, of course, vitamin D.

And there's plenty of calcium in these recipes as well—coming from greens, soybeans, seeds, sardines, cottage cheese, and many other foods you'll find in this section.

Also, the foods in these recipes are staples of the diets of the longest-lived people in the world, the people who inhabit the famed Blue Zones—Okinawa; Loma Linda, California; Ikaria, off the coast of Greece; Sardinia; and the Nicoya Peninsula of Costa Rica. Many of those people do not drink milk to any appreciable degree, and many of them have far less osteoporosis than we do, so they must be doing something right!

HOLDING BACK THE HORSEMEN

Bones and muscles are just as subject to the Four Horsemen of Aging as the rest of our bodies. Muscles, joints, and bones can be weakened by oxidation, harmed by stress (do you really feel physically strong when you're stressed to the max?), and significantly damaged by inflammation!

"Chronic, low-level inflammation is a component of many chronic diseases, including osteoporosis," says Keith McCormick, D.C., author of *The Whole-Body Approach to Osteoporosis* and an Ironman athlete who was himself diagnosed with osteoporosis. (If you haven't read about McCormick in *The Most Effective Ways to Live Longer*, let me just tell you, he's still competing!)

McCormick didn't follow the standard medical treatment for osteoporosis—drugs—and instead chose to get at the underlying causes of bone deterioration. He was one of my greatest influences when it came to exploring the ways diet can help us build and protect strong bones. That's why, in this section, you'll find recipes that are just teeming with natural anti-inflammatory properties. Foods such as cold-water fish, chia seeds, and nuts all contain omega-3s, the most potent anti-inflammatory agent I know of. And the only "side effect" of these bone protectors is that they also support your heart and your brain!

Speaking of McCormick, I'm a big fan of his other dietary recommendations for good bone health, and so is Chef Jeannette. That's why we've incorporated nearly all of his top-ten list of dietary strategies (found in his book) to protect and strengthen your bones (and your joints and muscles as well).

THE POWER OF PROTEIN

One of his strategies, and mine, worth noting is this one: Eat protein! Protein is incredibly important for the formation of the bone matrix. You'll find plenty of great sources here, especially from wild fish, naturally raised poultry, and grass-fed beef. One amino acid found in animal foods—lysine—is especially important for forming strong bones.

Leucine is another amino acid found in many of the protein foods in this section. Leucine has gotten a lot of research attention recently, especially in the fitness and bodybuilding worlds. Why should you care? Because there seems to be a direct correlation between how much leucine you take in and how well your muscles grow. (One bodybuilding site dramatically titled an article "Leucine: The Anabolic Trigger"!) You may not care much about "growing" new muscles. But I'll bet if you're reading this book, you care about keeping the ones you have. And as any bodybuilder or fitness person on the planet will tell you, you can't build and maintain good working muscles without enough protein!

Other great bone-building foods found in these pages include oranges, broccoli, and onions, all of which, according to McCormick, have bioactive compounds that have been found to increase bone density.

Of course, all of this wouldn't mean much to a cook if the recipes didn't taste amazing. If you're skeptical, I suggest you start with the Anti-Aging Apple-Pumpkin Ginger Soup.

Who knew building strong bones and joints could be this delicious?

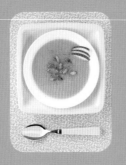 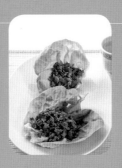

ENTRÉES

. . . .

Nutrient Blast Orange–Black Bean Soup

Anti–Aging Apple–Pumpkin Ginger Soup

An Ocean of Nutrition: Grilled Lobster and Mango with Coconut Cream

Fresh Caesar Salad with Mustard–Grilled Shrimp

Blood Orange–Scallop Salad with Feta and Macadamia

Protein Blast Asian Grilled Chicken

Bone–Building Bell Peppers Stuffed with Seafood Quinoa

Strengthening Mustard–Hoisin Lettuce Wraps

Better Butternut Flax Mac and Cheese

Leaner, Better Turkey–Basil Meat Loaf

Tangy Antioxidant Creole Seafood Stew

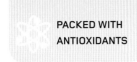
NUTRIENT BLAST ORANGE–BLACK BEAN SOUP

From Dr. Jonny: So what the heck is kombu, anyway? Glad you asked. It's a type of seaweed that's been used in traditional Japanese cooking for centuries, and it's rich in iodine, potassium, calcium, and iron, not to mention dietary fiber. Add it to this already stellar list of bone-building ingredients and you've got a superstar recipe that tastes amazing. Calcium from the oranges and yogurt mixes with a rich array of nutrients from the tomatoes, carrots, and peppers. The orange adds a surprising zest to this flavorful soup, enhanced by the onions, garlic, and cilantro. Cool and freeze the extra for a longevity "fast food" meal later on!

1 piece (1½ inches, or 4 cm) kombu

1 tablespoon (15 ml) olive oil

1 large sweet onion, diced

4 large cloves garlic, minced

2 cups (260 g) baby carrots

1 pound (455 g) black beans, presoaked*
(about 2½ cups [625 g] dried)

7 cups (1.7 L) no-sodium vegetable broth** or water

1½ teaspoons ground cumin

1 can (14.5 ounces, or 413 g) fire-roasted diced
tomatoes, undrained

2 medium red or yellow bell peppers, seeded and
chopped

¾ teaspoon salt

¼ teaspoon red pepper flakes

1 cup (235 ml) fresh-squeezed orange juice

1½ teaspoons orange zest

1½ cups (345 g) plain Greek yogurt

1 large garlic clove, minced

1½ tablespoons (25 ml) fresh-squeezed lime juice

⅓ cup (5 g) chopped fresh cilantro, packed

Soak the kombu in a small bowl of water for about 10 minutes until softened. Drain, mince, and set aside.

Heat the oil in a large soup pot over medium heat. Add the onion and sauté for 5 minutes. Add the garlic and sauté for 1 minute. Add the carrots and sauté for 2 minutes. Add the black beans and broth or water, increase the heat, and bring to a boil. Reduce the heat

to simmer, add the kombu and cumin, and cover and cook for about 75 minutes or until the beans are just tender to the squeeze.***

Add the tomatoes, bell peppers, salt, and red pepper flakes, and continue to simmer for 10 minutes. Add the orange juice and zest and purée 75 percent of the soup with an immersion blender (or in a blender), leaving some chunkiness and whole pieces. Return to low heat for an additional 10 minutes cook time.

In the meantime, in a small bowl thoroughly mix together the yogurt, garlic, lime juice, and cilantro.

Serve in soup bowls with a generous dollop of the yogurt mixture. Soup flavors will deepen over time.

Yield: 6 to 8 servings

Per Serving: 308 Calories; 4g Fat (12.5% calories from fat); 16g Protein; 53g Carbohydrate; 12g Dietary Fiber; 5mg Cholesterol; 266mg Sodium

* Presoaking beans shortens their cooking time and removes some of the bean sugars (oligosaccharides) that cause flatulence. To soak dry beans, pick them over for any small stones, then rinse them in a colander. In a large bowl, cover them with water, cover the bowl, and soak overnight. Drain and rinse.

** Salt and acid toughen beans and lengthen their cooking time, so don't use a cooking broth containing salt. No-salt veggie broths do make for a more flavorful soup, however, especially if you make it yourself from vegetable peels and scraps. Salt can be added once the beans are tender. Kombu contains a small amount of salt, but soaking removes most of it, and cooking the beans with minced kombu makes them more digestible.

*** Fresh, well-soaked dried beans will cook quickly, while older beans take a little longer. After the first hour, check beans every 10 minutes and make sure the liquid level is adequate, adding a little more broth if necessary. If you're short on time, substitute 2 cans rinsed and drained black beans and 3 large carrots cut into thin coins.

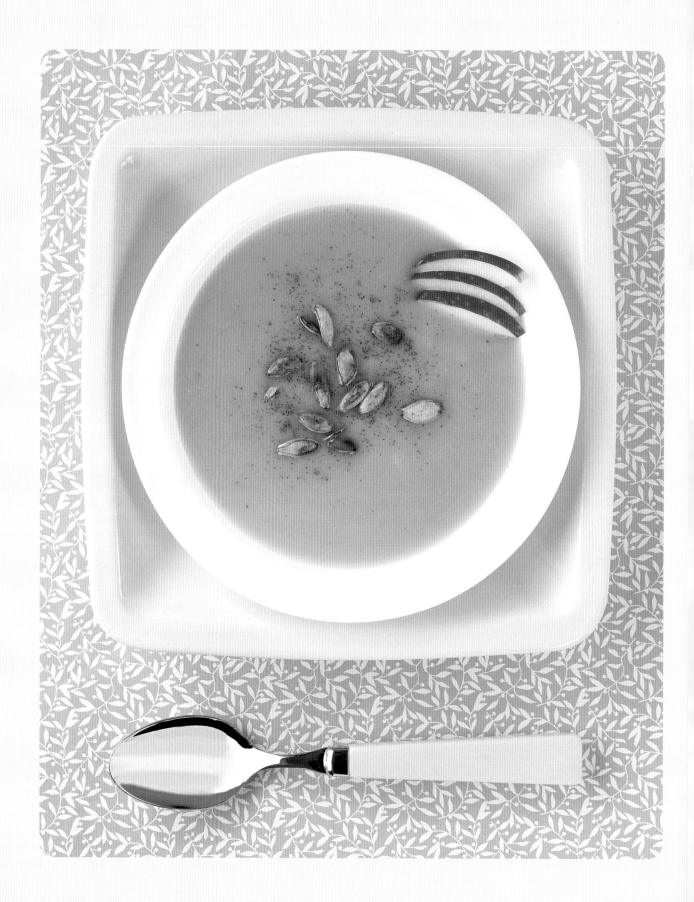

ANTI-AGING APPLE-PUMPKIN GINGER SOUP

From Dr. Jonny: There are so many anti-aging elements in this rich, luscious soup that I hardly know where to begin. Garlic lowers blood pressure, onions lower the risk of cancer, pumpkin seeds—with their calcium and magnesium—are great for the bones, and apples help fight inflammation. This is one of my favorite soups of all time: creamy and sweet but low calorie and all vegetable!

4 pounds (1¾ kg) sugar pumpkin (about 1 medium)

4 cooking apples, peeled, cored, and sliced

3 tablespoons (24 g) grated fresh ginger

1 garlic clove, minced

1 medium Vidalia onion, diced

4 cups (950 ml) vegetable or chicken broth

¼ cup (60 ml) frozen orange juice concentrate, thawed

Juice of ½ lemon

½ teaspoon ground cinnamon

½ teaspoon ground ginger

¼ teaspoon ground nutmeg

¼ teaspoon cayenne pepper

½ teaspoon salt

TOASTED PUMPKIN SEEDS

Seeds from pumpkin

1 teaspoon Bragg Liquid Aminos (or tamari)

MAKE THE SOUP

Wash the pumpkin and remove the stem. Using a heavy knife, cut the pumpkin vertically down the middle. Using a heavy spoon, scrape out all the seeds and fibers, reserving the seeds. Lay each half facedown on the cutting board and cut away the skins. Quarter each half of the skinned pumpkin.

Combine all soup ingredients in a slow cooker and cook for 7 hours on low or 4 to 5 hours on high (or until tender). Purée until smooth with an immersion blender or, once slightly cooled, in batches in a food processor or blender. Be careful when blending hot soups. Adjust seasonings as necessary.

PREPARE THE SEEDS

Preheat the oven to 200°F (93°C, or gas mark ¼).

Remove all vegetable fibers from the seeds and rinse.

Bring a couple of inches (5 cm) of water to boil in a small saucepan and add the seeds. Boil for 10 minutes to soften the hulls. Remove seeds, drain well, and pat dry with a clean dish towel. Toss with liquid aminos or tamari in a small bowl until the seeds are lightly coated. Spread the seeds into a single layer on a nonstick baking sheet (or use parchment paper on a regular baking sheet). Bake seeds for 20 to 30 minutes, stirring occasionally, until very lightly browned. (Do not burn!)

Sprinkle pumpkin seeds to taste on top of individual bowls of soup and serve.

Yield: about 6 cups (1.4 L)

Per Serving: 147 Calories; .4g Fat (3% calories from fat); 5g Protein; 35g Carbohydrate; 5g Dietary Fiber; 0mg Cholesterol; 850mg Sodium

FROM CHEF JEANNETTE:

In the wintertime and especially over the holidays, it's natural to crave something warming and sweet. If you incorporate naturally sweet, dense foods, such as pumpkin and winter squash, into your regular meals, they can help to satisfy and calm those cravings. A bowl of this rich, creamy soup is healthy and satisfying and can help you resist the urge for a big slice of conventional pie.

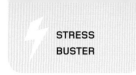

AN OCEAN OF NUTRITION: GRILLED LOBSTER AND MANGO WITH COCONUT CREAM

From Dr. Jonny: Some experts now think that a higher-protein diet actually can help prevent osteoporosis. And many people don't realize just how high in protein lobster actually is. One single lobster has a whopping 43 grams of the stuff! (One lobster also provides more than 100 mg of calcium, something not frequently found in a lot of protein foods.) The mango in this recipe contributes a healthy dose of potassium (323 mg per mango), an important nutrient for neutralizing acidity in the system. When the body is "acid," calcium will often be leached from the bones to buffer that acidity, meaning there's less of it in the bones where you need it to be! That alone makes potassium an important nutrient for bone health. The taste combo of mango, lobster, and the coconut milk dipping sauce makes for a rich and satisfying dish that won't leave you feeling uncomfortably stuffed.

4 live lobsters (1¼ to 1½ pounds [680 g] each)

1 cup (235 ml) light coconut milk

Juice of 2 limes

Juice of 1 lemon

1 tablespoon (20 g) agave nectar, or to taste

²/₃ cup (26 g) chopped fresh basil (or you can use cilantro, or a mix of both)

3 ripe mangoes, peeled

1 to 2 tablespoons (15 to 28 ml) melted coconut oil

Place the live lobsters in the freezer for at least 15 minutes to numb them (do not freeze and kill them). Fill a clean sink with ice water.

Bring a large lobster pot (or stockpot) filled ²/₃ of the way with water to a rolling boil over high heat. Place the lobsters in headfirst and parboil, covered, for 8 minutes.

Remove lobsters from cooking pot and plunge into ice bath in sink.

While lobsters are cooling, preheat your grill to medium-high heat.

In a small bowl, whisk together the coconut milk, citrus juices, agave, and chopped basil. Set aside.

Slice the 2 "cheeks" (broadsides of the pit) and 2 thinner sides (narrow sides of the pit) from each mango. Cut the mango into roughly even chunks and thread onto skewers.

Once lobsters are cool, shell them and remove pieces of meat, keeping them intact, where possible. Thread the lobster chunks carefully onto skewers. Drizzle coconut oil over mango and lobster skewers. Place them on the grill. Remove the lobster once hot and just-charred with grill marks, a minute or two per side. Do not overcook—the meat is already 90 percent cooked from parboiling.

Remove the mango once lightly charred, about 2 minutes per side.

Serve the grilled lobster and mango with bowls of coconut-basil dipping sauce on the side, or drizzle sauce over the top.

Yield: 4 servings

Per Serving: 442 Calories; 20g Fat (38.9% calories from fat); 31g Protein; 41g Carbohydrate; 6g Dietary Fiber; 143mg Cholesterol; 457mg Sodium

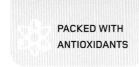
FRESH CAESAR SALAD WITH MUSTARD-GRILLED SHRIMP

From Dr. Jonny: If you don't love Caesar salad, you'll become a convert after you try this zippy version. Anchovies are a good source of calcium, iron, and phosphorus, and both anchovies and shrimp are terrific sources of protein. And while we're on the subject of protein, let's clear up a common misconception about bone health and protein. Years ago, some studies suggested that eating a lot of protein caused calcium to be secreted in the urine, so many health professionals believed that higher protein intakes weaken bones by causing calcium loss. But more current research points in the opposite direction. We now know that eating protein *increases* calcium absorption, so that extra calcium in the urine comes from increased absorption, not from being taken out of bones. "Most scientists now feel that a low-protein diet causes osteoporosis, while a high-protein diet may prevent it," says Gabe Mirkin, M.D. I agree.

GRILLED SHRIMP

3 tablespoons (45 g) Dijon mustard

¼ cup (60 ml) olive oil

Juice of 1 small lemon

1 teaspoon Sucanat

2 shallots, minced

1 pound (455 g) large shrimp, shelled and deveined

CAESAR SALAD

1 ½ tablespoons anchovy paste

2 cloves garlic, crushed

2 tablespoons (28 ml) fresh-squeezed lemon juice

1 raw or lightly poached egg (preferably organic)

1 teaspoon Dijon mustard

1 dash Worcestershire sauce, to taste (choose organic to avoid high-fructose corn syrup; we like Annie's)

⅓ cup (80 ml) olive oil

¼ cup (25 g) fresh-grated Parmesan cheese, plus extra for topping

¼ teaspoon each salt and fresh-ground black pepper

2 heads romaine lettuce, torn into bite-size pieces (about 8 cups, or 440 g)

Prepare the shrimp: In a medium bowl, whisk together the mustard, olive oil, lemon juice, Sucanat, and shallots. Stir the shrimp into the mustard mixture to evenly coat and marinate in the refrigerator for 4 to 6 hours.

Make the dressing: In blender or food processor, add anchovy paste, garlic, lemon juice, egg, mustard, Worcestershire sauce, olive oil, cheese, salt, and pepper, and process until blended.

Grill the shrimp: Preheat the grill to medium. Remove the shrimp from the marinade, drain well, and reserve marinade. Thread the shrimp evenly on 2 skewers. Grill, basting twice with marinade, until they just turn pink and are cooked through, about 3 minutes per side. Do not overcook.

In a large salad bowl, dress the lettuce to taste, add shrimp, and top with shaved Parmesan, if desired.

Yield: 4 servings

Per Serving: 352 Calories; 22g Fat (56.9% calories from fat); 30g Protein; 8g Carbohydrate; 1g Dietary Fiber; 231mg Cholesterol; 598mg Sodium

FROM CHEF JEANNETTE:

A classic Caesar is lettuce, dressing, Parmesan, and croutons. We skipped the croutons for this longevity version and added shrimp for protein. Feel free to add lots of other salad veggies too, if you'd like, to beef up the micronutrient content. Try shredded carrot, chopped tomato, sliced cucumber, and so on.

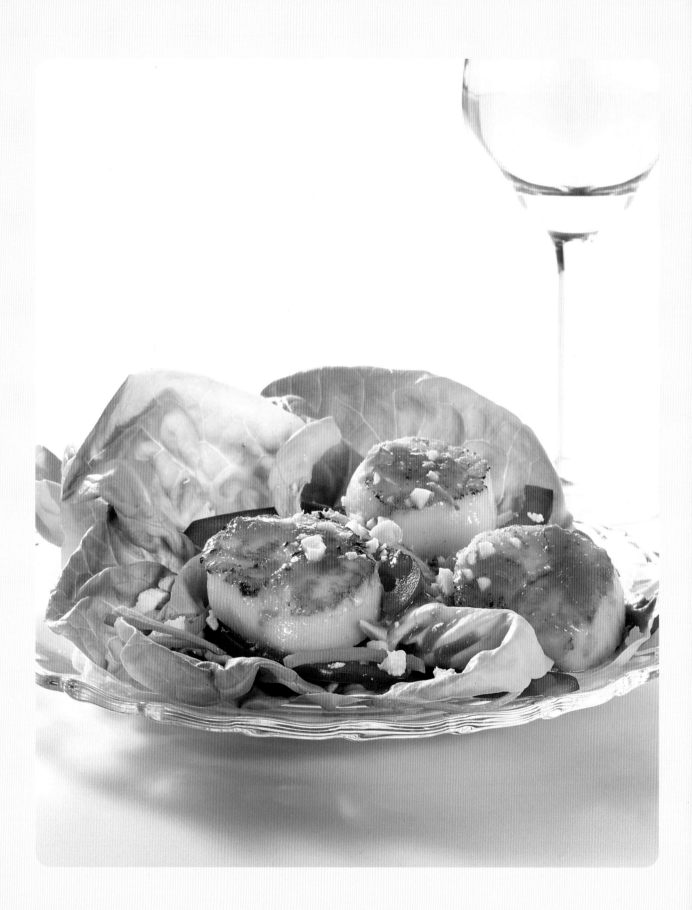

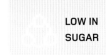

BLOOD ORANGE–SCALLOP SALAD WITH FETA AND MACADAMIA

From Dr. Jonny: One thing's for sure: You can't live the longevity lifestyle without strong bones. But everyone forgets that you can build bones very effectively without milk! There are more than 600 mg of calcium in this salad—more than twice the amount in a cup of milk—not to mention bone-building vitamin K and anti-inflammatory omega-9s from the macadamia nuts and olive oil. This unexpected treat, which combines the mildness of scallops with salty feta and the sweet tang of orange, makes for a fresh, light meal perfect for a summer dinner!

1 head sweet lettuce (butter or Bibb)

½ cup (55 g) finely grated carrot

½ red bell pepper, julienne cut

4 ounces (115 g) feta cheese, crumbled

Juice of 2 blood oranges

½ teaspoon blood orange zest

¼ cup (60 ml) champagne vinegar

Small shallot, diced fine

Small garlic clove, minced

1 teaspoon honey

¼ cup (60 ml) olive oil

1½ tablespoons (25 ml) macadamia nut oil

1½ pounds (710 g) fresh sea scallops

¼ cup (34 g) crushed roasted macadamia nuts

Make a bed of lettuce and scatter the carrots, julienned pepper, and feta over the top.

In a small bowl, whisk together the orange juice, orange peel, vinegar, shallot, garlic, and honey. Slowly drizzle in the olive oil, whisking to emulsify. (Alternatively, use an immersion blender to combine all dressing ingredients.)

Heat the macadamia oil in a large sauté pan over medium-high heat. Add the scallops and sear the tops and bottoms, cooking to desired doneness, about 2 to 4 minutes.

Scatter the cooked scallops over the salad, dress to taste, and toss gently to combine.

Sprinkle the macadamia nuts over all and serve.

Yield: 6 servings

Per Serving: 347 Calories; 23g Fat (57.5% calories from fat); 24g Protein; 13g Carbohydrate; 2g Dietary Fiber; 56mg Cholesterol; 410mg Sodium

PROTEIN BLAST ASIAN GRILLED CHICKEN

From Dr. Jonny: For years, the standard advice was that protein causes calcium to leach from the bones and that the more protein you eat, the weaker your bones will get. The truth is actually quite different. In one study, women aged 55 to 92 experienced a significant increase in bone density at the spine, neck, and hip for every 15-grams-per-day increase in animal protein they ate. Other studies have shown similar results. You need protein for strong bones, and here's a great way to get it. A snappy Japanese twist on the old American standby: chicken breast. For a tasty blast of protein anytime at all, grill some extra and freeze!

CHICKEN

½ cup (120 ml) sake (or you can use dry sherry)

2 tablespoons (28 ml) tamari

½ teaspoon honey

4 boneless, skinless chicken breasts

SAUCE

1 piece kombu (4 inches, or 10 cm), snipped into several pieces with scissors

1 cup (235 ml) water

½ cup (120 ml) unseasoned rice vinegar

2 tablespoons (40 g) honey

3 tablespoons (45 ml) tamari

1 teaspoon wasabi powder*

2 tablespoons (16 g) toasted sesame seeds

In a small bowl, whisk together the sake, tamari, and honey and set aside.

Rinse the chicken and pat it dry. If very thick, pound to about ½-inch (1-cm) thickness. Pierce the breasts several times with a fork and place in a shallow glass container, such as a pie plate. Pour the sake mixture over the breasts and allow to marinate for 1 to 2 hours in the fridge, turning occasionally.

In the meantime, in a small saucepan heat the kombu and water over high heat. Watch it closely and remove from the heat just before it starts to boil—you might see one or two bubbles. Cover the pan and let it steep while the chicken marinates.

To make the sauce, strain the kombu, reserving the broth, just before grilling the chicken. Finely mince ½ teaspoon of the kombu.

In a small bowl, whisk together the vinegar and honey until the honey is dissolved. Whisk in 2 tablespoons (28 ml) of the kombu broth, minced kombu, tamari, and wasabi powder. Set aside.

Grill the chicken on medium low for about 30 minutes or until cooked through (170°F or 77°C on an instant-read thermometer).* Slice thinly, sprinkle sesame seeds over individual portions, and serve with sauce.

FROM CHEF JEANNETTE:

For an even more nutritious meal, serve this chicken with a plate of lightly steamed or stir-fried bok choy.

You can buy toasted sesame seeds or toast them yourself: Place the desired quantity of raw seeds in a single layer in a small dry skillet and toast over medium heat, shaking occasionally to turn, for 2 to 3 minutes or until just starting to darken up—don't overbrown.

Yield: 4 servings

Per Serving: 392 Calories; 8g Fat (20.8% calories from fat); 54g Protein; 16g Carbohydrate; 1g Dietary Fiber; 144mg Cholesterol; 478mg Sodium

* Wasabi powder is a prepared Japanese radish powder used as a condiment. It is very pungent, with a biting quality like horseradish. Mixed with a little water, it forms the green paste used in sushi. Find it in Asian markets, macrobiotics sections of natural grocers, and large supermarkets.

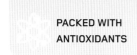

PACKED WITH
ANTIOXIDANTS

BONE-BUILDING BELL PEPPERS STUFFED WITH SEAFOOD QUINOA

From Dr. Jonny: Here's a hearty seafood dish that hits the "bones trifecta"—rich in bone-building nutrients, low in calories, big on taste. There's plenty of bone-protecting potassium in the vegetables and vitamin C in the mangoes and peppers. (Remember that potassium helps neutralize bone-depleting acids that are produced as part of everyday metabolism.) This is a truly delicious dish that satisfies without leaving you feeling heavy!

2 large red bell peppers

2 large yellow or orange bell peppers

3 cups (600 g) cooked small shrimp (thawed, if frozen)

2 tablespoons (28 ml) olive oil

1 sweet onion, diced fine

1 ripe mango, peeled, pitted, and diced fine

½ small jalapeño, seeded and minced, or to taste

1 can (6 ounces, or 170 g) white crabmeat, rinsed and drained

Juice of 1 large lime

Salt, to taste

Cracked black pepper, to taste

1 to 2 tablespoons (6 to 12 g) minced fresh mint, to taste

2 cups (370 g) cooked quinoa

Preheat the oven to 375°F (190°C, or gas mark 5).

Bring a large pot of lightly salted water to a boil over high heat. Slice the tops off the peppers and seed and core them.* Add the peppers to the pot of boiling water and cook for for 5 minutes. Drain well and set aside.

Place the cooked shrimp in a food processor, pulse 3 to 4 times until minced, and set aside.

Heat the oil in a large sauté pan over medium heat. Add the onion and sauté for 5 minutes. Add the mango and jalapeño and sauté for 1 minute. Add the minced shrimp and crabmeat and mix to combine. Add the lime, salt, and pepper, mix well, and warm for 1 minute. Fold in the mint and cooked quinoa and spoon mixture evenly into blanched peppers, packing well.

Wrap individual peppers tightly with aluminum foil and place upright on a baking sheet. Cook for about 15 minutes or until hot throughout.

Yield: 4 servings

Per Serving: 424 Calories; 10g Fat (21.9% calories from fat); 44g Protein; 39g Carbohydrate; 6g Dietary Fiber; 326mg Cholesterol; 474mg Sodium

* You can use a spoon for this or just clap their open ends together to get the seeds out and then pull the soft white veins out with your hands.

FROM CHEF JEANNETTE:

Don't need all four peppers at one meal? Just cool the extras in the fridge for about an hour, put them into a zip-closure freezer bag, press the air out, and store in the freezer. When you're ready to eat them, simply thaw them overnight in your refrigerator and cook as directed (it will probably take 5 or so minutes longer to reheat chilled peppers). Stuffed peppers are a lot of work, so it's worth it to make extra to freeze for later. One caveat: Seafood shouldn't be refrozen, so don't freeze these if you're working with frozen precooked shrimp.

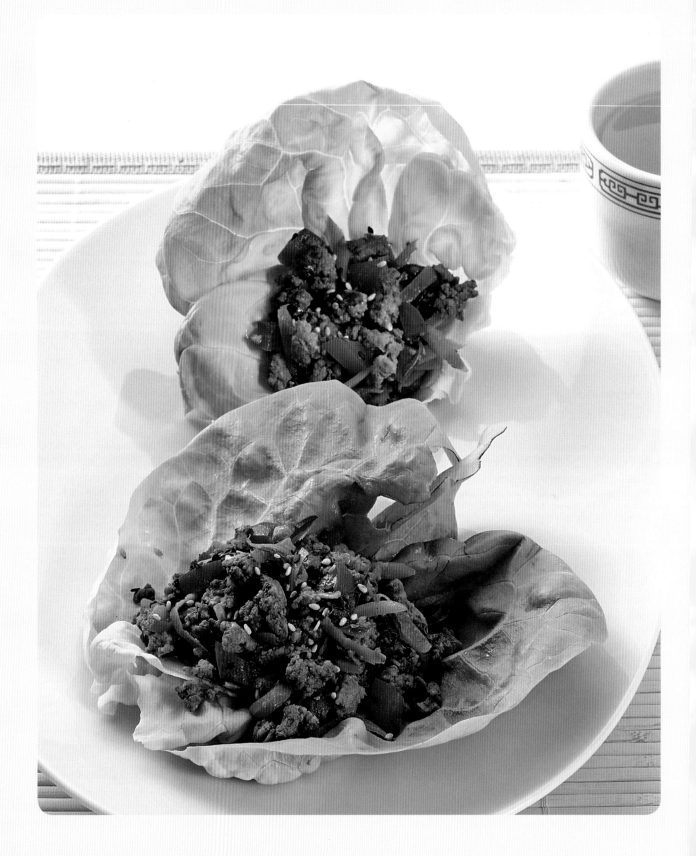

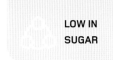

STRENGTHENING MUSTARD-HOISIN LETTUCE WRAPS

From Dr. Jonny: Though bodybuilders aren't always the most reliable source of information about nutrition, they're right about one thing: You need protein to build strong muscles. Now let me be clear: Just eating protein without working out isn't going to do it. A University of Arkansas study showed that eating meat helped older people grow stronger muscles as long as they also lifted weights. Remember, muscles are made primarily from amino acids—the "building blocks" of protein—and lean proteins such as turkey provide plenty of them. This recipe offers more than protein. It also offers a lot of calcium and vitamin K from the greens, both of which are essential for strong bones. Oh—and by the way—it also offers great taste. Personal note: Lettuce wraps are a great option for a reasonable-calorie meal when eating out at one of those chains that serve really huge portions of food such as Cheesecake Factory or P.F. Chang's.

---

1 head Boston or Bibb lettuce (or other type with large, pliable leaves)

1 tablespoon (15 ml) sesame oil

1 pound (455 g) lean ground turkey

1 tablespoon (15 ml) tamari

1 teaspoon mustard powder

1 small red bell pepper, seeded and diced fine

1 large carrot, peeled and grated

²/₃ cup (66 g) chopped scallions (about 1 bunch)

2 tablespoons (32 g) hoisin sauce

2 cups (60 g) mizuna greens* (or a mix of young mustard greens and baby spinach), chopped

1 teaspoon toasted sesame oil

¼ cup (32 g) black sesame seeds (or white sesame seeds, toasted)

---

* This delicious Asian salad green is a spring star in local farmer's markets. If you can't find it, make a mix of baby spinach and young mustard greens to taste or you can just use spinach. Mizuna has a light, peppery bite, sort of like mild arugula, and packs a nice dose of vitamin C, carotenes, calcium, and folic acid.

Core the lettuce and remove 12 to 16 large leaves, keeping them intact. Shred the remaining lettuce and set aside.

In a large skillet, heat the oil over medium heat. Add the turkey, tamari, and mustard powder, and cook, stirring frequently, until no pink remains, about 8 minutes. Drain any excess oil, add bell pepper, carrot, and scallions and cook for 3 minutes, stirring frequently. Stir in the hoisin sauce, mixing well, and greens, and cook until the greens are wilted, about 2 to 4 minutes. Remove from the heat and stir in the sesame oil and sesame seeds.

Make 4 piles of the shredded lettuce on 4 plates, placing 4 equal portions of meat onto each lettuce pile. Serve with 3 to 4 lettuce leaves each, with instructions to place a small scoop of meat and shredded lettuce into each whole leaf, roll up, and eat with fingers.

Yield: 4 servings

Per Serving: 283 Calories; 16g Fat (48.6% calories from fat); 26g Protein; 12g Carbohydrate; 3g Dietary Fiber; 74mg Cholesterol; 288mg Sodium

BETTER BUTTERNUT FLAX MAC AND CHEESE

From Dr. Jonny: True story: My business partner and master weight-loss coach Anja Christy is fond of telling people that when she first met me a decade ago she thought macaroni and cheese out of a box was a perfectly good meal. Regular mac and cheese is loaded with heavily processed "cheese food" (don't even call it cheese) and a ton of useless white pasta, hardly a recipe for living long. This version uses whole-grain macaroni and incorporates squash, which is rich in potassium, a mineral that nutritionist Susan Brown, Ph.D., aptly calls "the hidden bone guardian." Why? Because potassium neutralizes bone-depleting acids and prevents too much calcium from being excreted. Bonus points for the calcium in the real cheese! Best of all, this great dish still offers that comfort food feeling on a chilly evening.

Cooking oil spray

12 ounces (340 g) whole-grain elbow macaroni*

1 medium butternut squash, peeled, seeded, and cubed (about 4 cups)

2 tablespoons (28 ml) olive oil

1 large sweet onion, diced

1 teaspoon dry mustard

1 teaspoon tamari

1 tablespoon (16 g) mellow white miso

½ teaspoon salt

¼ cup (28 g) toasted sliced almonds

1 cup (120 g) grated sharp Cheddar cheese

½ cup (60 g) whole-wheat panko bread crumbs

¼ cup (25 g) ground flaxseed

½ cup (50 g) fresh-grated Parmesan cheese

* For gluten free, we like Tinkyada rice pasta best. But undercook it by about 3 minutes (for al dente) or it will fall apart when you mix it with the other ingredients.

Preheat the oven to 400°F (200°C, or gas mark 6). Lightly coat a 9 x 13-inch (23 x 33-cm) baking dish with cooking oil spray and set aside.

Cook the pasta al dente according to package directions.

While the pasta is cooking, steam the squash cubes for 15 minutes or until very soft.

In a medium skillet, heat the oil over medium heat and sauté the onion for 5 minutes.

In a large bowl, mix together the steamed squash, cooked onion, mustard, tamari, miso, and salt. Mix well or purée with an immersion wand. Fold in the almonds and cheese.

Gently fold in the pasta and spoon into a prepared baking pan.

In a small bowl, mix together the bread crumbs, flaxseed, and Parmesan. Spoon evenly over the top of the casserole and bake for 15 to 20 minutes or until lightly browned.

Yield: 6–8 servings

Per Serving: 439 Calories; 14g Fat (27.5% calories from fat); 17g Protein; 119g Carbohydrate; 9g Dietary Fiber; 21mg Cholesterol; 469mg Sodium

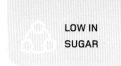
LEANER, BETTER TURKEY-BASIL MEAT LOAF

From Dr. Jonny: This great recipe was inspired by Heather Shannon-Short, who was the first cook to introduce Oprah to tofu in 1995. (There's a spicy tidbit for dinner conversation.) Your bones will love the lean protein, not to mention the vitamin-rich veggies. It's perfect for the whole family—even your kids will scarf it down. Heather has designed recipes for Barlean's Organic Oils and for an organic catering company (www.dining-details.com). If I wore a hat, I'd take it off to salute her for this inspiration. So will you after you taste it!

Olive oil

2 tablespoons (28 ml) organic coconut oil (such as Barlean's)

1 medium yellow onion, diced fine

1 stalk celery

2 small zucchini

3 cloves garlic, minced

¾ teaspoon dried oregano

½ teaspoon kosher salt

½ teaspoon cracked black pepper

¼ teaspoon cayenne pepper

1 large bunch fresh basil, chopped fine

¼ cup (15 g) chopped flat-leaf Italian parsley

2 pounds (900 g) ground turkey

1 cup (80 g) rolled oats (or soft, whole-wheat bread crumbs)

3 tablespoons (20 g) ground flaxseed (such as Barlean's Forti-Flax)

2 whole eggs (or 3 egg whites)

2 tablespoons (28 ml) Bragg Liquid Aminos (or tamari)

Preheat the oven to 350°F (180°C, gas mark 4).

Rub a small amount of olive oil on a broiler rack in the area where you'll place the meat loaf and set aside.*

In a large sauté pan over medium heat, melt the coconut oil and add the onion, sautéing for about 4 minutes or until it starts to soften.

While onion is cooking, add the celery and zucchini to a food processor until it is diced fine, but not puréed.

Add garlic to onion and cook 1 minute. Add processed celery and zucchini, oregano, salt, and peppers to the pan, sautéing until the veggies have softened, 6 to 7 minutes. Add the basil and parsley and sauté for 1 minute. Set aside and cool for 10 minutes.

In a large mixing bowl, gently mix together the turkey, oats, flaxseed, eggs, and liquid aminos or tamari. Gently mix together.** Fold in the sautéed vegetables and mix until just combined. Form mixture into a loaf and place onto prepared broiler rack. Bake for 40 to 50 minutes until completely cooked in the center (165°F, or 74°C, on an instant-read thermometer).

Yield: about 9 slices

Per Serving: 58.7 Calories; 3g Fat (47% calories from fat); 3.5g Protein; 5g Carbohydrate; 2g Dietary Fiber; 47mg Cholesterol; 380mg Sodium

* Using a broiler rack rather than the traditional loaf pan allows excess fat to drain off and forms a nice crust with a moist interior. You may also divide it into two smaller loaves for faster cooking.

** Do not overhandle the meat mixture or your meat loaf will get tough.

FROM CHEF JEANNETTE:

This is a mild flavored meat loaf that is great served hot for dinner and cold in sandwiches the next day. For an additional flavor zing, try it with a little high-quality ketchup or barbecue sauce.

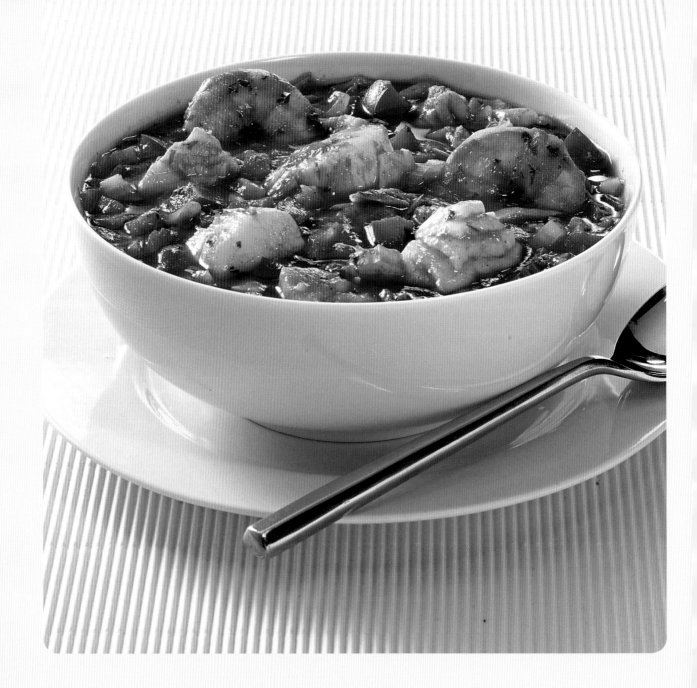

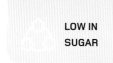

LOW IN SUGAR

TANGY ANTIOXIDANT CREOLE SEAFOOD STEW

From Dr. Jonny: I'm not quite sure where the expression "holy mackerel" comes from, but whoever made it up was on to something. An extraordinary range of nutrients is found in these fish, and many of them play a significant role in the health of your heart. (Not to mention your other parts!) Garlic lowers your blood pressure, onions supply important sulfur, the greens and tomato juice supply antioxidants, and the olive oil provides phenols and monounsaturated fat. All of which wouldn't mean much if this wasn't one of the spiciest and tangiest seafood stews you ever tasted—which it is. It'll also warm you right up on a winter day!

1½ tablespoons (25 ml) olive oil

1 yellow onion, diced

8 cloves garlic, minced

1 green bell pepper, seeded and diced

1 red bell pepper, seeded and diced

3 stalks celery, diced

1 bottle (32 ounces, or 905 g) high-quality vegetable tomato juice (we like Knudsen's Very Veggie)

1 bay leaf

¾ teaspoon paprika

¾ teaspoon cracked black pepper

½ teaspoon cayenne pepper, or to taste

½ teaspoon celery salt, or to taste

1 can (4³/₈ ounces, or 130 g) water-packed mackerel (we like Vital Choice), drained

8 ounces (225 g) medium shrimp

8 ounces (225 g) scallops, whole bay or halved sea scallops

8 ounces (225 g) halibut, cut into 1-inch (2.5-cm) pieces

½ bunch parsley, chopped

In a large stew pan, heat the oil over medium. Add the onion and sauté for 3 minutes. Add the garlic and sauté for 1 minute. Add the peppers and celery and sauté for 1 minute. Add the vegetable juice, bay leaf, paprika, black pepper, cayenne pepper, and celery salt, and increase the heat to bring the stew to a boil. Reduce the heat to a simmer, add the mackerel, cover, and simmer for 20 minutes.

Add the shrimp, scallops, and halibut and cook until the seafood is cooked through but not tough, about 5 minutes.

Stir in the parsley just before serving.

Yield: 4–6 servings

Per Serving: 344 Calories; 11g Fat (27.3% calories from fat); 41g Protein; 22g Carbohydrate; 5g Dietary Fiber; 145mg Cholesterol; 1368mg Sodium

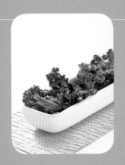

SIDE DISHES

· ·

A Sea of Nutrients: Cold Marinated Shrimp Salad
Vitamin Overload Stir-Fried Chard
Bone Up on Baked Okra
Krispy Kale: A Vitamin K Extravaganza
Not Your Average Green Beans

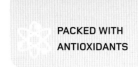
A SEA OF NUTRIENTS: COLD MARINATED SHRIMP SALAD

From Dr. Jonny: Shrimp is great to keep around in the freezer. It's a versatile source of protein, and with a mere fifteen minutes in a bowl of cold water it's ready to use in a variety of recipes. Shrimp's a great source of niacin, iron, phosphorus, and zinc and a terrific low-fat source of protein, which is absolutely necessary for strong bones. This zippy and incredibly light "Asian shrimp cocktail"—style recipe makes a great side dish or an appetizer. The cleansing daikon radish adds a lightly pungent note to the salad.

½ cup (120 ml) unseasoned rice vinegar

3 tablespoons (45 ml) tamari

Juice of 1 small lemon

2 teaspoons (14 g) honey, or to taste

¾ pound (340 g) cooked small shrimp

1 medium daikon radish, peeled and grated

1 medium carrot, peeled and grated

In a small saucepan over medium heat, combine the vinegar, tamari, lemon juice, and honey, stirring until the honey is dissolved and the marinade is hot but not boiling.

Add the shrimp to a glass storage container and pour the hot marinade over all, mixing gently to coat. Marinate 1 to 2 hours covered in the fridge until chilled.

Just before serving, roll the grated daikon into a clean dish towel and squeeze gently to remove excess moisture. Mix daikon and carrot and make 4 salad beds on small serving plates. Spoon a bit of the marinade over the grated veggies to taste and divide the shrimp evenly to top 4 plates. Serve cold.

Yield: 4 servings

Per Serving: 125 Calories; 1g Fat (10.5% calories from fat); 18g Protein; 11g Carbohydrate; 1g Dietary Fiber; 129mg Cholesterol; 320mg Sodium

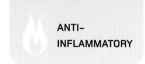

VITAMIN OVERLOAD STIR-FRIED CHARD

From Dr. Jonny: In *The 150 Healthiest Foods on Earth* I wrote that when I first checked the nutritional data on Swiss chard I practically did a double take—I simply couldn't believe that this unappreciated vegetable came so "fully loaded" with so many vitamins and minerals for such a ridiculously low calorie cost! But it does. It's a powerhouse of bone-building nutrients such as magnesium, which helps your body to use calcium, and potassium, which protects your bones by neutralizing bone-robbing acids. Stir-frying in coconut oil imparts a nice nutty flavor, though the almond or avocado oil will also serve you well. Great selection of pungent spices gives this dish an Indian flair.

1½ tablespoons (25 ml) coconut oil (or almond or avocado)

1 teaspoon cumin seeds

1 teaspoon mustard seeds

½ teaspoon red pepper flakes

1 teaspoon minced ginger

2 pounds (900 g) Swiss chard, heavy stems removed, leaves chopped into 2- to 3-inch (5- to 7.5-cm) pieces

½ teaspoon salt

3 tablespoons (12 g) fresh parsley, minced

Heat the oil in a large skillet or wok over medium high. Add the seeds and fry, stirring, for 1 minute. Add the pepper flakes and ginger and fry for 1 minute. Add the chard and salt and stir-fry for 3 to 5 minutes or until desired doneness. Stir in the parsley for the last minute of cook time.

Yield: 4 servings

Per Serving: 101 Calories; 7g Fat (51.8% calories from fat); 4g Protein; 9g Carbohydrate; 4g Dietary Fiber; 0mg Cholesterol; 672mg Sodium

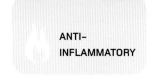
BONE UP ON BAKED OKRA

From Dr. Jonny: We've been (wrongly) taught, mostly through the efforts of the dairy industry, that the only way to get our calcium is through milk. Well, what if you don't like the stuff? Or what if, like most of the world, you're lactose intolerant? How do you get your calcium? There are many ways to get it, and here's one of them: okra. Every 100-calories' worth of this fantastic vegetable provides a whopping 350 mg of calcium, not to mention half as much magnesium (a perfect ratio for bone health), and about ⅓ more potassium than a medium-size banana. Many people avoid okra because the seeds can give it a gummy texture, but this light, baked version is miles away from a gelatinous gumbo.

---

1 pound (455 g) young okra

4 cloves garlic, crushed and sliced

2 tablespoons (28 ml) olive oil

¼ teaspoon salt, plus a sprinkle

Sprinkle cracked black pepper

4 heirloom tomatoes, quartered

1 tablespoon (14 g) ghee*

½ teaspoon fennel seeds

½ teaspoon cumin seeds

¼ teaspoon red pepper flakes

¾ teaspoon Sucanat

¼ cup (10 g) fresh basil, chopped

---

* Ghee is simply clarified butter, the milk solids and water boiled away. It is used a lot in Indian cuisine and healing diets. It has a distinct, nutty flavor and is very stable; you can cook with it at high temperatures and it doesn't need refrigeration for storage. Look for it on the oil shelves of high-end grocers or natural food stores.

Preheat the oven to 400°F (200°C, or gas mark 6).

Carefully trim the stalk end of the okra, leaving the body intact (no seeds exposed). In a large bowl, toss the okra with the garlic, olive oil, a sprinkle of salt, and pepper to coat. Lay them in a roasting pan and bake for about 15 to 20 minutes or until they start to become tender.

In the meantime, lightly blend the tomatoes in a blender or food processor until just coarsely puréed and set aside.

Heat the ghee over medium heat in a large saucepan and add the fennel and cumin seeds, cooking until fragrant, about 3 minutes. Pour the tomatoes into the pan, add the remaining ¼ teaspoon salt, red pepper flakes, and Sucanat, and cook for about 10 minutes. Add the roasted okra and basil to the tomato sauce and mix gently. Correct for acidity, if necessary, with salt or Sucanat, cook for another minute, and serve.

Yield: 4 servings

Per Serving: 174 Calories; 11g Fat (52.9% calories from fat); 4g Protein; 18g Carbohydrate; 5g Dietary Fiber; 9mg Cholesterol; 150mg Sodium

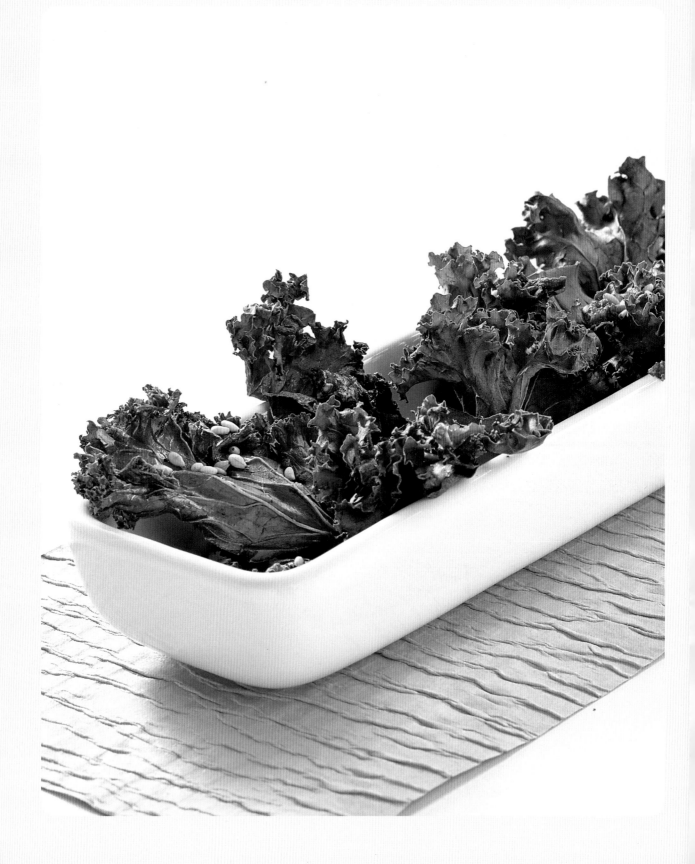

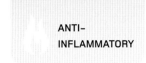

ANTI-
INFLAMMATORY

KRISPY KALE: A VITAMIN K EXTRAVAGANZA

From Dr. Jonny: Kale is one of my favorite vegetables, ever since I stumbled on the delicious raw kale salad in the prepared foods section of Whole Foods. Whoever put that salad together was on to something—it combines kale with pine nuts and dried cranberries and coats the whole thing with a light oil, blending sweet, bitter, and nutty to produce a sensational blend that continues to be one of their best sellers today. And if you haven't tried it, trust me, you should. Besides the fact that it tastes way better than you might imagine from looking at it, it's a veritable feast for your bones, containing—in addition to the usual suspects calcium and magnesium—a whopping 547 micrograms of vitamin K. Low levels of this vitamin are linked with low bone density, and a Harvard study showed that women who get at least 110 micrograms of vitamin K are 30 percent less likely to fracture a hip! If you're not one to scarf up a big plate of greens, try this simple recipe anyway. The roasting changes the fibrous texture into a rich, crispy-chewy one. You'll love it. So will your bones!

2 bunches curly kale

2 tablespoons (28 ml) olive oil, divided

1 tablespoon (15 ml) tamari

4 cloves garlic, minced

⅛ teaspoon red pepper flakes

1 tablespoon (15 ml) red wine vinegar

¼ teaspoon cracked black pepper

Preheat the oven to 375°F (190°C, or gas mark 5).

Rinse and spin the kale in a salad spinner (or drain well and pat dry). Cut or pull the thick central ribs off the leaves and discard. Tear or chop the leaves into 2- to 3-inch (5- to 7.5-cm) pieces.

In a large bowl, whisk together 1 tablespoon (15 ml) of the olive oil, the tamari, the garlic, and red pepper flakes. Add the kale and toss to coat. Spread the kale out evenly on a large, shallow roasting pan. Bake for 15 minutes, stirring 2 or 3 times, or until desired doneness. (If you like your kale crispier, just cook it for a longer period until it reaches the texture you're looking for. Just watch it closely to prevent scorching.)

In the meantime, in a small bowl, whisk together the remaining tablespoon of olive oil, red wine vinegar, and black pepper. Dress the cooked kale to taste, toss, and serve.

Yield: 4 servings

Per Serving: 82 Calories; 7g Fat (68.9% calories from fat); 1g Protein; 5g Carbohydrate; 1g Dietary Fiber; 0mg Cholesterol; 77mg Sodium

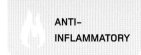
NOT YOUR AVERAGE GREEN BEANS

From Dr. Jonny: These just might be the tastiest green beans you've ever eaten. No kidding. And let me just say three things about why they make for strong bones: calcium, magnesium, vitamin K. The hazelnuts deliver the first two and the beans are good for the third. Remember to crush the garlic before slicing so you get the heart-healthy *allicin* that forms when the garlic is smashed. The macadamia nut oil adds a nice clean taste note.

1½ pounds (710 g) haricots verts, stems removed, or trimmed green beans

4–6 shallots, sliced lengthwise and separated*

4 large cloves garlic, crushed and quartered

2 tablespoons (28 ml) macadamia nut oil

½ teaspoon salt

½ teaspoon cracked black pepper

3 tablespoons (45 ml) balsamic vinegar**

⅓ cup (77 g) roasted hazelnuts, coarsely chopped

* If you don't have shallots on hand, you can substitute half of a Vidalia onion, sliced thin.

** The balsamic vinegar gives the dish a sweet flavor. You can also try a good red wine vinegar for an Italian flair and a healthy Blue Zone staple.

Preheat the oven to 450°F (230°C, or gas mark 8).

Line a large baking sheet or shallow baking pan with aluminum foil.

In a large bowl, gently toss the haricots verts with the shallots, garlic, oil, salt, and pepper to evenly coat. Spread the mixture in an even layer in the prepared pan. Roast, stirring every 10 minutes, for 30 minutes or until the beans are tender and shallots are soft and lightly caramelized. Gently toss the cooked beans with vinegar and sprinkle nuts over the top before serving.

Yield: Just under 6 cups (600 g) or about 4 servings

Per Serving: 206 Calories; 19g Fat (79.4% calories from fat); 3g Protein; 9g Carbohydrate; 2g Dietary Fiber; 0mg Cholesterol; 270mg Sodium

FROM CHEF JEANNETTE:

Haricot vert (pronounced ar-ee-koh vare) is French for "green bean." They are slender and more tender than conventional green beans, and deep green.

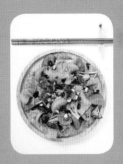

SALADS

· ·

Bone–Building Mandarin–Broccoli Salad
Fabulous Fruit–and–Veg Vitamin C Salad

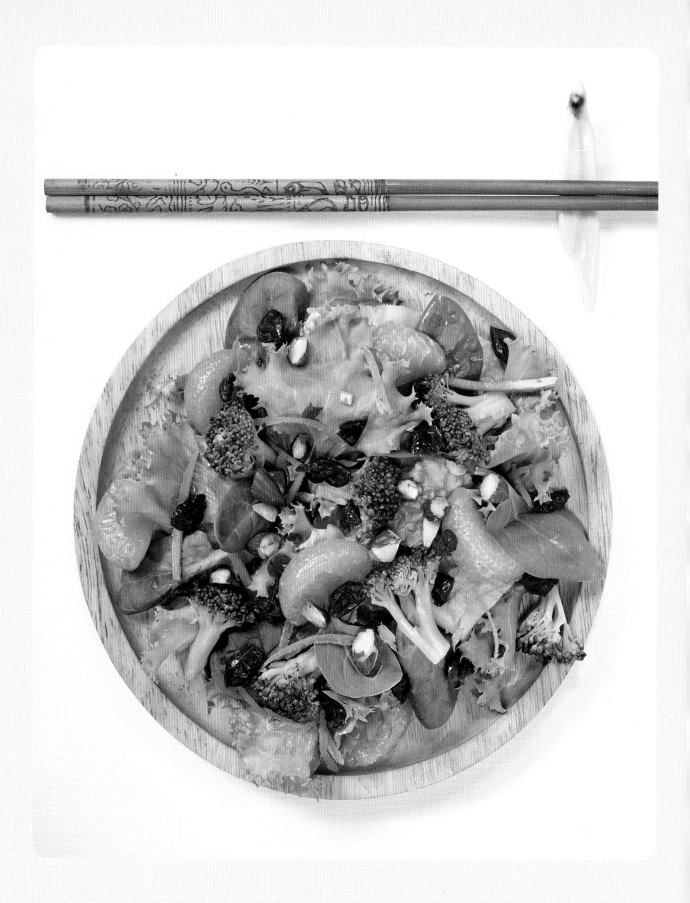

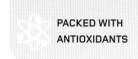
BONE-BUILDING MANDARIN-BROCCOLI SALAD

From Dr. Jonny: This recipe contains a mix of ingredients that help you build bones and lower inflammation, such as spinach and broccoli, both of which are terrific sources of vitamin K, an important nutrient for bone health. Olive oil adds a strong anti-inflammatory component to this fresh-tasting dish of sweet and acidic flavors.

2 cups (142 g) broccoli florets, cut to the size of quarters

6 tablespoons (90 ml) tarragon vinegar

2 tablespoons (28 ml) sherry

2 teaspoons (12 g) Dijon mustard

2 tablespoons (28 ml) olive oil

1 tablespoon (6 g) finely grated orange zest

1 can (11 ounces, or 313 g) mandarin oranges, drained, juice reserved

5 cups (275 g) baby romaine lettuce

1 cup (30 g) baby spinach

1 head endive, chopped

1 cup (110 g) shredded carrots

½ cup (60 g) dried cranberries

⅓ cup (48 g) tamari almonds, chopped roughly (or roasted almonds)

You can prepare the broccoli and dressing ahead of time, if desired.

Steam the broccoli florets over boiling water for 3 minutes. Remove the broccoli and shock it for 30 seconds in a large bowl of cold water. Drain well. Set aside in a medium bowl.

In a small bowl, whisk together the vinegar, sherry, mustard, olive oil, zest, and 2 tablespoons (28 g) of the reserved mandarin juice.

Pour about half the dressing over the broccoli florets and toss to combine. Refrigerate the florets to chill, if desired.

Just before serving, drain the broccoli florets and toss the greens together in large salad bowl to combine.

Sprinkle the carrots over the greens, the broccoli over the carrots, and nestle orange slices into the salad. Sprinkle cranberries on top and pour the remaining dressing to taste over salad.

Garnish with chopped almonds and serve.

Yield: about 4 servings

Per Serving: 192 Calories; 10g Fat (45.3% calories from fat); 5g Protein; 23g Carbohydrate; 10g Dietary Fiber; 0mg Cholesterol; 103mg Sodium

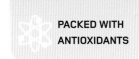

FABULOUS FRUIT-AND-VEG VITAMIN C SALAD

From Dr. Jonny: This unique salad will definitely spark some conversation. Guests will compliment you on the unexpected combination of tastes and textures. The avocados add a creamy smoothness to the peppery, tart bite of the calcium-rich dark leafy greens and grapefruit. Rich in vitamin C, this salad also provides bone-building vitamin K and the healthy fat you need to absorb it. Some recent research suggests that extracts from pomegranate may help prevent bone loss. Little known fact: Avocados are loaded with fiber. Didn't know that, did you?

1 pink grapefruit, peeled, with pith removed

1 large ripe Hass avocado, peeled and pitted

¼ cup (60 ml) fresh-squeezed pink grapefruit juice

1 tablespoon (15 ml) champagne vinegar

1 tablespoon (15 ml) almond oil (or lightly flavored vegetable oil)

¼ teaspoon salt

4 cups (120 g) spinach, well washed and chopped into bite-size pieces

2 cups (40 g) arugula, well washed

¼ cup (32 g) pomegranate seeds

In a small bowl whisk together the grapefruit juice, vinegar, oil, and salt. Set aside.

In a large salad bowl, toss together the spinach and arugula.

Segment the grapefruit and slice the segments into bite-size pieces. Spread over the salad bed. Cut the avocado into long, thin slices. Arrange the slices over the grapefruit. Lightly dress the salad to taste and top with pomegranate seeds.

Yield: 4 servings

Per Serving: 152 Calories; 11g Fat (62.4% calories from fat); 3g Protein; 13g Carbohydrate; 3g Dietary Fiber; 0mg Cholesterol; 164mg Sodium

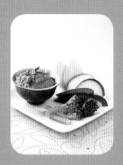

BREAKFASTS and SNACKS

· ·

Better Bones Muffins

Potassium-Powered Raw Muesli

**Sweet and Savory Magnesium-Calcium
Combo Snacks**

Bone-sational Mexi-Tofu Dip

Easy Edamame Hummus

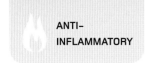

BETTER BONES MUFFINS

From Dr. Jonny: Chef Jeannette originally created this delicious recipe for R. Keith McCormick, D.C., author of *The Whole-Body Approach to Osteoporosis*. McCormick knows what it takes to build and maintain strong bones—he's an Ironman athlete who was diagnosed with osteoporosis while still a young man. McCormick's personal journey led him to discover that contrary to popular perception, there is much more to healing osteoporosis than simply filling up on calcium. Strong bones require a mix of important minerals (including magnesium), vitamins like vitamin K and D, and proper amounts of high-quality protein. There's also an inflammatory component to weak bones, so lowering inflammation, which can be seriously aggravated by too much sugar and high-glycemic foods, is a high priority as well. (By the way, McCormick continues to compete—and practice healing—today.) McCormick's directions to Chef Jeannette were to find a way to combine protein (whey powder), fiber (flaxseed and vegetables), low-glycemic sweeteners, and good sources of both calcium (molasses and whey) and magnesium (dark chocolate) for the ultimate "strong bone" snack. This absolutely delicious and freezable snack fills the bill perfectly and is a great example of how favorite foods like muffins can be made into longevity powerhouses!

1¼ cups (150 g) whole-wheat pastry flour

¼ cup (25 g) wheat or oat bran

¼ cup (32 g) whey protein powder

2 tablespoons (13 g) ground flaxseed

1 teaspoon ground cinnamon

¼ teaspoon ground nutmeg

½ teaspoon baking soda

¼ teaspoon baking powder

2 eggs

½ cup (120 g) xylitol

2 tablespoons (40 g) blackstrap molasses

2 tablespoons (28 ml) melted orange or apple juice concentrate

⅓ cup (80 ml) virgin coconut oil, melted

1 cup (113 g) grated zucchini, unpeeled*

½ cup (55 g) peeled and grated sweet potato

½ cup (72 g) chopped nuts, optional (almonds, walnuts, pecans, etc.)

½ cup (85 g) dark chocolate chips, optional

* For moister muffins, purée the zucchini in a food processor to ¾ cup (180 g) at applesauce consistency. You'll need about 1 small zucchini.

Preheat the oven to 325°F (170°C, or gas mark 3) and line 12 muffin cups with paper liners.

In a large bowl, combine the flour, bran, protein powder, flaxseed, cinnamon, nutmeg, baking soda, and baking powder. Stir gently until well mixed. Beat the eggs in a mixer for about 2 minutes until they are light and foamy. Add the xylitol, molasses, juice concentrate, and coconut oil, and blend on low until combined. Stir in the zucchini and sweet potato.

Gently fold the wet mixture into the dry until just combined. Add the nuts and chocolate chips, if using, and stir once or twice to mix. Scoop the batter into prepared muffin tins, filling each cup about ¾ full.

Bake for about 20 minutes (test centers for doneness with a toothpick). Cool on a wire rack. These muffins freeze well.

Yield: 1 dozen muffins

Per Serving: 450 Calories; 13g Fat (19.7% calories from fat); 7g Protein; 114g Carbohydrate; 4g Dietary Fiber; 36mg Cholesterol; 95mg Sodium

FROM CHEF JEANNETTE:

You may have to look to your local health food store to find whole-wheat pastry flour and xylitol. The flour is whole grain, but milled very finely so it has a nice light texture compared to regular whole-wheat flour, which has too heavy a feel for some baked goods.

Xylitol is one of the sugar alcohols (look for the "ol" at the end of the word: maltitol, sorbitol, etc.). Sugar alcohols aren't actually digested by the body but pass right through without elevating insulin levels—that makes them an ideal sweetener for type 2 diabetics and others trying to keep their blood sugar levels stable, a key longevity practice. They can cause mild digestive discomfort if consumed in high amounts, so keep your portions in check! We like xylitol and erythritol the best, and both come in a granulated form similar to sugar. They aren't as sweet as sugar, and erythritol has a "cool" feeling when you eat it, so it works great in frozen treats. You can find both of these products in your natural food stores and some higher-end grocers.

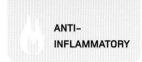

ANTI-
INFLAMMATORY

POTASSIUM-POWERED RAW MUESLI

From Dr. Jonny: Muesli is one of my favorite out-of-the-box cereals, but I stopped buying it long ago because it was so much easier and cheaper to make my own. Truthfully, though, this recipe beats the pants off my low-tech version (throw some raw oats together with some nuts, soak in raw milk, and eat). The prunes and/or figs are absolutely loaded with potassium, a nutrient you may not think of when you think about bone strengthening, but you should. One study showed that post-menopausal women with low bone density significantly improved the density of their spine and hip bones when they went on potassium citrate supplements. And, potassium helps neutralize the acid produced by a typical American diet. Just for good measure there's some protein, calcium, and magnesium in the nuts and seeds. Plus, you can customize this fiber-filled nutritious base recipe with any fresh, seasonal fruit for any time of year.

FRESH ALMOND MILK

1½ cups (217 g) raw almonds

4½ cups (1 L) water, divided

½ teaspoon vanilla extract

DRY GRAIN AND NUT MIX*

1 ½ cups (120 g) rolled oats

¼ cup (34 g) chopped raw Brazil nuts

¼ cup (28 g) chopped raw almonds

½ cup (72 g) raw sunflower seeds

2 tablespoons (16 g) raw sesame seeds

½ cup (40 g) coconut chips

½ teaspoon ground cinnamon

DRIED FRUIT

6 prunes OR 4 dried figs, soaked 10 minutes and chopped

3 dates, pitted and chopped

Make the almond milk: Soak the raw almonds overnight in water to cover.** Drain and add soaked almonds to blender with 2 cups (475 ml) of the (fresh) water and blend until the almonds are completely incorporated. Add the remaining 2 ½ cups (475 ml) water and vanilla and blend until smooth. Drain the almond milk through a fine mesh sieve (or cheesecloth or nut milk bag, if you have either) and discard the nut meal. Set the almond milk aside.

Make the dry grain and nut mix: In a large bowl, stir together the oats, nuts, seeds, coconut chips, and cinnamon to combine well.

Make the muesli: Add prunes or figs and dates to dried mix and stir well to incorporate. Divide among 4 bowls. Divide almond milk and pour out evenly over 4 bowls. Top with fresh seasonal fruit, if desired, and enjoy.

Yield: 6 servings

Per Serving: 515 Calories; 38g Fat (62.3% calories from fat); 16g Protein; 35g Carbohydrate; 11g Dietary Fiber; 0mg Cholesterol; 9mg Sodium

FROM CHEF JEANNETTE:

If desired, sweeten the muesli by stirring a little maple syrup into the almond milk before pouring over the dry mix, but it will have a better longevity impact if you just sweeten it with fresh fruit, such as sliced bananas or ripe peaches.

You can pour the nut milk over the cereal the night before and leave it overnight in the fridge. This turns it into a kind of "raw oatmeal" with a denser texture. It's easier to digest, too.

 * This dry grain and nut mix will store well in your pantry for a few weeks or your fridge for a few months.

** To save time, make almond milk with unsoaked raw almonds (1 portion nuts to 2 portions water) in the same way, but soaking them makes them more digestible.

SWEET AND SAVORY MAGNESIUM-CALCIUM COMBO SNACKS

From Dr. Jonny: The thing that many people—including, sadly, many doctors—don't understand about calcium and bones is this: You can throw all the calcium you like at the body, but if it doesn't get into the bones it's not doing what you need it to be doing. You need magnesium (not to mention vitamin D) for your body to fully metabolize and utilize calcium. Some people feel that the ideal ratio of calcium to magnesium is 1:1, but the general consensus is that 2:1 is fine also. This great combination of yogurt, cottage cheese, and nuts provides a wonderful blend of calcium and magnesium, while the apricots provide a big fat dose of potassium, an important mineral the body uses to neutralize bone-robbing acids. Plus the snack is ridiculously easy to prepare and can easily be customized by creating your own flavor combos.

BASE MIX

2 cups (460 g) plain yogurt

2 cups (450 g) plain cottage cheese

SWEET COMBO

Base mix (see above)

2 tablespoons (40 g) honey, or to taste (or use xylitol or a few drops of liquid stevia)

1 drop vanilla extract

½ teaspoon cardamom

¼ teaspoon ground cinnamon

4 large fresh apricots, pitted and diced, OR ½ cup (65 g) dried apricots, chopped

½ cup (62 g) toasted pistachios

In a medium bowl stir together the yogurt and cottage cheese. Mix in the honey, vanilla, cardamom, and cinnamon until well incorporated. Fold in the apricots and sprinkle with pistachios.

Yield: 4 servings

Per Serving: 314 Calories; 14g Fat (39.8% calories from fat); 22g Protein; 26g Carbohydrate; 2g Dietary Fiber; 24mg Cholesterol; 512mg Sodium

SAVORY COMBO

Base mix (see above)

¼ cup (4 g) fresh cilantro or parsley (15 g), chopped

Juice of 1 lime

1 clove garlic, finely minced

½ teaspoon salt, or to taste

¼ teaspoon cracked black pepper

½ red bell pepper, diced fine

1 stalk celery, trimmed and diced fine

¾ cup (113 g) cherry tomatoes, quartered

⅓ cup (45 g) toasted pine nuts

In a medium bowl stir together the yogurt and cottage cheese. Mix in the cilantro, lime juice, garlic, salt, and black pepper until well incorporated. Gently stir in bell pepper, celery, and tomatoes, and sprinkle with pine nuts.

Yield: 4 servings

Per Serving: 241 Calories; 10g Fat (38.3% calories from fat); 22g Protein; 16g Carbohydrate; 1g Dietary Fiber; 24mg Cholesterol; 791mg Sodium

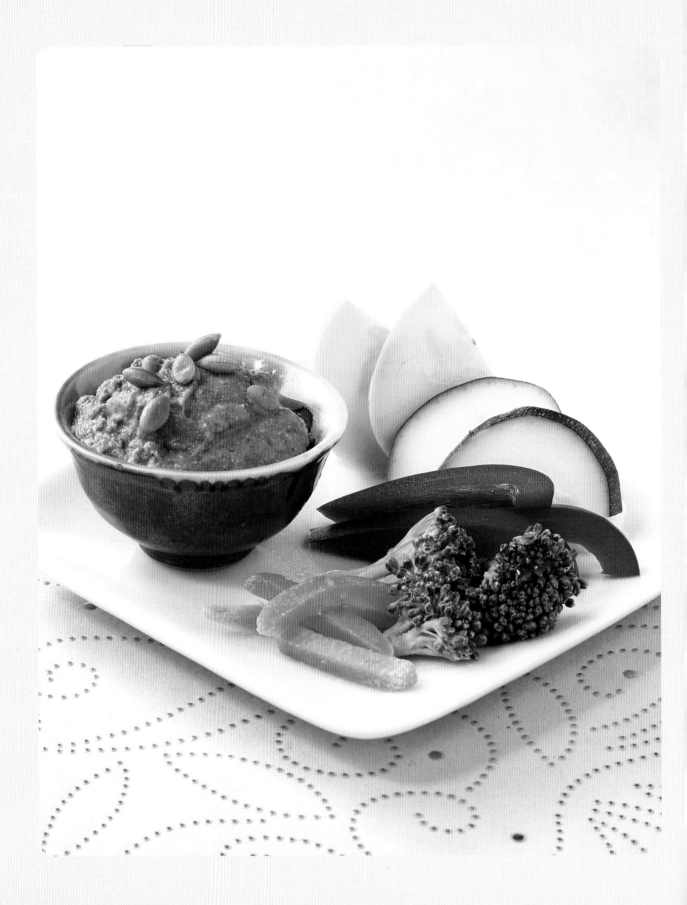

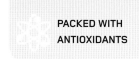
BONE-SATIONAL MEXI-TOFU DIP

From Dr. Jonny: Here's an interesting factoid for you: Many Asian cultures have way lower rates of osteoporosis than Americans do and guess what—they don't drink milk. Maybe they do just fine getting their calcium (and vitamin D) from other sources such as the small bones in fish . . . and from calcium-rich tofu. In any case, this dish gives you plenty of calcium along with magnesium—calcium's partner in bone health—provided courtesy of the toasted pepitas. Tip: For extra calcium, look for tofu prepared with calcium sulfate. You'll get more nutritional bang for your buck!

1 cup (460 g) firm silken tofu

1 can (14.5 ounces, or 413 g) black beans, drained and rinsed

¼ cup (28 g) oil-packed sun-dried tomato strips, drained

¾ cup (195 g) salsa (see recipe on page 255 or use prepared)

¼ cup (4 g) cilantro

3 cloves garlic, minced

²⁄₃ teaspoon ground cumin

½ teaspoon dried oregano

½ teaspoon salt, or to taste

Cracked black pepper, to taste

⅛ teaspoon chipotle pepper, optional

¼ cup (35 g) toasted pepitas (pumpkin seeds)

Blend the tofu in a food processor until smooth, about 5 seconds. Add the beans and process until smooth. Add the tomatoes and process until broken up. Add the salsa, cilantro, garlic, cumin, oregano, salt, and peppers, and blend until smooth, scraping down the sides as necessary. Garnish with pepitas before serving.

Yield: about 3 ½ cups (875 g)

Per Serving: 60 Calories; 1.4g Fat (20% calories from fat); 5g Protein; 8g Carbohydrate; 2.4g Dietary Fiber; 0mg Cholesterol; 237mg Sodium

FROM CHEF JEANNETTE:

Add a squeeze or two of fresh lime or lemon juice to really pop the flavors. For longevity duos, try this with vegetable sticks, baked corn chips, or mixed into a salad. Or try mixing it with cooked ground turkey and lettuce to make a great taco or corn wrap.

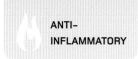
EASY EDAMAME HUMMUS

From Dr. Jonny: When I first introduced my friend Anja Christy to edamame, she had trouble pronouncing it. Whenever we'd go to a Japanese restaurant, she'd kiddingly say, "Let's order some of that Eddy's Mommy." And that's how I think of these boiled green soybeans, which used to be one of the best-kept nutritional secrets on the planet till they became a staple at sushi restaurants. And if you don't happen to frequent sushi bars, then let me let you in on the secret now. One tiny half-cup of shelled edamame beans has an incredible 9 grams of fiber and 11 grams of protein. Edamame beans are a great way to get protein in your diet without any of the drawbacks of factory-farmed meat. Just for good measure, the Greek yogurt adds some extra calcium to the mix, one of the most important nutrients for bone health. This light, bright, high-fiber/bone-healthy spread can be enjoyed as a dip with vegetable crudités, or as a life-enhancing mayo alternative on your sandwiches.

2 cups (236 g) frozen shelled, cooked edamame beans, thawed (or use frozen raw and cook according to package directions)

½ cup (115 g) plain Greek yogurt

Juice of 1 lemon

2 cloves garlic, minced

½ teaspoon curry powder

½ teaspoon ground cumin

½ teaspoon salt

Process the thawed edamame in a blender until smooth, scraping down the sides as necessary. Add the yogurt and blend into a purée. Add lemon juice, garlic, curry, cumin, and salt, and process until well incorporated.

Yield: about 2 cups (520 g)

Per Serving: 31 Calories; 1g Fat (32% calories from fat); 2.5g Protein; 3.4g Carbohydrate; 1.4g Dietary Fiber; .5mg Cholesterol; 80mg Sodium

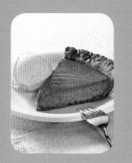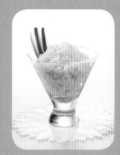

DESSERTS

· ·

Not Your Mother's Pumpkin Pie
Gingered Mango and Green Tea Freeze

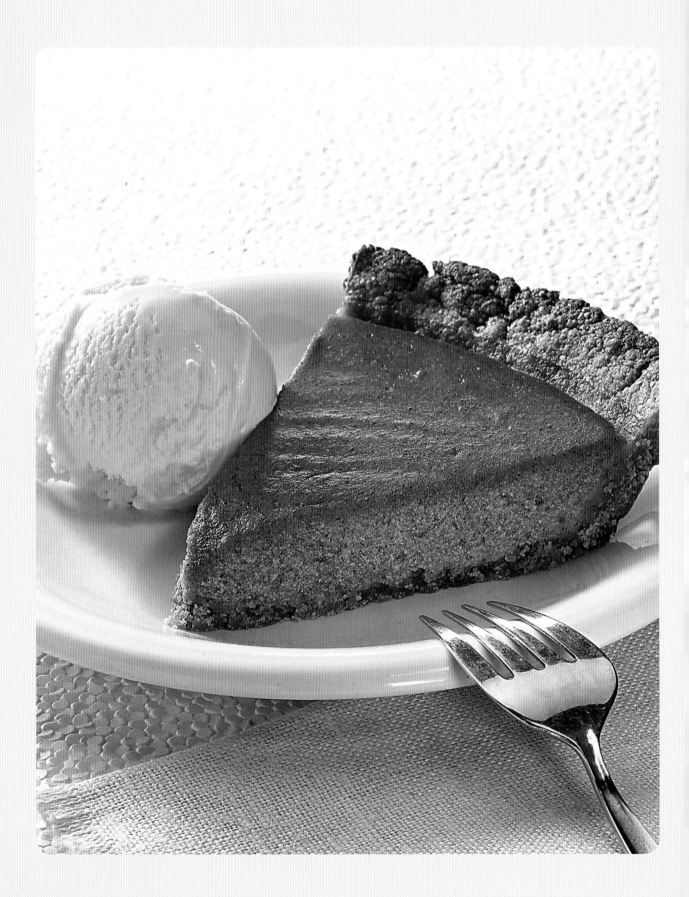

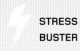
NOT YOUR MOTHER'S PUMPKIN PIE

From Dr. Jonny: This is a fantastic alternative to conventional pumpkin pie—you trade out the life-shortening heavy crust for a fiber-rich substitute. It's filled with omega-3 oils that strengthen everything—the brain, heart, and bones—and reduce inflammation, one of the Four Horsemen of Aging. Plus, no butter or cream, lowering calories but without compromising taste. Seriously! The spiced flavor gives it a nice warming quality. You'll never want to go back to store bought!

CRUST

Unflavored cooking oil spray

½ cup (65 g) unsulphured dried apricots (or dates)

½ cup (70 g) roasted, salted pepitas (pumpkin seeds)

½ cup (60 g) whole-wheat pastry flour

½ cup (47 g) almond flour (or finely processed raw almonds)

½ cup (60 g) oat flour (or finely processed rolled oats)

¼ cup (60 ml) almond oil (or any unflavored oil)

2 tablespoons (40 g) maple syrup

FILLING

1 package (12.3 ounces, or 340 g) extra-firm silken tofu (or 1½ cups)

1 can (15 ounces, or 425 g) pumpkin purée

⅔ cup (230 g) maple syrup or agave nectar

1 teaspoon vanilla or orange extract

2 teaspoons ground cinnamon

2 teaspoons ground ginger

¼ teaspoon cloves

¼ teaspoon allspice

Preheat the oven to 350°F (180°C, or gas mark 4).

Coat a 9-inch (23-cm) deep-dish pie plate with cooking oil spray to lightly coat.

Soak the apricots in enough hot water to cover for 10 to 15 minutes.

Grind the pepitas in a food processor until the seeds resemble a coarse, uniform meal. Remove the ground seeds and wipe out the processor.

Drain the apricots, reserving the soaking liquid, and place the apricots in the food processor. Process the apricots until they are nearly a paste, about 30 seconds. Add the ground pepitas, wheat flour, almond flour, oat flour, oil, and maple syrup and process well, scraping down the sides periodically. If the mixture is too dry, add the apricot soaking liquid 1 teaspoon at a time until the mixture forms a moist dough that holds together well.

Press the crust dough into the oiled pie plate, distributing evenly. Bake for 10 minutes and set aside.

While baking, clean and dry the food processor. Drain the tofu and process in the food processor until it reaches the consistency of thick, smooth yogurt. Add the pumpkin purée, maple syrup or nectar, extract, and spices, and process, scraping down the sides periodically, until the mixture is smooth and creamy. Pour the mixture into the prepared pie crust and place a ring of foil around the upper edges of the crust. Bake for 40 to 45 minutes until the filling is set. The pie will continue to firm somewhat as it cools. Serve warm or chilled.

Yield: 8 pieces

Per Serving: 352 Calories; 15g Fat (35.6% calories from fat); 9g Protein; 50g Carbohydrate; 7g Dietary Fiber; 0mg Cholesterol; 13mg Sodium

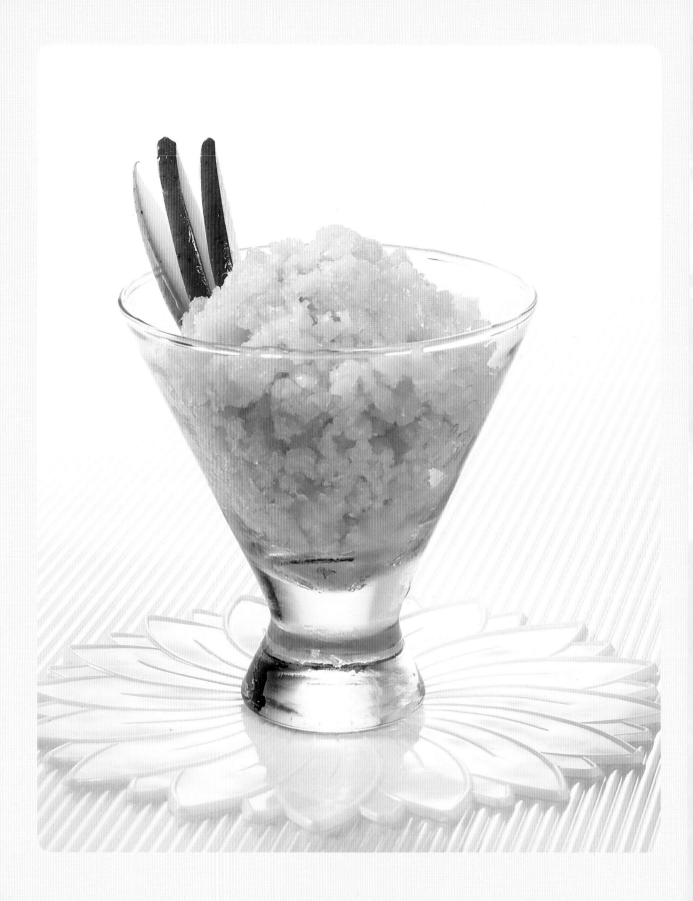

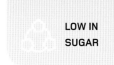

GINGERED MANGO AND GREEN TEA FREEZE

From Dr. Jonny: Green tea, ginger, and mango—the very sound of it is intriguing. It is deep orange in color, and the light ginger notes help showcase the creamy, rich flavor of fresh mango—more like ice cream than a sorbet. This is a bone builder if there ever was one. Green tea is packed with healthy compounds from the plant kingdom known as *polyphenols*, and the fruit is loaded with antioxidants and minerals. Best of all, it's sweetened with one of the healthiest, noncaloric natural sweeteners around—erythritol. It's fresh and tropical, and you'll find yourself swirling it around in your mouth before swallowing!

½ cup (75 g) dried mangoes, chopped*

2 tablespoons (6 g) loose green tea leaves (about 4 bags' worth)**

½ cup (120 ml) boiling water

¼ cup (60 g) erythritol***

⅓ cup (40 g) grated ginger

3 cups (525 g) mangoes (about 4), peeled, pitted, and cut into chunks

* Dried mango is tough and leathery. It's easier to use kitchen shears than a knife to snip it into pieces.

** Look for loose tea leaves, because there isn't enough water in the recipe for the required number of bags. If you can only find bags, just tear them open and use the leaves. Strain the tea gently without pressure.

*** Erythritol has a grainy texture that disappears when you boil it. Because of its "cooling" quality, it is an ideal sweetener for iced treats. You will find it bagged in most natural food stores and many high-end grocers. If you don't have any on hand, use any dry sweetener (such as xylitol) or a few drops of liquid stevia in its place.

**** Freezing for 2 hours will give you a slushier consistency more like a thick frappé. Freezing for the full 4 will give you a consistency more like a sorbet. If you refreeze processed portions, just wait 10 minutes before serving. If you're impatient, you can also eat it immediately as a pudding without freezing at all!

In a small bowl, cover the dried mangoes with water and soak while you prepare the tea, about 10 minutes.

Place the tea leaves in a mug and pour boiling water over all. Set a plate on the top to cover and let it steep for 5 minutes. Remove the cup and strain the tea gently through a double-mesh strainer into the smallest saucepan you have. Whisk in the erythritol and place over medium-high heat. Bring to a boil and whisk until the erythritol is completely dissolved, about 20 seconds.

Remove from the heat and squeeze the grated ginger with your hand so that the juice runs into the tea. Cool the tea in the fridge for 15 to 20 minutes until lukewarm.

Drain the dried mango.

Once the tea is cooled, in a food processor combine the soaked dried mango and fresh mango and process until smooth, scraping down the sides as necessary. Pour the tea into the purée and process until smooth and well incorporated.

Pour evenly into a deep-dish pie plate and cover tightly with a layer of microwave-safe plastic wrap. Freeze for 2 to 4 hours, depending on preferred consistency.****

To serve, let it sit on a counter for about 5 minutes until you can remove the mango from the pie plate. Break up into large chunks with a heavy knife and process again until smooth, about 20 seconds. Serve immediately.

Yield: about 4 servings

Per Serving: 165 Calories; 1g Fat (3.2% calories from fat); 1g Protein; 55g Carbohydrate; 4g Dietary Fiber; 0mg Cholesterol; 16mg Sodium

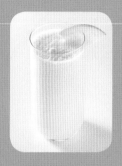

DRINKS

· · · · · · · · · · · · · · · · · · · ·

Creamy Green Smoothie
Day-at-the-Park Dreamsicle Shake
Carrot-Orange Juice for Strong Bones
Antioxidant Almond Nog

CREAMY GREEN SMOOTHIE

From Dr. Jonny: Here's a delicious shake that'll give your bones a boost with a double dose of calcium courtesy of the winning duo of tofu and milk. (Where I live I can get raw organic milk, which is definitely my preference, but any of Chef Jeannette's options will work just fine.) A mere tablespoon of spirulina has an amazing 4 grams of protein, 2 grams of iron, and virtually as much potassium as a potassium supplement pill! It will also turn anything you mix into it green—great on Halloween!

2 frozen bananas, or more to taste

3½ cups (805 ml) milk (cow's or unsweetened vanilla soy, almond, or hemp)

¾ cup (345 g) soft silken tofu

2 tablespoons (9 g) raw almond or cashew butter*

1 tablespoon (15 g) sweetener, optional (maple syrup, xylitol, etc.)

1 tablespoon (8 g) spirulina powder

Pinch fresh-grated nutmeg

Add all ingredients to a blender and process until smooth. Add additional milk to thin, or ice cubes to chill, if desired.

Yield: 4 servings

Per Serving: 277 Calories; 13g Fat (38.6% calories from fat); 16g Protein; 29g Carbohydrate; 3g Dietary Fiber; 28mg Cholesterol; 137mg Sodium

* Or you can just add ¼ cup (36 g) raw almonds or cashews.

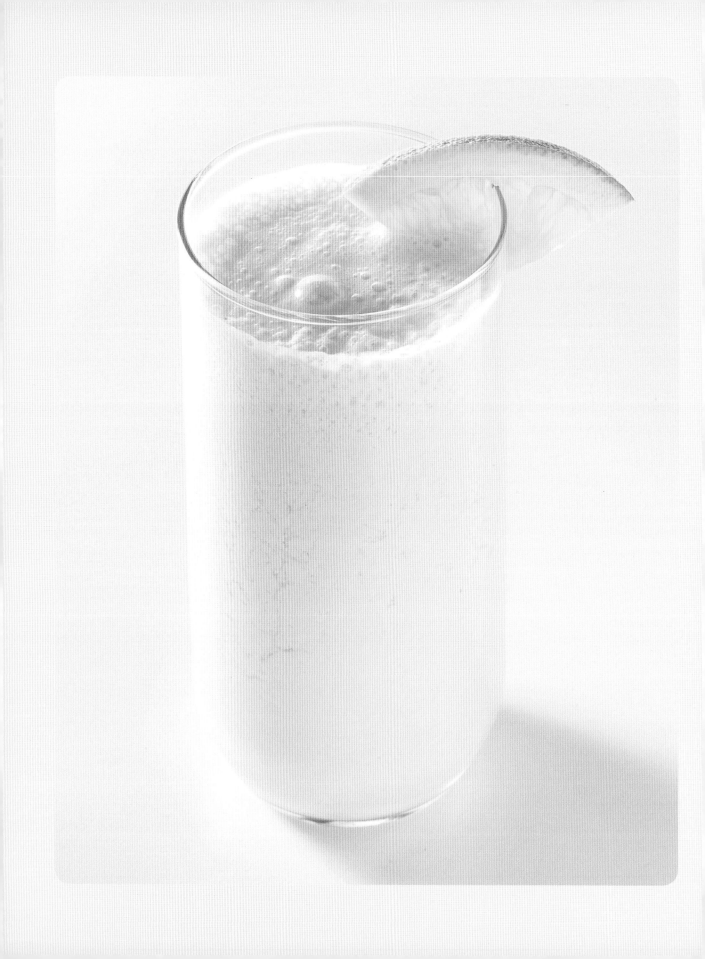

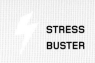

DAY-AT-THE-PARK DREAMSICLE SHAKE

From Dr. Jonny: I admit to being biased toward this recipe and here's why: When I grew up, the Good Humor man used to drive around our neighborhood with his ice-cream truck, and that meant I was going to get to eat a Creamsicle! To me the combination of orange sherbet and vanilla ice cream was exquisite. So I love this recipe because you get the taste of the old Creamsicles in a nutrient-rich blend of high-calcium and bone-building foods such as yogurt and orange juice. And this one gets its delicious rich taste from actual food, not artificial flavors.

2 oranges, peeled

⅓ to ½ cup (80 to 120 ml) calcium-fortified frozen orange juice concentrate, thawed, to taste

2 cups ice cubes

1 cup (230 g) plain yogurt

2 cups (475 ml) milk (cow's, unsweetened vanilla, almond, or soy milk)

1 teaspoon vanilla extract

Place all ingredients into a powerful blender (we like Vitamix) and blend until smooth.

Adjust concentrate for sweetness and ice cubes for frozen consistency.

Yield: about 4 small glasses

Per Serving: 202 Calories; 6g Fat (26.7% calories from fat); 7g Protein; 30g Carbohydrate; 2g Dietary Fiber; 24mg Cholesterol; 88mg Sodium

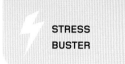
CARROT-ORANGE JUICE FOR STRONG BONES

From Dr. Jonny: Strong bones are one of the foundations of a healthy body, and a healthy body—and mind, of course—is the foundation for long life! This fresh, tasty drink is a bone-strengthening powerhouse. There's a ton of calcium, especially since Chef Jeannette left the peels of the orange intact, and the carrots, orange, and apple more than compensate for any bitterness in the calcium-rich greens. A clever concoction that works for breakfast or as a late afternoon pick-me-up.

5 large carrots, unpeeled

2 leaves curly kale

2 small collard leaves

¼ cup (15 g) parsley

1 small organic orange or clementine, unpeeled

½ apple, stemmed and unpeeled

Wash all produce thoroughly, cut it into large chunks, and run through a juicer.

Stir gently to combine and drink immediately.

Yield: 1 large or 2 small glasses

Per Serving: 176 Calories; 1g Fat (5.5% calories from fat); 6g Protein; 40g Carbohydrate; 11g Dietary Fiber; 0mg Cholesterol; 103mg Sodium

FROM CHEF JEANNETTE:

The skins of oranges are loaded with calcium, but they are often too thick for most juicers to handle and are typically very bitter and loaded with pesticides. Instead, look for organic, thin-skinned versions (such as clementines rather than navel) to power your bone juice.

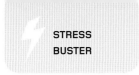

ANTIOXIDANT ALMOND NOG

From Dr. Jonny: Traditional eggnogs are made with loads of sugar and brandy, eggs, and cream—not exactly a recipe for long life. (Note that it's not the eggs that are the problem—it's the huge sugar and alcohol load!) This tasty twist on the nog is low in alcohol and sugars and high in nutrition. Almonds are rich in magnesium, potassium, manganese, copper, the antioxidants vitamin E and selenium, and bone-building calcium. Best of all, this baby can be served chilled on a warm night or cold on a hot one. Enjoy!

---

²/₃ cup (97 g) raw almonds*

3 cups (710 ml) milk (cow's, unsweetened vanilla soy, or almond)

¼ teaspoon vanilla

¼ teaspoon ground cinnamon

3 tablespoons (45 ml) blackstrap rum (or use ¼–½ teaspoon rum extract for alcohol-free version)

1 tablespoon (20 g) raw honey

½ teaspoon fresh-ground nutmeg

* Using whole raw almonds means that your drinks will contain the fibrous almond skins (and all their nutrients and fiber). For a smoother cocktail, use blanched, skinless almonds.

In a small skillet, dry toast the almonds over medium heat until they are lightly browned, about 5 minutes. Once they begin to brown, watch them closely because they can become overcooked very quickly. Remove from the pan, cool slightly, and grind to a powder in a food processor.*

Add the almond powder, milk, vanilla, cinnamon, rum, and honey to a blender and blend until well mixed. Warm over medium-low heat (for cold weather) or chill for 1 hour in the refrigerator (for warm weather) and divide among 4 mugs or glasses.

Sprinkle nutmeg onto tops of drinks and serve.

Yield: 4 servings

Per Serving: 270 Calories; 19g Fat (59.7% calories from fat); 11g Protein; 18g Carbohydrate; 3g Dietary Fiber; 24mg Cholesterol; 90mg Sodium

FROM CHEF JEANNETTE:

You can also substitute seeds scraped from half a Madagascar vanilla bean for the vanilla extract for a richer flavor. If you want to beef up the protein, iron, and other minerals, add 2 teaspoons of nutritional yeast to replace the eggs in a classic nog.

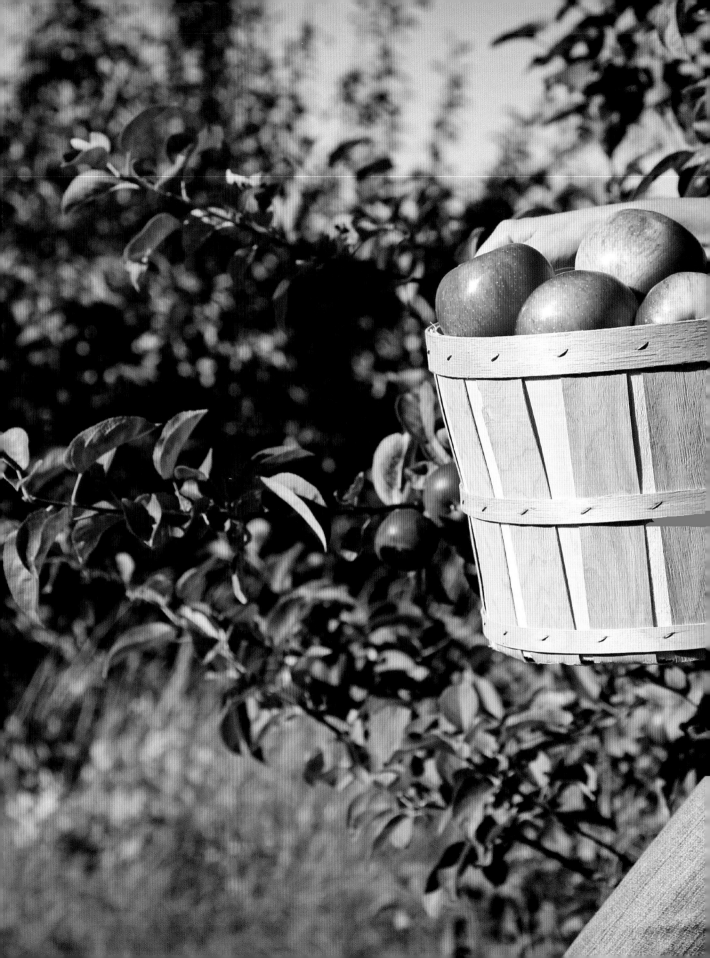

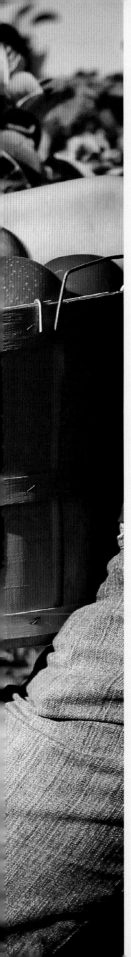

Chapter IV
Eat an Apple a Day—and These Meals—to Keep the Doctor Away

. . . .

ENTRÉES

From A to C Cream of Coconut and Butternut Soup

Immune Boon Kung Pao Chicken Soup

Feel-Good Chinese Mushroom Stew

Powerhouse Portobellos with Manchego Cheese over Wilted Spinach

Zinc-C Fest: Savory Succotash with Ground Beef

Lean and Mean Beef and Veggie Stir-Fry

Strengthening Shrimp, Soba Noodle, and Roasted Shiitake Salad

Potent Polenta Pie with Sun-Dried Tomato Pesto and Grilled Summer Veggies

Shake-Off-the-Chills with Tofu-Cremini Chili

SIDE DISHES

Grandma's Good-for-You Sauerkraut

Beta-Carotene Apple–Winter Squash Bake

Feisty Fungi: Green Beans with Sautéed Cremini Mushrooms

Ayurvedic Asparagus and Tomatoes

SALADS

Chopped Antioxidant-Rich Artichoke-Tomato Salad

Grated Beta-Carotene Salad

BREAKFASTS

Right Start Apricot-Prune-Walnut Breakfast Bread

A.M. Antioxidant Smoothie

SNACKS AND DESSERTS

Immune-Strengthening Shiitake Broth

Chocolate–Vitamin C Fruit Salad

Mighty Melon-Berry Madness

Longevity Fruit Gels—Not Just Jell-O

Smooth Move Comforting Fruit Compote

DRINKS

Toasted Chai Latte for Long Life

Juicy, Stress-Bustin' Ginseng Ale

Fresh Start Strawberry-Mint Fizz

Green Pineapple Pleaser

The Potassium Powerhouse: Fruit-Potato Juice

I know this is a cookbook, and this is the place we're supposed to talk about food and immunity, but I have to be honest—it's really hard to talk about the immune system without mentioning our thoughts and feelings.

Don't worry, I'm not going to go all Oprah on you and talk about "the Secret" and how you can "think" yourself well, but I will tell you this: What we do, think, and feel profoundly influences the operation of our immune system.

As does our food, which we'll get to in a moment.

To understand exactly how our thoughts and feelings (and yes, our foods!) influence immunity, it might be best to do a short review of exactly what the immune system is and what it does for a living.

The primary job of the immune system boils down to one thing: keep the bad guys out—the bad guys being microbes, viruses, bacteria, and the like. So this giant network of organs, hormones, the lymphatic system, white blood cells, and all the other components of the immune system have ultimately one shared purpose, and that is to keep out of the body what doesn't belong. The immune system acts like a giant bouncer at a nightclub. It looks for riffraff, which can be any kind of microbe or pathogen that might be up to no good, and then it attempts to evict them from the premises.

Okay, so far so good.

A MICROBIAL ARMY OF BOUNCERS

The immune system is made up of a whole network of tissues, cells, and organs that work together as a unit. The cells involved are white blood cells. So when your doctor tells you your white blood cell count is high, it often means you have an infection. White blood cells are the army of bouncers the body sends out when it senses there's a problem (like an invasion by a virus or bacteria). These white blood cells are called leukocytes, and they're stored in many different locations in the body, the primary locations being the lymphoid organs, including the thymus gland, spleen, and bone marrow. Leukocytes are also stored in clumps of lymphoid tissue such as the lymph nodes. (Now you know why when you were a kid and you were sick, you often had swollen lymph glands!)

Leukocytes come in two flavors: phagocytes, which act like little Ms. Pac-Men, running around and chewing up invading organisms, and lymphocytes, which are cells that allow the body to remember and recognize previous invaders—and help the body destroy them. These cells circulate throughout the body via lymphatic vessels (and blood vessels).

Lymphocytes also come in two flavors of their own: B-cells and T-cells. (You may have heard of T-cell count. It's often used as an indicator of how sick or healthy a person is when suffering from a systemic virus such as HIV.) B-cells and T-cells have different purposes. B-cells are like the scouting officers in the army, seeking out targets and then sending in the troops to lock onto those targets. The T-cells are like the soldiers, destroying the bad guys that the B-cells just told them about.

Okay, we're almost done now, and you've done a great job hanging in. I just want to tell you about one more component of the immune system, and then I'll show you how it all hangs together.

There's a special kind of T-cell, a subclass of T-cell, if you will, known as NK cells. NK stands for natural killer! But these cells aren't like the bad guys in the Halloween slasher movies. They're more like the Terminator, going in after the bad guys with big guns. They play a major role in the rejection of tumors and viruses. They work by injecting a kind of material that acts like rat poison to invading bad guys, causing the target cells to die. If you want a top-of-the-line-functioning immune system, which is clearly one of the keys to a healthy long life, you definitely want a nice active bunch of NK cells on your team.

It's really hard to talk about the immune system without mentioning our thoughts and feelings.

So guess what increases NK activity?

Satisfying personal relationships. Social support. Personal sharing. Humor. Laughter. Pursuing your bliss. Relaxation. Physical exertion and aerobic exercise.

I told you it was impossible to talk about immunity without talking about your thoughts and actions!

All the things mentioned above have been shown in research to increase not only NK cells but also overall lymphocyte function and activity. In fact, a study published as long ago as 1984 clearly showed that negative states (such as bereavement, academic stress, loneliness, depression, and so on) all decreased lymphocyte activity and specifically NK cell number and activity. Conversely all the good stuff listed above increased NK cell activity as well as other measures of a healthy, robust immune system.

So there, that's my plug for the mind–body connection. (After all, it wouldn't be a Jonny book if I didn't mention how all this stuff was related!)

Now we can move on to food.

IMMUNE–ENHANCING EDIBLES

Many specific nutrients in food have direct influences on immune system functions. For example, low levels of vitamin B_6 have been associated with impaired immune function, especially in the elderly. Low B_6 intake decreases the production of lymphocytes, which, you'll remember, are the class of cells that include T-cells and B-cells. You'll find plenty of vitamin B_6 in all the protein dishes featured in this section, such as Immune Boon Kung Pao Chicken Soup and Lean and Mean Beef and Veggie Stir-Fry.

Vitamin A, found in all the red vegetables and fruits that you'll frequently be using in the recipes that follow, such as the A.M. Antioxidant Smoothie and the Grated Beta-Carotene Salad, has been shown to be an immune enhancer that actually increases antibody response. (A little interesting factoid: Vitamin A supplementation significantly decreases death rates from infectious diseases among children who have acute measles or who are from areas in which vitamin A deficiency is common.)

Then there's the old standby, vitamin C, found in abundance throughout this section in recipes such as the Chocolate–Vitamin C Fruit Salad and the Green Pineapple Pleaser. Vitamin C does two amazing things (which you're actually going to understand better than most people, since you stuck with me and read the above paragraphs). Number one, vitamin C increases phagocytosis, which is the long technical name for the process by which those specialized immune-system cells (the ones that are like miniature Ms. Pac-Men) actually "eat up" the bad guys. The more vitamin C, the more ravenous those Ms. Pac-Men become! And vitamin C

Remember, shared and loving experiences, such as meals, are just as powerful a booster of immune function as the other nutrients mentioned in this section.

also increases—wait for it, now—chemotaxis, which is the rate of speed with which those white blood cells get to the site of an infection. (So you can think of vitamin C as a kind of high-octane gas that the white blood cells use to travel to their destination.)

You'll also find plenty of probiotics in this section (from foods such as pickles and sauerkraut), and here's why. Probiotics help with immunity in a big way. Remember, your gastrointestinal tract functions as a "first-defense" barrier against bacteria and other microorganisms, and how good a job it does depends largely on the population of "good" bacteria in your gut. (Those good bacteria are called probiotics.)

The bottom line is that many nutrients—the aforementioned plus omega-3 fats, zinc, and the vast array of antioxidants—all play a part in keeping your immune system healthy and strong. And the recipes in this section are loaded with those nutrients.

To come full circle, it's good to remember that food isn't just a delivery system for nutrients. It's also something to be shared with family and friends. The very act of preparing it, lovingly and mindfully, can reduce stress, one of the Four Horsemen of Aging and one that has a profoundly depressing effect on immunity.

So, enjoy the recipes in this section knowing that they give you a ton of the nutrients that turbocharge that complex web we know as immunity.

Remember, shared and loving experiences, such as meals, are just as powerful a booster of immune function as the other nutrients mentioned in this section.

Luckily you don't have to choose—you can have both! Enjoy!

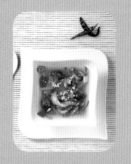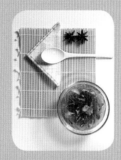

ENTRÉES

· ·

From A to C Cream of Coconut and Butternut Soup
Immune Boon Kung Pao Chicken Soup
Feel-Good Chinese Mushroom Stew
Powerhouse Portobellos with Manchego Cheese over Wilted Spinach
Zinc-C Fest: Savory Succotash with Ground Beef
Lean and Mean Beef and Veggie Stir-Fry
Strengthening Shrimp, Soba Noodle, and Roasted Shiitake Salad
Potent Polenta Pie with Sun-Dried Tomato Pesto and Grilled Summer Veggies
Shake-Off-the-Chills with Tofu-Cremini Chili

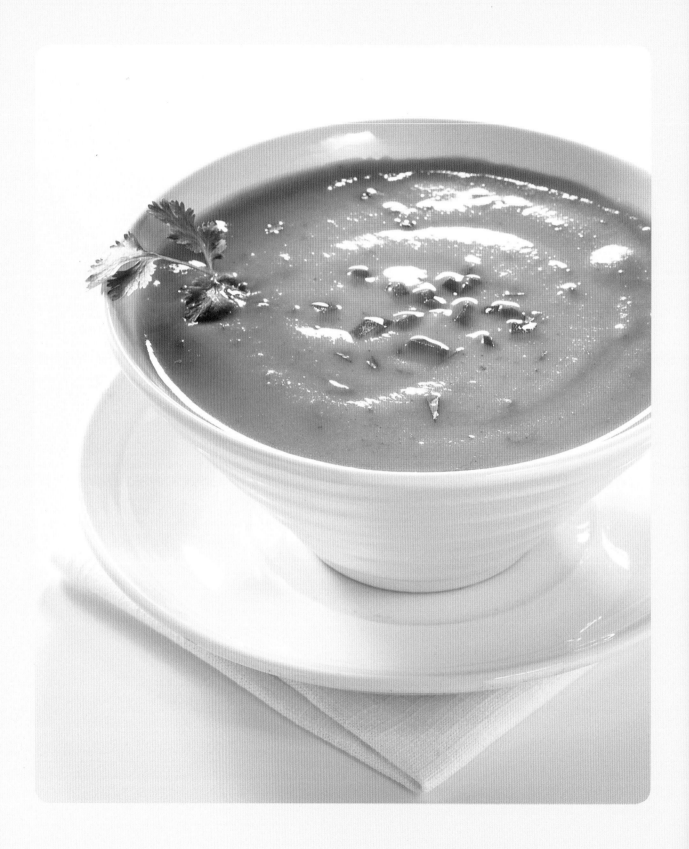

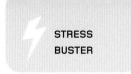

FROM A TO C CREAM OF COCONUT AND BUTTERNUT SOUP

From Dr. Jonny: A great recipe for building the immune system. The red peppers are loaded with vitamin C, the butternut squash is full of vitamin A, and the coconut oil is antimicrobial. The soup is rich and warming with a surprisingly fresh "bite" from the lime and cilantro. I especially love the way Chef Jeanette has made the recipe customizable for protein and fat content.

1 tablespoon (15 ml) coconut oil (or unflavored vegetable oil)

1 large sweet onion, diced

3 large cloves garlic, minced

3 tablespoons (18 g) minced gingerroot

1 teaspoon salt

2½ teaspoons (7.5 g) ground cumin

1 tablespoon (6 g) coriander

¼ teaspoon cayenne

1 red bell pepper, seeded and diced

1½ pounds (710 g) butternut squash, peeled, seeded and cubed (about 1 large squash)

4 cups (950 ml) vegetable broth

1 can (13.5 ounces or 384 g) coconut milk*

Juice of 1 lime

1 bunch fresh cilantro, chopped

* You can customize this soup for fat and protein content, if desired. Use full-fat coconut milk for the richest soup. If you prefer lower fat and higher protein, use low-fat coconut milk and add one 12.3-ounce (340-g) block of firm silken tofu: Drain the tofu and purée in a blender until smooth and creamy. Add to the puréed soup and cook for 10 minutes more before adding the lime and cilantro.

In a heavy-bottom soup pot, heat the oil over medium heat. Sauté the onion until soft but not burned, about 7 minutes. Add the garlic, ginger, salt, cumin, coriander, and cayenne, stirring to combine well. Sauté for 1 minute. Add the bell pepper and squash, stirring well to coat, and sauté for about 3 minutes. Add the broth and coconut milk, increase the heat to high, and bring the soup to a boil. Reduce the heat to a low simmer, cover, and cook for 20 to 25 minutes or until all vegetables are very tender.

Remove from the heat and purée the soup with an immersion blender until very smooth.

Return the soup to the burner and heat on low for 5 minutes. Remove from the heat and stir in the lime and cilantro.

Yield: about 8 cups (1.9 L)

Per Serving: 338 Calories; 19g Fat (47% calories from fat); 7g Protein; 41g Carbohydrate; 6.2g Dietary Fiber; 1.7mg Cholesterol; 1493mg Sodium

FROM CHEF JEANNETTE:

To save time, you can purchase butternut squash prepeeled and even precut.

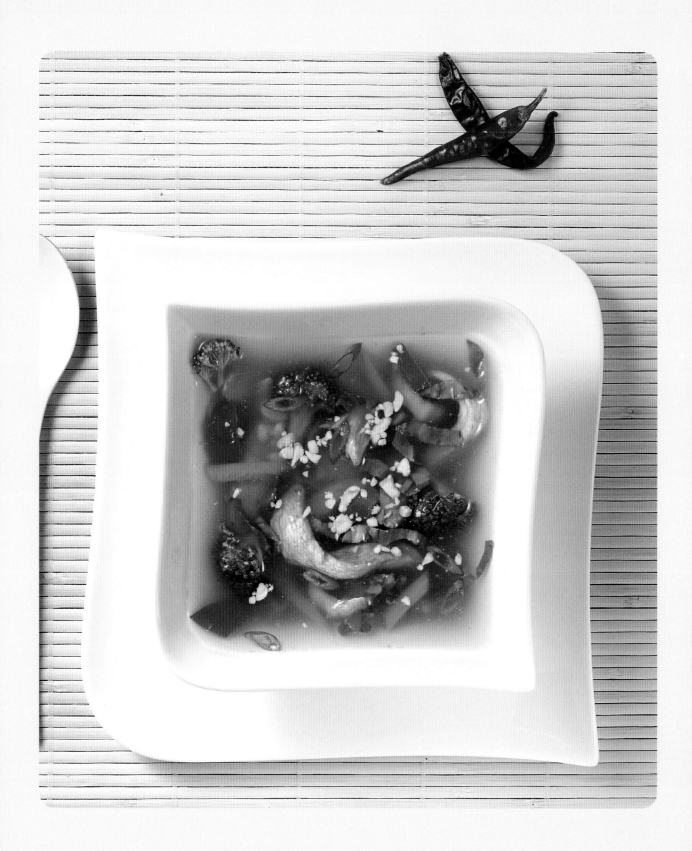

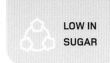

IMMUNE BOON KUNG PAO CHICKEN SOUP

From Dr. Jonny: If you've ever ordered kung pao chicken from the average Chinese takeout, I have some bad news for you. It's one of the highest-calorie take-out dishes around—with the average serving weighing in at more than 1,000 calories without the rice, noodles, or side dishes—and the ingredients are, shall we say, not designed to extend your life. Cheap oils, factory-farmed chicken, a ton of sugar in the sauce. As my grandmother used to say, "Don't ask!" Grandma also touted chicken soup for every ailment, and recent research indicates that she was right! Here's a way to get your kung pao fix in a spicy chicken soup that will warm you right up. Garlic boosts immunity, as do the sulfur compounds in onions, the vitamin A in carrots, and of course the myriad nutrients in the broccoli, especially cancer-fighting indoles. Together these make this satisfying Asian soup a boon for your immune system.

2 boneless, skinless chicken breasts, sliced (about ½ inch, or 1 cm, wide x 2 inches, or 5 cm, long)

2 tablespoons (28 ml) dry sherry or sake, plus 2 tablespoons (28 ml) dry sherry or mirin

2 tablespoons (28 ml) plus 1 teaspoon tamari, divided

2 tablespoons (28 ml) peanut oil

3 cloves garlic, minced

1 red bell pepper, seeded and chopped

2½ cups (178 g) small broccoli florets (¾ inch, or 2 cm; about 2 crowns)

½ cup (65 g) julienne-cut carrots (or thick-grated)

1 tablespoon (6 g) minced ginger

½ cup (50 g) sliced scallions

3 or 4 whole dried red chiles, or to taste*

4 cups (950 ml) chicken broth

2 tablespoons (28 ml) unseasoned rice vinegar (or white wine vinegar), divided

2 teaspoons Sucanat

4 heads baby bok choy, coarsely chopped**

½ cup (75 g) roasted peanuts, crushed

Place the chicken breasts in a shallow glass container or a zip-closure plastic storage bag.

In a small bowl, whisk together the 2 tablespoons (28 ml) sherry or sake and 1 teaspoon tamari and pour over the sliced chicken, mixing to coat. Marinate the chicken for about 20 minutes.

In a large soup pot, heat the oil over medium. Stirring continuously to prevent sticking, add the garlic and sauté 1 minute. Add the bell pepper and sauté 1 minute.

Add the broccoli and sauté 1 minute.*** Add the carrots and sauté 1 minute. Add the ginger, scallions, and chiles and sauté 1 minute. Pour the broth over all and stir in the remaining tamari and sherry, 1 tablespoon (15 ml) vinegar, and the Sucanat. Increase the heat and bring to a simmer. Lower the heat and simmer, covered, for about 10 minutes. Drain the chicken and add to the soup, continuing to simmer for about 5 minutes or until the chicken is almost cooked. Stir in the bok choy and simmer for about 3 more minutes or until wilted and chicken is cooked through (no pink but still juicy). Stir in the second tablespoon (15 ml) of vinegar and serve with peanuts sprinkled on top.

Yield: about 6 servings

Per Serving: 305 Calories; 13g Fat (39.7% calories from fat); 27g Protein; 16g Carbohydrate; 3g Dietary Fiber; 45mg Cholesterol; 829mg Sodium

* Substitute ½ to ¾ teaspoon red pepper flakes or to taste.

** Substitute chopped mature bok choy. The greens will cook very quickly, but the white ribs will need a full 3 to 4 minutes in the soup to soften.

*** The broccoli cooks for so long that it becomes a little grayish in color. The flavor is great, but if you'd like a prettier visual presentation and crispier broccoli, make your florets a little larger, remove the broccoli after stir-frying, and set aside. Then just add it to the soup a minute or so before adding the bok choy.

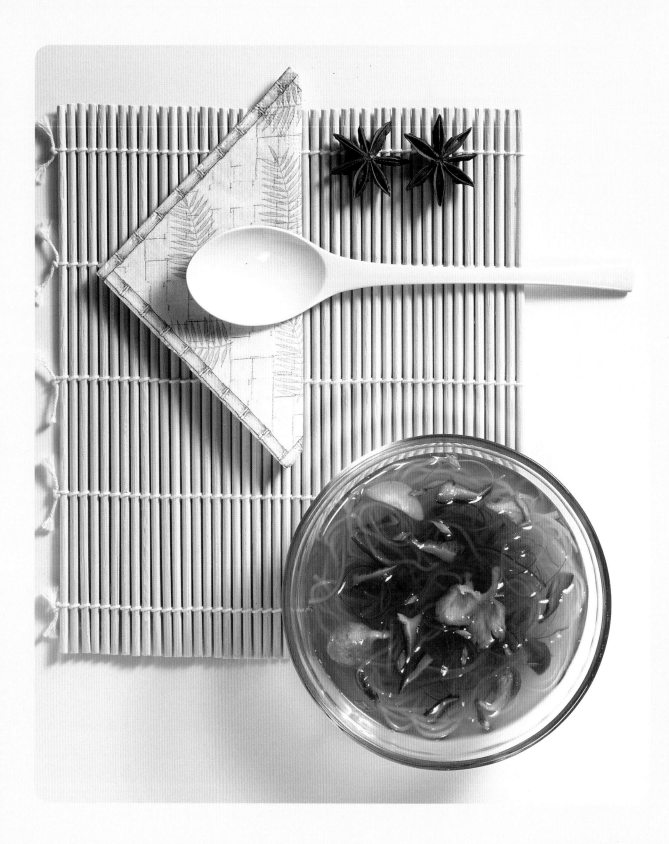

FEEL-GOOD CHINESE MUSHROOM STEW

From Dr. Jonny: Medicinal mushrooms have been used in folk medicine for thousands of years, and the ability of some mushrooms to inhibit tumor growth and enhance aspects of the immune system have been a subject of research for approximately 50 years. Chef Jeannette used an interesting trilogy of mushrooms for this light and healing stew, all of which have individual selling points. Flavor-rich black mushrooms contain polysaccharides, which are thought to boost the immune system. Shitake mushrooms are a great source of beta glucans, which elicit a strong immune response from cells, including T-cells, says Robert Rountree, M.D., author of *Immunotics.* "No one knows precisely why immune cells respond to beta glucans, but some scientists think that beta glucans 'trick' immune cells into thinking they are under attack." The third mushroom—the regular, plain-old button oyster mushroom known as cremini—is a decent source of zinc, one of the most important nutrients for the immune system.

1 ounce (28 g) dried black mushrooms

2 cups (475 ml) water

2 cups (475 ml) vegetable broth, plus more if necessary

½ cup (120 ml) rice wine (or sake or dry sherry)

1½ (25 ml) tablespoons tamari

2 star anise pods

1 cup (70 g) sliced fresh oyster mushrooms

1 cup (70 g) sliced and stemmed fresh shitake mushrooms

½ cup (58 g) shredded daikon radish, optional

¾ cup (120 g) sliced green onions

2 tablespoons (20 g) shredded wakame

4 ounces (115 g) clear bean threads (also called cellophane or glass noodles)

1 tablespoon (15 ml) mirin

1 tablespoon (15 ml) water

1 tablespoon (8 g) kudzu

1 tablespoon (15 ml) unseasoned rice vinegar

Soak the black mushrooms in 2 cups (475 ml) of hot water for 20 to 30 minutes or until plump and tender.

Remove stems and slice the mushrooms, reserving the soak water. Carefully pour the soak water into a large soup pot, leaving any sandy sediment behind. Add the sliced black mushrooms, vegetable broth, rice wine, star anise, oyster mushrooms, shitake mushrooms, and daikon, if using. Mix gently and bring to a boil over high heat. Lower the heat and simmer, covered, for about 25 minutes until all mushrooms are tender, adding more broth if level gets too low.

Toward the end of cook time, prepare the bean threads according to the package directions, usually soaking in boiling water for 5 minutes, then draining and rinsing.

Stir in wakame and prepared bean threads.

Immediately mix the mirin, water, and kudzu in a small cup until kudzu is dissolved, stir into the stew, and simmer for a minute or two until slightly thickened. Remove the star anise, stir in the rice vinegar, and serve.

Yield: 4–6 servings

Per Serving: 223 Calories; 2g Fat (8.7% calories from fat); 8g Protein; 41g Carbohydrate; 5g Dietary Fiber; 1mg Cholesterol; 1222mg Sodium

FROM CHEF JEANNETTE:

For a deeper flavor, use oyster sauce in place of the wine, 1–2 tablespoons (15–30 ml) or to taste.

You need the dried mushrooms to help make the broth, but you can use any combination of fresh mushrooms you like for this soup, including all one type.

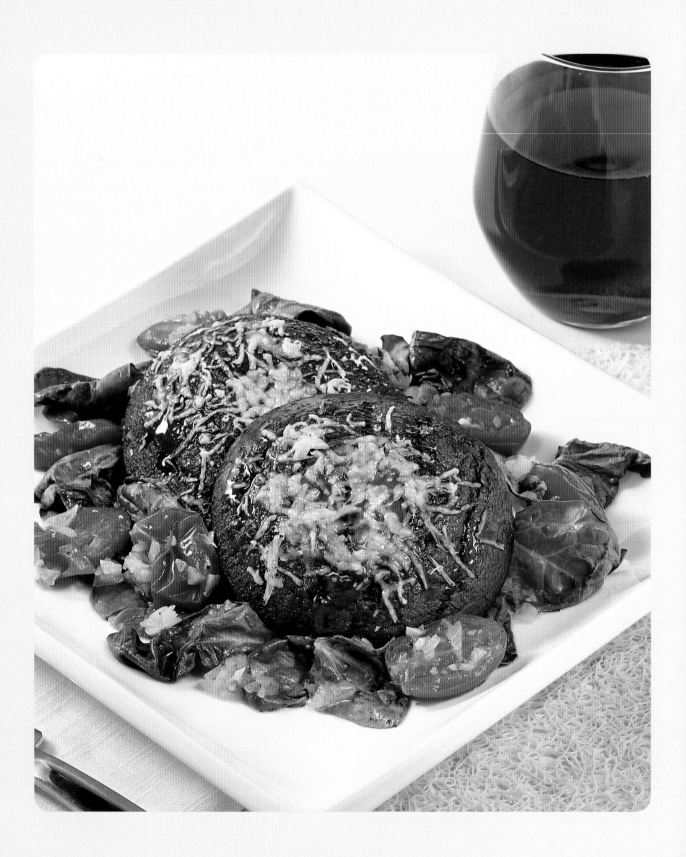

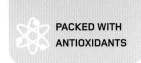

PACKED WITH ANTIOXIDANTS

POWERHOUSE PORTOBELLOS WITH MANCHEGO CHEESE OVER WILTED SPINACH

From Dr. Jonny: Mushrooms have long been known to enhance the immune system. Though the most famous of the "immunity mushrooms" are reishi, shiitake, and maitake, the fact is that mushrooms of all shapes and size—including the delicious portobello—are great for the immune system. Portobellos are surprisingly high in fiber and protein and loaded with immune-boosting niacin. They're basically white button mushrooms on steroids and they teem with antioxidants and polysaccharides, nutrients that seem to have anticancer properties. With even more nutrients from the spinach and tomatoes, this recipe offers a great combination of immune boosters.

¾ cup (175 ml) white wine

3 tablespoons (45 ml) white wine vinegar

1½ tablespoons (25 ml) olive oil

4 cloves garlic, minced

1 teaspoon dried thyme

4 large portobello caps, cleaned and stemmed*

⅓ cup (40 g) grated Manchego cheese

In a small bowl, whisk together the wine, vinegar, olive oil, garlic, and thyme. Place the mushroom caps upside down in an 8 x 8-inch (20 x 20-cm) baking dish or an 8-inch (20-cm) cake pan and carefully pour the marinade over them to coat. Let the mushrooms marinate for 20 minutes.

While the mushrooms are marinating, prepare the spinach and dressing.

Preheat the grill to medium or broiler to high if cooking indoors.

Once marinated, grill the mushrooms for 10 to 12 minutes until tender, turning once or twice for even cooking; or place the mushrooms on an ungreased broiler pan 6 inches (15 cm) below the heating element and cook for 2 to 3 minutes per side, watching carefully to prevent burning.

Sprinkle cheese evenly over gill side of mushrooms and return to grill or broiler for 30 to 60 seconds or until cheese is melted.

(continued on next page)

* To clean a portobello mushroom, gently wipe any dirt away with a soft cloth or brush. Do not rinse in water, as water makes mushrooms a little slimy. To remove any remaining stem, you can slice it cleanly off at the base with a sharp knife or grasp the stem at its base with your fingers and twist the cap with your other hand until it separates.

FROM CHEF JEANNETTE:

Manchego cheese is a creamy sheep's cheese—the molecules are smaller than those in cow cheese, and many people digest it better. It's made from pasteurized milk and has a rich, creamy texture with a flavor somewhat similar to feta. There are three types: fresco (fresh), curado (about 3 months old), and viejo (aged more than 3 months). You can find it in most large grocery stores.

187

WILTED SPINACH WITH WARM TOMATO VINAIGRETTE:

6 cups (180 g) baby spinach, washed and trimmed

2 tablespoons (28 ml) olive oil

2 shallots, minced

1 clove garlic, minced

2 cups (300 g) cherry tomatoes, halved, divided

1 cup (235 ml) dry white wine

Pinch Sucanat

½ teaspoon salt

½ teaspoon cracked black pepper

2 tablespoons (28 ml) high-quality white wine vinegar

Arrange the spinach into a bed in a large salad bowl.

In a large saucepan heat the oil over medium. Add the shallots and sauté for 3 minutes. Add the garlic and sauté for 1 minute. Add 1 cup (150 g) of the tomatoes and the wine, Sucanat, salt, and pepper, and increase heat, if necessary, to bring to a low simmer.

Simmer for 10 minutes or until most of the wine is cooked off and the tomatoes have mostly broken down.

Stir in the remaining tomatoes and the vinegar, tossing to combine, and heat for 1 to 2 minutes until warmed throughout. Cover to keep warm until portobellos are ready.

Spoon warm vinaigrette over the spinach to wilt and place the cooked mushrooms in the spinach.

Serve immediately.

Yield: 4 servings

Per Serving (excluding unknown items): 296 Calories; 17g Fat (60.6% calories from fat); 8g Protein; 16g Carbohydrate; 4g Dietary Fiber; 11mg Cholesterol; 321mg Sodium. Exchanges: 0 Grain(Starch); 3 Vegetable; 2½ Fat; 0 Other Carbohydrates

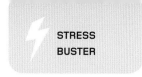

ZINC-C FEST: SAVORY SUCCOTASH WITH GROUND BEEF

From Dr. Jonny: When it comes to building immunity, most people think of vitamin C. What we often forget is that the real engine of the immune system is zinc. And the best source of zinc is beef (as well as certain seafood). This savory dish is loaded with zinc from the (hopefully grass-fed) beef, as well as being loaded with our old standby, vitamin C courtesy of the lima beans, spinach, and corn. Speaking of lima beans, they have one of the greatest all-around nutritional résumés on the planet—9 grams of fiber, 12 grams of protein, and even some vitamin A, a great immune system booster. You'll also get beta-carotene—a vitamin-A precursor—from the carrots, bell peppers, and parsley. Vitamin A helps regulate the immune system and also helps *lymphocytes*, a type of white blood cell, fight infections more effectively. Succotash is often a simple side dish, but this hearty version makes a "meaty" one-pot meal!

1 cup (250 g) dried baby lima beans, soaked*

1 bay leaf

½ teaspoon dried thyme

1¾ teaspoon salt, divided

1 tablespoon (15 ml) plus 2 teaspoons (10 ml) olive oil, divided

3 shallots, diced

2 cloves garlic, minced

1 pound (455 g) leanest ground beef (96 percent)

½ teaspoon cracked black pepper

1 tablespoon (15 ml) olive oil

1 red bell pepper, diced fine

¾ cup (83 g) finely grated carrots

1 can (14.5 ounces or 413 g) diced tomatoes, undrained

1 ½ cups (195 g) frozen corn, thawed

2 packed cups (60 g) baby spinach

¼ cup (15 g) parsley, chopped

¾ teaspoon lemon zest

1 or 2 squeezes fresh lime juice, optional

* To save time, you can also use thawed frozen lima beans instead of cooking dried beans from scratch. Because most vegetables are flash-frozen very soon after being picked, they retain a high nutrient content, nearly as high as fresh versions, and significantly more than canned or jarred versions.

Drain and rinse the soaked beans and cover generously with water in a soup pot. Add the bay leaf and thyme and bring to a boil over high heat. Reduce the heat and simmer, covered, for 30 to 45 minutes until beans are just tender. Add ¾ teaspoon salt for the last 5 minutes of cooking time. Drain, discard the bay leaf, and set aside.

Heat 2 teaspoons of oil in a large skillet over medium heat. Add the shallots and sauté for 2 to 4 minutes until translucent. Add the garlic and sauté 1 minute. Add the ground beef, ½ teaspoon salt, and pepper and cook, stirring occasionally, until browned completely, about 8 to 10 minutes. Drain and set aside.

While the beef is browning, heat remaining tablespoon (15 ml) olive oil in a soup pot or Dutch oven over medium heat. Add the bell pepper and sauté for 5 minutes. Add the carrots and sauté for 2 to 3 minutes. Stir in the lima beans, browned beef, tomatoes, corn, and remaining ½ teaspoon salt, stirring gently to combine. Simmer for 5 to 7 minutes until the veggies are tender and everything is heated through, adding a little vegetable broth if too dry. Stir in the spinach and cook for 1 minute or until lightly wilted. Stir in the parsley, zest, and lime juice, if using, just before serving.

Yield: 4 to 6 servings

Per Serving: 441 Calories; 20g Fat (39.7% calories from fat); 26g Protein; 42g Carbohydrate; 11g Dietary Fiber; 52mg Cholesterol; 702mg Sodium

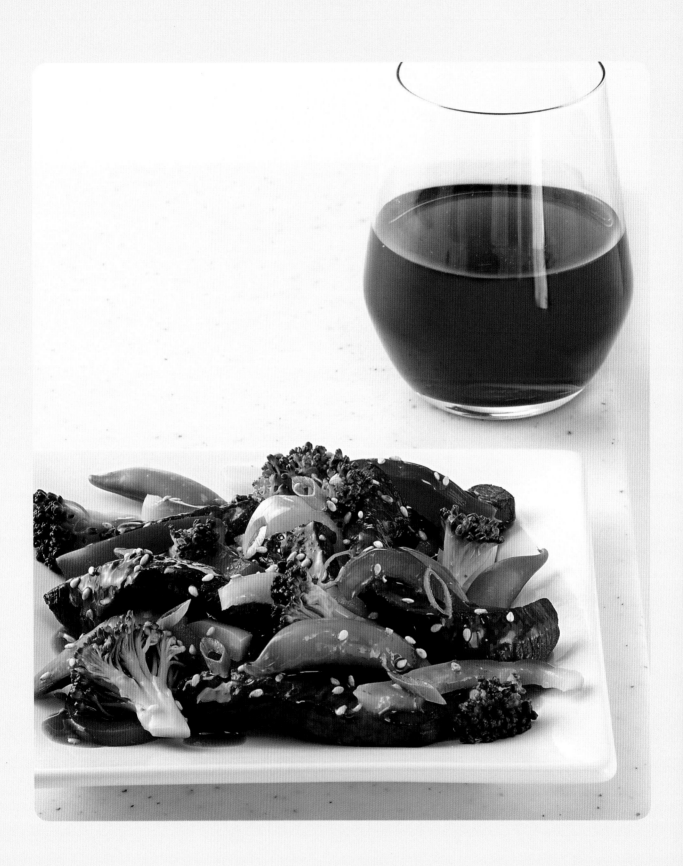

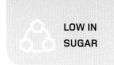

LEAN AND MEAN BEEF AND VEGGIE STIR-FRY

From Dr. Jonny: Vitamins, minerals, antioxidants, phytochemicals, proteins—they all contribute to the efficient machinery we call the immune system, and this recipe delivers a high-octane tankful of them. Protein from the steak balances nicely with the alkalizing vegetables. The vegetables, in turn, are loaded with an array of vitamins and minerals that power the immune system engine in more ways than we can count. And the steak is a great source of iron and B_{12}, both of which are needed to make you feel your best!

STEAK MARINADE

Juice of 1 orange

2 tablespoons (28 ml) tamari

1 clove garlic, minced

1 pound (455 g) boneless top sirloin or flank steak, fat trimmed and cut into ¼ inch (0.5 cm)–thick slices, 2 to 3 inches (5 to 7.5 cm) long

SAUCE

⅓ cup (80 ml) chicken or vegetable broth

3 tablespoons (45 ml) oyster sauce

1 tablespoon (15 ml) sherry (or sake, if you have it)

1 teaspoon tamari

2 teaspoons (14 g) honey

1 teaspoon toasted sesame oil

1 teaspoon orange zest

1 teaspoon kudzu

2 teaspoons broth or water

STIR-FRY

2 teaspoons high-heat (refined) sesame or peanut oil, divided, plus a few extra drops

2 cups (142 g) bite-size broccoli florets

1 large red or yellow bell pepper, seeded and julienned

1 cup (75 g) snow or sugar snap peas, trimmed, strings removed

5 cloves garlic, minced

2 tablespoons (12 g) minced ginger

⅓ cup (33 g) sliced scallions

2 tablespoons (16 g) toasted sesame seeds, optional

Pour juice and tamari into a gallon-size zip-closure bag, add garlic, and mix with your hands. Add steak strips and move around to coat with the marinade. Refrigerate for 15 minutes to overnight. Drain marinade and set beef aside.

To make the sauce: In a small bowl, whisk together the vegetable broth, oyster sauce, sherry, tamari, honey, sesame oil, and zest, and set aside.

Place the dry kudzu into a small cup and set aside.

For stir-fry: In a large skillet, heat 1 teaspoon of the oil over medium-high heat for 1 minute. Add steak strips and sauté, turning frequently, for 3 to 5 minutes or until cooked to desired doneness. Remove steak with tongs and set aside. Add remaining teaspoon of oil to pan and add broccoli and bell pepper, sautéing for about 2 minutes. Add peas and sauté for 2 to 3 more minutes or until vegetables are cooked to desired doneness. Remove veggies from pan and set aside with steak.

Pour a few drops of oil into the pan and add garlic, ginger, and scallions, and sauté for 1 minute. Pour sauce into pan—it will come to a quick simmer. Immediately add 2 teaspoons broth to kudzu in cup and mix to dissolve. Pour kudzu mixture into sauce and stir for about 20 seconds or until slightly thickened. Add meat and veggies back to the pan and stir to coat with sauce and rewarm, about 1 minute.

Sprinkle with sesame seeds before serving.

Yield: 4 servings

Per Serving: 358 Calories; 20g Fat (51.4% calories from fat); 25g Protein; 19g Carbohydrate; 4g Dietary Fiber; 71mg Cholesterol; 353mg Sodium

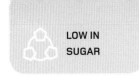
STRENGTHENING SHRIMP, SOBA NOODLE, AND ROASTED SHIITAKE SALAD

From Dr. Jonny: When holistic health practitioners think "food for immunity," they almost always think of mushrooms. Mushrooms are a great source of *beta-glucans*, special sugar molecules that elicit a strong immune response. Keith Martin, Ph.D., of Arizona State University calls mushrooms "powerhouses for boosting the immune system." Robert Rountree, M.D., author of *Immunotics*, says shiitakes work best for people at high risk for colds and the flu. They also taste terrific. Mixed with fortifying protein from the shrimp, this light meal is absolutely perfect for lunch or a hot evening. If you haven't tried roasted shiitake mushrooms, you're in for a treat. They are rich and earthy with a nice smoky quality.

ROASTED SHIITAKES

1 tablespoon (15 ml) olive oil

1 tablespoon (15 ml) tamari

½ pound (225 g) shiitake mushrooms, stems removed and caps thinly sliced (about ⅓ inch or 0.7 cm)

SOBA NOODLES

½ pound (225 g) dried soba noodles (Japanese buckwheat noodles)

Dressing

½ cup (130 g) smooth natural peanut butter (unsweetened)

⅔ cup (160 ml) light coconut milk

2 cloves garlic, minced

1 tablespoon (6 g) minced ginger

2 tablespoons (40 g) honey

¼ cup (4 g) fresh cilantro

Juice of 1 lime

2 tablespoons (28 ml) tamari

½ teaspoon sambal oelek, or to taste

SALAD BASE

1 cup (110 g) grated carrots

1 red bell pepper, seeded and diced fine

1 English cucumber, diced or julienned

½ cup (8 g) cilantro, chopped

½ cup (20 g) fresh Thai basil, julienned (or regular basil if you can't find Thai)

2 cups (140 g) shredded Napa cabbage, optional

12 large peeled, deveined, cooked shrimp

Preheat the oven to 375°F (190°C, or gas mark 5).

For roasted shiitakes: In a large bowl, whisk together the olive oil and tamari. Add sliced shiitakes and toss together to coat. Spread the shiitakes out in a single layer on a parchment-lined baking sheet and roast for about 35 minutes, turning at 15 minutes, until the mushrooms have browned and are starting to crisp but are not scorched.

For soba noodles: While shiitakes are cooking, boil the soba noodles in a large pot of salted water for 8 minutes or until al dente. Drain and immediately rinse with very cold water or immerse in an ice water bath. When cool, drain well and set aside.

For the dressing: Add the peanut butter, coconut milk, garlic, ginger, honey, cilantro, lime, tamari, and sambal oelek to a food processor and blend until smooth, scraping down the sides as necessary.

To make the salad: In a large bowl, gently toss together the carrots, bell pepper, cucumber, cilantro, basil, and cabbage. Stir in the noodles and shrimp and dress to taste, gently mixing to coat. Top with shiitakes and serve.

Yield: 6 servings

Per Serving: 483 Calories; 16g Fat (26.7% calories from fat); 19g Protein; 79g Carbohydrate; 9g Dietary Fiber; 18mg Cholesterol; 569mg Sodium

FROM CHEF JEANNETTE:

This shiitake presentation comes from Myra Kornfield's genius concept (www.myrakornfield.com). I like to double the recipe and keep leftovers in the fridge to add to later salads or sandwiches or to top a cup of miso or winter squash soup. This whole recipe is, in fact, an homage to her fabulous "spring roll salad," longevity-style! Within this recipe, as with many Asian dishes, all the major flavor receptors are tweaked: salt, sour, sweet, bitter, and even pungent, generating a deep level of satisfaction that can make it easier to feel satisfied with less—a long-life bonus.

Sambal oelek is a very spicy chile paste that originated in Indonesia. Some natural and Asian markets will carry it, and you can often find it in the "ethnic" or gourmet sections of large grocery stores. If you can't find it, you can substitute ½ teaspoon of cayenne pepper.

To cook shrimp, use one of these healthy cooking methods: grill raw shrimp over medium heat on a skewer (1 to 2 minutes per side); stir-fry them over medium-high heat in a small amount of sesame oil (about 3 minutes); or poach them in simmering lemon water for 3 to 4 minutes. You can also use precooked frozen shrimp: Just thaw under cold water. This salad works with the shrimp at both hot and cold temperatures, cook's choice.

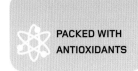

PACKED WITH ANTIOXIDANTS

POTENT POLENTA PIE WITH SUN-DRIED TOMATO PESTO AND GRILLED SUMMER VEGGIES

From Dr. Jonny: Mashed potatoes are not on anyone's list as a longevity food, no matter how hard you squint. So what to do when you want a little starch? Try this great longevity substitution: cornmeal polenta, a great alternative to any of the usual, life-shortening empty calories from rolls, white rice, or mashed potatoes. Sun-dried tomato pesto adds a healthy dose of antioxidants to fight aging cell damage, while raw garlic and calcium-rich Parmesan cheese give your immune system a nice boost. Did I mention it tastes better than potatoes, too?

POLENTA

Olive oil cooking spray

1½ tablespoons (25 ml) olive oil

1 small red onion, diced fine

2 cloves garlic, minced

3 cups (710 ml) water or vegetable broth

1 teaspoon salt

1 cup (140 g) cornmeal

FROM CHEF JEANNETTE:

Corn, from which polenta is derived, is a rich source of B vitamins, especially thiamin, pantothenic acid, and folate.

This recipe has three components, so it's not a super-quick one. To shorten prep time, use prepared polenta or prepared pesto, but take the time to grill the veggies for that fabulous summer barbecue flavor. If corn is in season, try stirring a few cobs' worth of grilled corn kernels (cut them off first!) into the polenta just before pouring into the pie plate to set.

This works as a great side dish to grilled fish or chicken or can serve as a summer entrée with a generous green salad.

Coat a 9-inch (23-cm) deep-dish pie plate with olive oil spray. Set aside.

In a large saucepan heat the oil over medium. Add the onion and sauté for 5 minutes. Add the garlic and sauté for 1 minute. Add the water, increase heat, and bring to a boil. Once the water is boiling, reduce the heat to medium, add salt, and very gradually stir in the cornmeal, whisking constantly to prevent lumps until the mixture starts to thicken.* Cook, whisking frequently, until very thick, 10 to 12 minutes, adjusting heat up or down as necessary to maintain a low simmer.

Remove from the heat and pour evenly into prepared plate. Put aside to set and prepare the pesto.

* If the mixture forms stubborn lumps, remove the pan briefly from the heat and zap the mixture with an immersion blender to break up lumps and create a smooth consistency.

SUN-DRIED TOMATO PESTO

½ cup (55 g) julienne-cut, oil-packed sun-dried
  tomatoes, drained

3 tablespoons (45 ml) olive oil, plus extra if needed

1 tablespoon (15 ml) balsamic vinegar

1 clove crushed garlic

2 tablespoons (18 g) toasted pine nuts

¼ cup (10 g) basil leaves

⅓ cup (33 g) fresh-grated Parmesan cheese, divided

¼ teaspoon salt

¼ teaspoon black pepper

In the food processor, pulse together tomatoes, olive
oil, vinegar, garlic, pine nuts, basil, ¼ cup (25 g) of
the Parmesan, salt, and black pepper until smooth,
scraping down the sides as necessary. Drizzle extra oil
a teaspoon at a time if mixture is too dry. Set aside and
grill squash.

GRILLED SUMMER VEGGIES

1 small zucchini

1 small yellow summer squash

1 red bell pepper, seeded

1 tablespoon (15 ml) olive oil

½ teaspoon salt

½ teaspoon black pepper

Preheat grill to medium.

Slice unpeeled zucchini and squash lengthwise into thin
slices (about ¼ inch, or 0.5 cm, thick). Slice bell pepper
into thin rings or strips.

In a large bowl toss veggies with oil, salt, and black
pepper to coat.

Grill veggies for 3 to 4 minutes per side or until soft and
lightly browned (squash).

Assemble the pie: Spread the pesto evenly over the
prepared polenta and arrange the vegetables on the
pesto. Sprinkle the remaining cheese over all, cut into
wedges, and serve.★★

Yield: 4 to 8 slices

Per Serving: 213 Calories; 13g Fat (54.2% calories from
fat); 5g Protein; 20g Carbohydrate; 3g Dietary Fiber;
3mg Cholesterol; 567mg Sodium

★★ Pie is great served just warm, but if you prefer it hot, pop assembled
  pie into a 375°F (190°C, or gas mark 5) oven for 10 minutes.

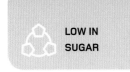

SHAKE OFF THE CHILLS WITH TOFU-CREMINI CHILI

From Dr. Jonny: It's hard to think of a more perfect combination of ingredients for the immune system than this new spin on chili, which is perfect for warming you up on a cold winter day. Mushrooms give the immune system a nice big boost when it comes to attacking foreign invaders. And interestingly enough, the plain old garden-variety white button mushrooms known as cremini have stronger immune-boosting effects than their more exotic and pricey cousins. Mushrooms, fresh vitamin-rich vegetables, and lean protein—what could be better for keeping you healthy?

2 tablespoons (28 ml) olive oil

1 large yellow onion, diced

1½ cups (105 g) cremini mushrooms, stems trimmed and sliced

6 cloves garlic, minced

1 red bell pepper, seeded and diced

1 yellow squash, diced

½ cup (55 g) grated carrot

½ cup (120 ml) dry red wine

2 cups (475 ml) vegetable or chicken broth

2 cans (14.5 ounces, or 413 g, each) fire-roasted diced tomatoes, undrained

3 tablespoons (48 g) tomato paste

1 pound (455 g) extra-firm tofu, drained well, diced

2 cans (15 ounces, or 425 g, each) white kidney beans (or red or pink), drained

1 teaspoon ground cumin

1 teaspoon dried oregano

2 tablespoons (15 g) chili powder, or to taste

½ teaspoon salt

Cracked black pepper, to taste

½ teaspoon chipotle pepper (or cayenne), or to taste

½ cup (8 g) chopped fresh cilantro

In a large sauté pan or Dutch oven, heat the oil over medium heat. Add the onion and sauté 3 minutes. Add creminis and sauté 4 minutes. Add the garlic and sauté 1 minute. Add the bell pepper, squash, carrot, and red wine and simmer, stirring gently, for about 4 minutes. Add the broth, tomatoes, tomato paste, tofu, beans, cumin, oregano, chili powder, salt, and peppers and stir gently to combine. Bring to a low simmer and cook, uncovered, for about 30 minutes or until all veggies are soft. Stir in the cilantro just before serving.

Yield: about 6 servings

Per Serving: 367 Calories; 10g Fat (25.6% calories from fat); 18g Protein; 50g Carbohydrate; 16g Dietary Fiber; 1mg Cholesterol; 1321mg Sodium

FROM CHEF JEANNETTE:

If you'd prefer to use lean meat rather than tofu, brown a pound of lean ground turkey with the onion instead—just don't forget to drain any extra liquid fats after cooking to keep your chili healthy. For extra heartiness—and fiber—throw in a half cup of rinsed quinoa when you add the broth. Squeeze a little fresh lime juice into the chili just before serving for a bright finishing note.

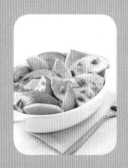

SIDE DISHES

Grandma's Good-for-You Sauerkraut
Beta-Carotene Apple–Winter Squash Bake
Feisty Fungi: Green Beans with Sautéed Cremini Mushrooms
Ayurvedic Asparagus and Tomatoes

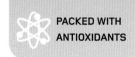

PACKED WITH ANTIOXIDANTS

GRANDMA'S GOOD-FOR-YOU SAUERKRAUT

From Dr. Jonny: So before we talk about sauerkraut, let me first tell you about cabbage and how we found out that it was so amazingly good for you. It all started when researchers noticed that women in Poland hardly ever got breast cancer. But when they moved to the United States, they suddenly started getting breast cancer at about the same frequency as their American counterparts. After digging around a bit, researchers found that the likely explanation was the amount of cabbage Polish (and eastern European) women ate when in their native lands. Further exploration revealed compounds in cabbage—in fact, in the entire brassica vegetable family—called *indoles*, which are potent modifiers of hormones that could be carcinogenic. So we know cabbage is a great food, and what happens when you take that great food and make it even better by naturally fermenting it? You get . . . (drum roll, please) . . . sauerkraut. Which is cabbage plus the wonderful probiotics (healthy bacteria) that result from the natural fermenting process. Specifically bacteria of the *Lactobacillus* genus help improve immune function, not to mention digestion and the absorption and assimilation of nutrients. The key, of course, is natural fermentation, which is very doable when you follow the directions below. The result is a fresh, delicious kraut for immune health.

BRINING WATER*

3 cups (710 ml) water

1 tablespoon (19 g) kosher salt

SAUERKRAUT

1 large green or white cabbage, outermost leaves removed, cored and quartered (about 3 pounds [1¼ kg] with core, to total 2½ pounds [1 kg] shredded)

2 tablespoons (38 g) kosher salt

2 teaspoons (4.2 g) caraway seeds, optional

Boil water for 20 seconds, remove from heat, and stir in salt to dissolve. Set aside or refrigerate to cool completely.

Sterilize a large mixing bowl (glass or enamel; avoid aluminum or other metals), fermenting crock and lid (or large glass/enamel bowl and fitted plate), and an 8- to 10-pound (3.5- to 4.5-kg) rock in the dishwasher.**

Wash your hands thoroughly before handling sterilized items and proceeding with recipe.

* If you'd like to use bagged brining water as opposed to sterile weights, prepare more at the same ratio (3 cups, or 710 ml, water to 1 tablespoon, or 19 g, kosher salt).

** To make your own fermented vegetables, which we highly recommend as a longevity and general nutritional health practice, invest in a stoneware crock that's made for the purpose. They are usually cylindrical and taller than they are wide. They are relatively inexpensive, and you can find them at hardware stores or any shop that carries canning and pickling supplies. If you just want to try it once, use a glass or ceramic bowl, but you'll need a plate that fits very snugly just inside the bowl's edges and a towel to cover it to keep it from light exposure.

FROM CHEF JEANNETTE:

If you have a large crock or wish to make more at one time, just maintain the ratio of 2 ½ pounds (1 kg) shredded cabbage to 2 tablespoons (38 g) kosher salt.

Slice the cabbage quarters finely, widthwise, to get thin strips, approximately ¼ inch (0.5 cm) wide by 2 to 3 inches (5 to 7.5 cm) long. You should end up with about 7 cups (420 g). (You can use the slicing attachment on your food processor to speed this process, but make sure the strips are no thicker than ¼ inch [0.5 cm] and your processor bowls and blades have been sterilized in the dishwasher.)

Combine the cabbage and salt in a sterilized bowl and mix well until the cabbage is thoroughly coated and juice begins to form. Mix in the caraway seeds, if using, and pack the cabbage and all juices into the sterilized crock or bowl. Pour enough cooled brining water into the crock to cover the cabbage completely by ½ inch (1 cm). (If your cabbage is super-fresh, it may generate enough juice on its own from the salting to do this.) Cover snugly and weight the cover: Use a sterile lid or plate that fits just inside the edges of your container and top with your sterile weight. If you can't find a heavy rock or other weight, you can fill a new (clean) gallon-size zip-closure bag ¾ full with cooled brining water. Tightly seal another bag around the first to prevent leakage (using brine ensures that if it does leak, it won't ruin your salt ratio). Using a "water bag" will also help seal the edges of your crock to keep it airtight.

Use plastic wrap to seal the entire top and cover with a heavy dish or hand towel.

Allow the mixture to sit, undisturbed, in an area out of direct sunlight that ranges from 65°F to 70°F (18°C to 21°C; no warmer or your kraut may spoil) for 2 weeks.

Check at 10 days (if you like it less tart) or 2 weeks for flavor strength (use a sterile set of nonreactive tongs to extract enough to taste). If you want it stronger, carefully replace all coverings for another week or so (warmer temps generate faster fermentation, while cooler temps generate slower).

Once your kraut reaches desired strength, store covered but unweighted in its brine in the fridge. Serve cold or at room temperature.

Yield: about 6 cups (825 g) sauerkraut

Per Serving: 6 Calories; trace Fat (17.8% calories from fat); trace Protein; 1g Carbohydrate; 1g Dietary Fiber; 0mg Cholesterol; 2384mg Sodium

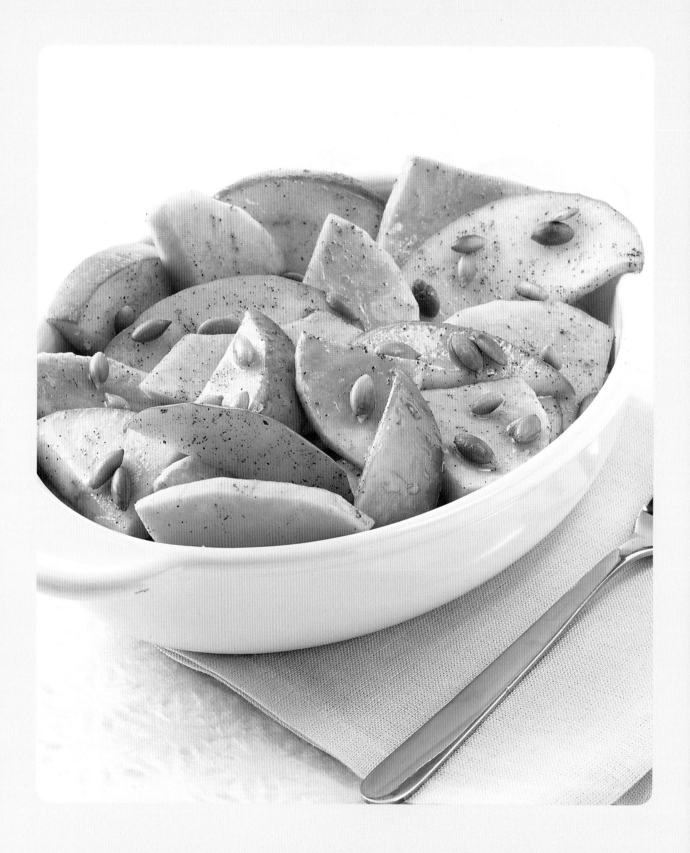

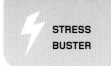

BETA-CAROTENE APPLE—WINTER SQUASH BAKE

From Dr. Jonny: "Take two portions and call me in the morning!" This delicious recipe is bound to turbocharge your immune system; the beta-carotene and vitamin A in the squash are natural immunity boosters. And apples are one of the best sources of the anti-inflammatory flavonoid *quercetin*. Fragrant and sweet, this dish works equally well as a side dish or a snack. Try it for breakfast on a cold morning!

Cooking oil spray

1½ pounds (710 g) winter squash*

½ teaspoon ground cinnamon

½ cup (120 ml) apple cider

½ cup (120 ml) orange juice

1 tablespoon (15 ml) almond oil

1 tablespoon (20 g) maple syrup

3 green apples, unpeeled, cored, and sliced thick

¼ cup (28 g) sliced almonds or pepitas (roasted pumpkin seeds, 35 g)

* Butternut squash works well.

Preheat the oven to 350°F (180°C, or gas mark 4). Coat a 9 x 13-inch (23 x 33-cm) baking dish with cooking oil spray. Set aside.

Peel, seed, and quarter the squash (if using butternut, 1½ pounds (710 g) is about 2 small squash). Slice width-wise into thin pieces, about ¼ inch (0.5 cm).

In a large bowl, whisk together the cinnamon, cider, orange juice, oil, and syrup. Add the squash and apple slices and stir gently to coat. Pour the mixture into the prepared baking dish and cover tightly with aluminum foil. Bake for about 45 minutes or until the squash is fork-soft. Sprinkle the nuts over the top and serve.

Yield: about 6 servings

Per Serving: 161 Calories; 5g Fat (27.4% calories from fat); 3g Protein; 29g Carbohydrate; 4g Dietary Fiber; 0mg Cholesterol; 6mg Sodium

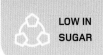

FEISTY FUNGI: GREEN BEANS WITH SAUTÉED CREMINI MUSHROOMS

From Dr. Jonny: Our friend, recipe designer Heather Short, contributed this fabulous mushroom-rich recipe, which features one of the best foods I know for the immune system—organic coconut oil. I live on this stuff and use it to stir-fry veggies and scramble eggs. Coconut oil is rich in lauric acid and caprylic acid, fatty acids that have known antimicrobial activity. Mushrooms are one of the best immune-system-boosting foods on the planet. Even though they're often overshadowed by their more exotic relatives, shiitake and reishi, creminis (ordinary button mushrooms) are also nutritious and much easier to find. The green beans contribute vitamins C and A, both great for immunity. This dish is easy to make even for a bachelor like me. A great side dish!

4 cups (400 g) green beans, washed, trimmed, and cut into 2-inch (5-cm) pieces

2 tablespoons (28 ml) organic coconut oil (such as Barlean's)

1 package (8 ounces, or 225 g) cremini mushrooms, cleaned and sliced

Salt and cracked black pepper, to taste

½ cup (70 g) toasted pepitas (pumpkin seeds)

Fill a large mixing bowl to the halfway mark with ice and water. Set aside.

Bring a large pot of salted water to a boil over high heat. Add the green beans and boil for 2 minutes until they are a bright green color. Quickly drain them and plunge them into the prepared ice water to stop the cooking. Once they are cool (about 2 minutes), drain and set aside.

In a large sauté pan over medium heat, melt the coconut oil. Add sliced creminis to the hot oil, sprinkle with salt and pepper, and sauté, turning occasionally, for about 5 minutes.* Add the green beans, mix gently, and sauté for about 3 minutes more. Top with pepitas and serve.

FROM CHEF JEANNETTE:

For variety, you may also substitute blanched broccoli florets or thin zucchini rounds for the green beans in this recipe. Try the broccoli version with toasted almond slices and the zucchini with toasted pecan pieces. If you have some on hand, you can also try adding a couple of tablespoons of port to the mix when you add the green beans for a more robust flavor.

Yield: 4 servings

Per Serving: 173 Calories; 10g Fat (48.2% calories from fat); 6g Protein; 18g Carbohydrate; 5g Dietary Fiber; 0mg Cholesterol; 12mg Sodium

* As Julia Child tells us, the secret to getting mushrooms to brown properly is not to crowd them in the pan!

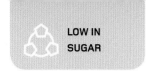

LOW IN SUGAR

AYURVEDIC ASPARAGUS AND TOMATOES

From Dr. Jonny: In Ayurvedic medicine, asparagus is believed to help develop peace of mind, a loving nature, and a calm spirit—every one of which boosts immunity through the interaction of mind and body (the science of which is called psychoneuroimmunology, but I digress). There's some science behind these traditional uses. Asparagus root contains compounds that actually affect hormone production and possibly influence emotions (which in turn strengthens immunity). But enough of the science. Asparagus tastes good, especially when baked with tomatoes to keep it moist and mellow. This simple and elegant dish, loaded with vitamins A, C, and K, is a great-tasting way to boost your immune system—the light, salty Parmesan and fresh bite of basil give it the perfect finish.

1 tablespoon (15 ml) olive oil

1 pound (455 g) asparagus, peeled and trimmed

½ stalk celery, minced

1 shallot, minced

2 heirloom tomatoes, sliced

¼ teaspoon salt

¼ teaspoon white pepper

½ teaspoon dried thyme

½ cup (20 g) fresh basil

¼ cup (25 g) freshly shaved Parmesan cheese

Preheat the oven to 350°F (180°C, or gas mark 4).

Spread oil around bottom of a small baking pan (7 x 11 inches, or 18 x 28 cm). Lay the asparagus in the pan and spread the celery and shallot over all. Lay the tomato slices over the asparagus and sprinkle with salt, pepper, and thyme. Snip the basil into strips with scissors or cut chiffonade style and sprinkle over the seasoned tomatoes. Top with Parmesan and bake for 30 minutes or until asparagus is fork-tender.

Yield: 4 servings

Per Serving: 95 Calories; 6g Fat (51.4% calories from fat); 5g Protein; 7g Carbohydrate; 2g Dietary Fiber; 5mg Cholesterol; 258mg Sodium

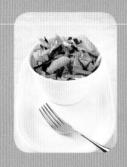

SALADS

· ·

Chopped Antioxidant–Rich Artichoke–Tomato Salad
Grated Beta–Carotene Salad

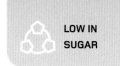
CHOPPED ANTIOXIDANT-RICH ARTICHOKE-TOMATO SALAD

From Dr. Jonny: The mix of artichokes and tomatoes makes this an unusually delightful salad you won't find in restaurants. It's absolutely loaded with antioxidants plus a few extras such as balsamic vinegar (which helps with your blood sugar), flaxseed oil (immune-boosting lignans and omega-3s), lycopene-rich tomatoes, and sulfur-rich onions. Beauty! The garlic and lemon juice give it a tangy overtone. This fresh-tasting salad, adapted from the wonderful Heather Short, feels like you should be eating it at an outdoor café in Italy!

6 cups (330 g) mixed Italian salad greens (romaine, spinach, radicchio, endive, etc.), chopped

2 large Roma tomatoes, chopped

1 can (14 ounces, or 400 g) artichoke hearts, rinsed, drained, and chopped

1 medium red bell pepper, chopped

1 medium yellow bell pepper, chopped

1 medium red onion, chopped

2 teaspoons (3 g) capers

¼ cup (10 g) chopped fresh basil

1 tablespoon (15 ml) balsamic vinegar

2 teaspoons (10 ml) fresh-squeezed lemon juice

2 tablespoons (28 ml) flaxseed oil (such as Barlean's)

1 garlic clove, minced

1 teaspoon dried oregano

Pinch salt

Fresh-ground black pepper to taste

In a large salad bowl, make a bed of the chopped salad greens.

In another large bowl, add the tomatoes, artichoke hearts, bell peppers, onion, capers, and basil, and toss together gently to combine. In a small bowl, whisk together the vinegar, lemon juice, flaxseed oil, garlic, oregano, and salt. Pour over veggies and toss gently to combine. Spoon veggies over chopped salad and grind pepper over all, to taste.

Yield: 4 servings

Per Serving: 175 Calories; 8g Fat (35.9% calories from fat); 6g Protein; 25g Carbohydrate; 9g Dietary Fiber; 0mg Cholesterol; 157mg Sodium

FROM CHEF JEANNETTE:

Heather's original concept was to use this as a bruschetta topping on a grilled baguette. We converted it to a longevity salad to avoid the extra starch, but it sure is tasty that way! Another thought if you'd like to keep the bruschetta feel with fewer carbs, is to make a small amount of grilled whole-grain bread "croutons" and toss them over the top. To make a simple crouton, preheat the broiler and cut the top and sides off of a slightly stale whole-wheat or sourdough peasant loaf. Tear the crusts into strips, rub them with a crushed garlic clove, and brush them lightly all over with olive oil. Lay the strips onto a broiler rack or baking sheet and broil very briefly (might take only a minute) to toast and make them crispy (remove any blackened edges before serving). Top the salad with as many as you'd like and serve immediately.

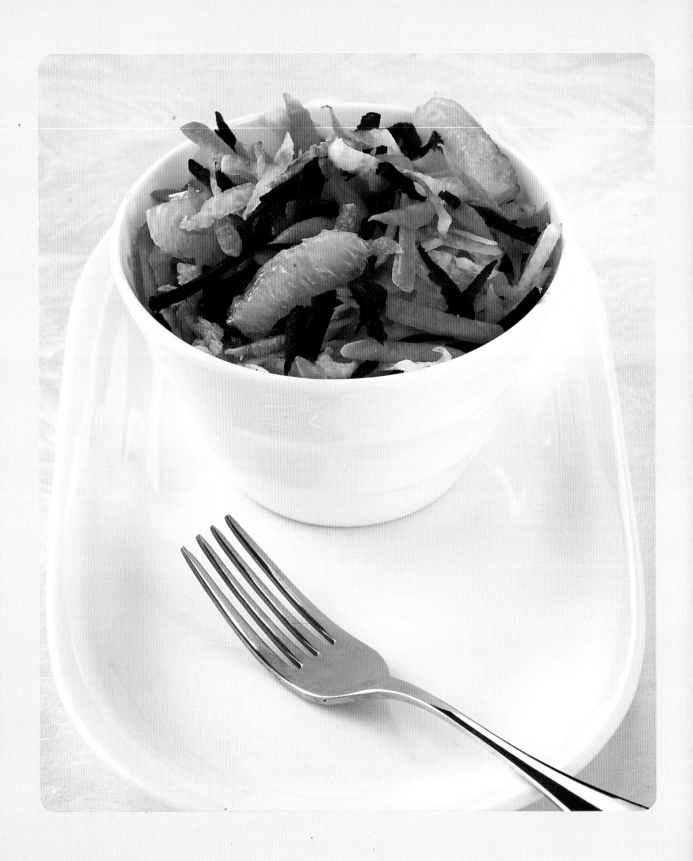

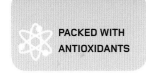

PACKED WITH ANTIOXIDANTS

GRATED BETA-CAROTENE SALAD

From Dr. Jonny: Forget potato salad for a minute—it's so yesterday. Jicama will make you forget you ever loved it. Juicy, crunchy, and lightly sweet, it's kind of a cross between a really good apple and a white potato, with a tan skin the color of a baked potato. The orange color of the carrots and orange is a reminder that this salad is loaded with beta-carotene and vitamin A, both known immune system boosters. "Regular" potato salad can't hold a candle to this zippy, nutritious, and low-calorie dish, which functions equally well as a light summer lunch or a side salad for a hearty dinner. Hint: It's especially good with the optional nuts.

2 cups (220 g) peeled and grated carrots
(about 3 large)

1 cup (225 g) peeled and grated fresh beet
(about 1 medium or 2 small)*

1 cup (130 g) peeled and grated jicama
(part of 1 small jicama)**

2 fresh oranges, peeled, segmented, and segments
cut into bite-size pieces

2 tablespoons (28 ml) fresh-squeezed orange juice

1 tablespoon (15 ml) fresh-squeezed lemon juice

½ teaspoon lemon zest

2 teaspoons (14 g) raw honey

Pinch salt

In a large bowl, gently toss together grated carrots, beet, jicama, and oranges to combine.

In a small bowl, whisk together the orange juice, lemon juice, zest, honey, and salt.

Dress salad to taste. The longer it rests, the deeper the flavors will be. Toss gently just before serving. Garnish salad with toasted nuts or seeds, if desired.

Yield: 4 servings

Per Serving: 97 Calories; trace Fat (2.3% calories from fat); 2g Protein; 23g Carbohydrate; 6g Dietary Fiber; 0mg Cholesterol; 85mg Sodium

* Look for young, fresh beets with smooth skin. Young beets are juicy, and the juice stains everything. It will even color your other salad ingredients pink, so be prepared!

** If you can't find jicama, substitute an equal amount of peeled grated firm, crisp apple.

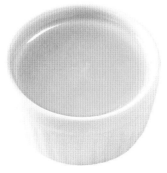

FROM CHEF JEANNETTE:

If you'd prefer a savory salad, omit the orange and dress with 1½ tablespoons (25 ml) almond oil, 1½ tablespoons (25 ml) apple cider vinegar, 1 small clove minced garlic, a teaspoon of Dijon mustard, a pinch of chipotle or cayenne pepper, and salt to taste.

You can use a hand grater for everything or, for speed, use the grater attachment on a food processor.

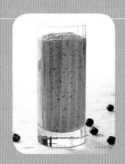

BREAKFASTS

. . . .

Right Start Apricot–Prune–Walnut Breakfast Bread
A.M. Antioxidant Smoothie

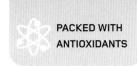

PACKED WITH ANTIOXIDANTS

RIGHT START APRICOT-PRUNE-WALNUT BREAKFAST BREAD

From Dr. Jonny: Potassium is the third most abundant mineral in the body. It's almost impossible to keep your immune system healthy without an adequate supply of this mineral, and most of us don't get nearly enough. (In 2004, the Institute of Medicine set the adequate intake of potassium at 4,700 mg a day for any adult over 19 years old. More than 90 percent of Americans don't meet this recommendation.) This rich, dark brown bread bursts with potassium, which helps neutralize the body acids that can cripple the immune system. And blackstrap molasses, long one of my favorite foods, is a great source of iron. "We need iron for strength and vigor," says the Penn State University Online Research website, adding that iron plays a key role in DNA and enzyme synthesis and other basic life processes. And, apple cider vinegar is a wonderfully alkalizing food that helps further balance an overly acidic body. Soy milk and cider vinegar replace fat-laden buttermilk with the same overall effect: a dense, satisfying, high-fiber bread that's a great way to start the day.

Cooking oil spray

¾ packed cup (131 g) prunes

¼ cup (33 g) dried apricots

1 tablespoon (15 ml) apple cider vinegar

1 cup (235 ml) unsweetened plain soy milk

1¾ cups (210 g) whole-wheat pastry flour

2 tablespoons (13 g) ground flaxseed

¼ cup (35 g) cornmeal

1 teaspoon baking powder

½ teaspoon baking soda

½ teaspoon ground cinnamon

½ teaspoon salt

¼ cup (60 g) xylitol

½ cup (60 g) walnuts, chopped (or ½ cup [55 g] sliced almonds)

¼ cup (85 g) blackstrap molasses

Preheat the oven to 350°F (180°C, or gas mark 4).

Coat a standard loaf pan with cooking oil spray.

Combine the prunes and apricots in a small bowl and cover with warm water. Set aside to soak for 10 minutes while you prepare the other ingredients.

Pour the cider vinegar into the soy milk, stir gently, and set aside.

In a large bowl, combine the flour, flaxseed, cornmeal, baking powder, baking soda, cinnamon, salt, xylitol, and walnuts and whisk gently to mix.

Drain the prunes and apricots and combine them in a food processor or strong blender with the soy milk mixture and molasses. Process until nearly smooth, scraping down the sides as necessary, about 1 minute off and on. Pour the wet mixture into the dry and mix until just combined. Pour into the prepared loaf pan and bake for 55 minutes to 1 hour or until a knife comes out clean and top is dry and lightly browned. Let the bread rest for 5 minutes and turn out to cool completely on a rack.

Yield: 1 loaf

Per Serving: 148 Calories; 2g Fat (12% calories from fat); 4.8g Protein; 32g Carbohydrate; 4.6g Dietary Fiber; 0mg Cholesterol; 269mg Sodium

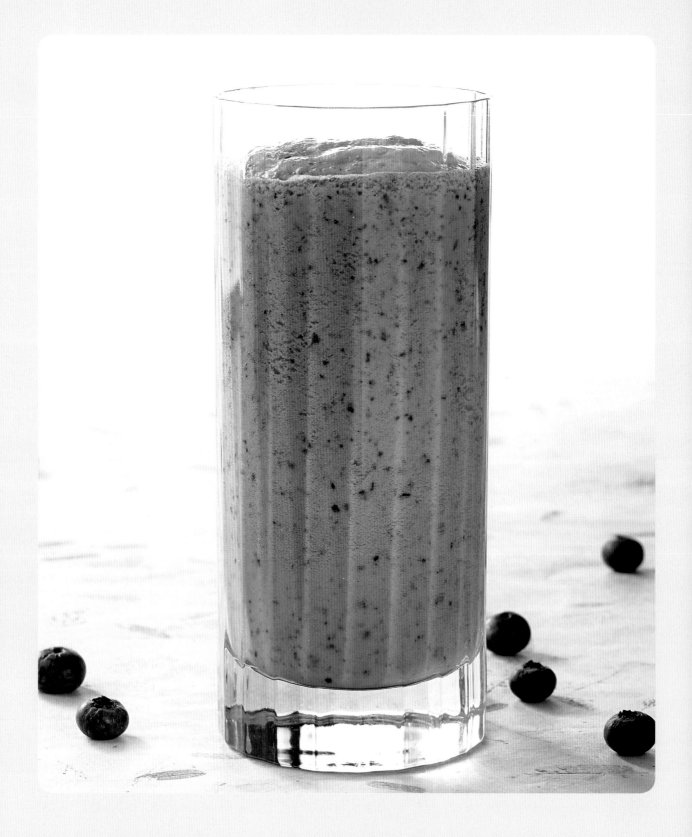

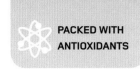

**PACKED WITH
ANTIOXIDANTS**

A.M. ANTIOXIDANT SMOOTHIE

From Dr. Jonny: Flu, shmu! Start drinking smoothies like this and your immune system will be so strong everyone in the office will wonder how come you never get sick! You'd have to take two handfuls of vitamin supplements to get all the antioxidants and phytochemicals in this delicious smoothie! Açai berries make everyone's list of top superfoods; pomegranate juice has been found in research to be helpful for blood pressure, atherosclerosis, prostate health, diabetes, and even erectile function. But wait, there's more! In addition to these antioxidant-loaded fruits, you've got whey protein! It's an unbeatable combination. The açai berry's intense earthy (and somewhat tart) taste is beautifully balanced by the sweetness of the frozen banana. This drink's one of my faves!

2 cups (475 ml) almond milk (or cow's, hemp, soy, etc.)

2 scoops vanilla whey powder (or other protein powder)

½ cup (120 ml) 100 percent açai juice, unsweetened (we like the Sambazon Açai frozen organic smoothie packs)

½ cup (120 ml) 100 percent pomegranate juice, unsweetened

1 cup (155 g) frozen blueberries

1 frozen or fresh banana, peeled and halved

Blend all ingredients together in blender until smooth.

Yield: 2 large or 4 small servings

Per Serving: 339 Calories; 6g Fat (13.9% calories from fat); 33g Protein; 44g Carbohydrate; 7g Dietary Fiber; 3mg Cholesterol; 206mg Sodium

FROM CHEF JEANNETTE:

Feel free to play with this base mix: Add more banana if you like your smoothies creamier and sweeter; add some plain yogurt for a dose of acidophilus and a bit more protein; add ice cubes to make it slushier, or more milk to make it more liquid; or add a tablespoon (15 ml) of flaxseed oil to keep everything moving.

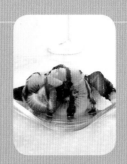

SNACKS and DESSERTS

··

Immune-Strengthening Shiitake Broth
Chocolate–Vitamin C Fruit Salad
Mighty Melon–Berry Madness
Longevity Fruit Gels—Not Just Jell-O
Smooth Move Comforting Fruit Compote

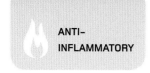

ANTI-INFLAMMATORY

IMMUNE-STRENGTHENING SHIITAKE BROTH

From Dr. Jonny: If you feel a cold coming on, grab some of this soup immediately. (Even if you don't, it'll give your immune system a shot in the arm!) Shiitake mushrooms are one of the most potent stimulators of immunity in the mushroom kingdom. According to the American Cancer Society, studies in animals have found antitumor, cholesterol-lowering, and virus-inhibiting effects in compounds in shiitake mushrooms. Of course, that doesn't guarantee that the same effects will be found in people, but mushrooms have been a traditional healing food for thousands of years, and I'm of the opinion that if something's been used that long as a remedy, there's usually a good reason. Mushrooms aren't the only immune system booster in this light, Asian-flavored broth. Seaweed (wakame) and collard greens are also loaded with antioxidants and phytochemicals that help the immune system work better. This is a light, cleansing, and uplifting macrobiotic broth and is the perfect thing if you're feeling under the weather. It's also ideal when you're feeling over the weather, too!

---

8 dried shiitake mushrooms (we like the donko variety)

3 pieces (2 inches, or 5 cm, each) wakame, rinsed, optional

1 cup (70 g) shredded collard greens

1 cup (116 g) grated daikon

1 cup (110 g) grated carrot

1 small pickled umeboshi plum, diced fine (or 1 teaspoon paste, or 1½ teaspoons ume plum vinegar)

1 teaspoon Bragg Liquid Aminos (or tamari), or to taste

Soak the dried mushrooms for 6 to 12 hours, covered, in 7 cups (1.7 L) of water.* After soaking, keep the soaking water, remove and discard the mushroom stems, and slice the caps thinly. Place the soaking water and sliced caps in a pot over medium-high heat. Bring just to a boil, cover, and reduce the heat to a low simmer for 20 minutes. Add the wakame for the last 5 minutes of simmer time and the collards for last 3 minutes. Remove from the heat and stir in the daikon, carrot, plum, and liquid aminos or tamari.

Yield: 4 servings

Per Serving: 8 Calories; trace Fat (4.1% calories from fat); 2g Protein; 11g Carbohydrate; 3g Dietary Fiber; 0mg Cholesterol; 277mg Sodium

* You can set this up in the morning for an afternoon snack or at night for a healthy, alkalizing a.m. breakfast or snack.

FROM CHEF JEANNETTE:

Bragg Liquid Aminos is a handy and nutritious seasoning to keep on hand all the time. Similar in taste to tamari and soy sauce, but unfermented, it's actually a combination of liquid amino acids, the building blocks of protein. It is high in sodium, so use it sparingly, but the flavor is intense so you don't need much. I like to buy the version in the spray bottle so I can quickly "spritz" veggies or eggs for a flavorful extra protein boost. You can find this product in all natural food stores and many high-end grocers as well.

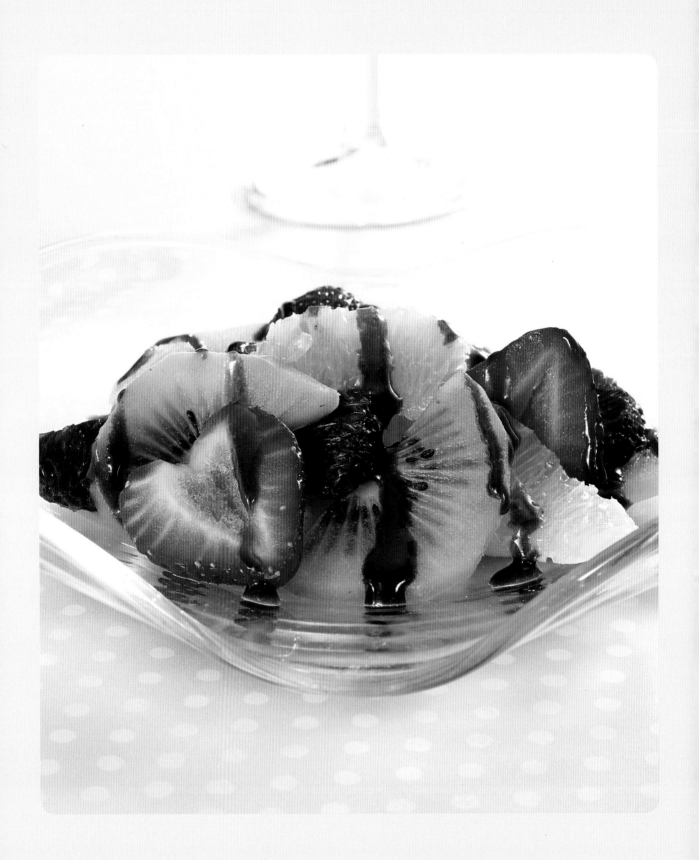

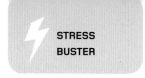
CHOCOLATE—VITAMIN C FRUIT SALAD

From Dr. Jonny: I have a dear friend, Oliver Beaucaup, who teaches tennis full time in St. Martin. As you can imagine, spending eight hours a day on the tennis court keeps him in great shape. At sixty-three, he looks and acts like a man half his age, which helps him keep up with his gorgeous eight-year-old daughter. But I digress. When I first met Oliver so many years ago, we talked at one time about how he stays so incredibly healthy. He told me his secret was that he ate one to two whole kiwis every day. I always thought this was interesting but far from scientific, till I started researching my book *The 150 Healthiest Foods on Earth* and found that kiwis have the highest amount of vitamin C of any fruit. No wonder Oliver never got sick! But enough about kiwis—let's talk about this "to die for" dressing! When served over this fruit salad, it works as a great life-lengthening snack or dessert when you need something sweet, salty, and chocolaty. Enjoy—I know you will!

---

1 seedless blood orange (or navel)

3 fresh kiwifruits, peeled, halved lengthwise, and sliced into half moons

3 cups (435 g) stemmed and halved fresh strawberries (or sliced if large)

½ cup (67 g) roasted salted macadamia nuts (or ½ cup [55 g] sliced almonds)

Sprigs fresh mint or basil, optional, for garnish

DRESSING

1½ tablespoons (25 ml) macadamia nut oil (or almond)

1 tablespoon (15 ml) champagne vinegar

1½ tablespoons (30 g) raw honey (or orange blossom—divine!)

1½ teaspoons high-quality cocoa powder (we like Ghirardelli)

Pinch salt

Slice the top and bottom off of the orange and set it on one of the flat ends. Using a sharp paring knife, cut away both the peel and the white pith, exposing the pulp. It's easiest to do this top to bottom, rather than around the middle. Slice the orange into thin rounds and quarter each slice. In a medium salad bowl, combine the prepared orange, kiwi, and strawberries, mixing gently, and set aside.

In a small bowl, whisk together the oil, vinegar, honey, cocoa, and salt until well incorporated. Drizzle over the fruit to taste, sprinkle with macadamias, and garnish with herb sprigs, if using.

Yield: 4 servings

Per Serving: 238 Calories; 14g Fat (47.9% calories from fat); 4g Protein; 29g Carbohydrate; 7g Dietary Fiber; 0mg Cholesterol; 39mg Sodium

FROM CHEF JEANNETTE:

I was horsing around with cocoa dressings to satisfy a craving when I came up with the concept for this recipe. Another version I loved was to use raspberry vinegar in place of the champagne vinegar. I tried it as a dressing over my all-time favorite salad (featured in *The Healthiest Meals on Earth*) with baby spinach, chèvre, fresh raspberries, and toasted, nutrient-rich sliced almonds. If you are an adventurous culinarian, give it a try—it was out of this world!

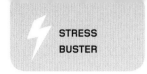

MIGHTY MELON-BERRY MADNESS

From Dr. Jonny: Funny thing about the immune system—it's deeply influenced by your mood. Sharing, family connections, support systems, exercise—all of these literally boost the activity of some of your body's most powerful weapons against microbial invaders! So on taste alone, this fruity, frothy drink should boost immunity. It's enough to raise your serotonin by itself! But the thing of it is, there's good nutritional support for the immune system hidden in all that taste. Protein from the eggs provides amino acids that are the building blocks for all the neurotransmitters and other biochemicals that make your mind sharp; flaxseed oil provides anti-inflammatory action, and the red fruits are filled with vitamin A. You win on both counts with this drink—taste and nutrition!

2 cups (310 g) peeled and chopped fresh cantaloupe
(or frozen, thawed)

2 cups (290 g) stemmed and halved fresh strawberries,
(or frozen, thawed)

¾ cup (95 g) fresh raspberries (or frozen, thawed)

1 cup (243 g) lightly pasteurized egg whites

¼ cup (24 g) mint, optional

1–2 tablespoons (14–28 ml) high-lignan flaxseed oil
(such as Barlean's) to taste

1 tablespoon (15 g) xylitol, or to taste
(or use 4 drops liquid stevia, or to taste)

Combine fruit, egg whites, and mint, if using, in a blender and process until smooth. Add the oil and xylitol and blend briefly until well incorporated.

Yield: 4 glasses

Per Serving: 150 Calories; 7g Fat (42.2% calories from fat); 8g Protein; 16g Carbohydrate; 4g Dietary Fiber; 0mg Cholesterol; 106mg Sodium

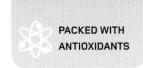

LONGEVITY FRUIT GELS—NOT JUST JELL-O

From Dr. Jonny: While classic Jell-O is indeed fairly low-cal, so is dirt, but that doesn't mean I want to eat it! Now compare regular Jell-O to Chef Jeannette's longevity gels, which are just as sweet and light, even fruitier, and loaded with nutrients that are conspicuously absent from any commercial Jell-O I've ever seen. The base is a Japanese gelatin called agar agar, and it's made from—get this—red seaweed. But don't worry; in its flake form it doesn't taste anything like fish! The flavor is neutral, like Western gelatin. It's a great vegan alternative to animal-derived gelatin and is a fine source of iodine, calcium, iron, phosphorus, and vitamins, all of which help keep your immune system in top shape!

BASE GEL

4 cups (950 ml) low-acid fruit juice (or half juice, half water for less sugar)

4 tablespoons (14 g) agar flakes

2 cups (about 350 g) chopped fruit

To make Japanese gelatin, pour the juice into a large saucepan and add the agar flakes. Bring to a boil over medium-high heat, reduce the heat to medium, and simmer until the flakes are completely dissolved, usually 5 to 6 minutes. Stir in fruit, pour into a glass storage container, and refrigerate for 1 to 2 hours until set.

Gel Ideas

STRAWBERRY POM

2 cups (475 ml) apple juice

1 cup (235 ml) pomegranate juice

1 cup (235 ml) water

2 cups (340 g) sliced strawberries

½ cup (48 g) sliced mint leaves

BERRY BLAST

4 cups (950 ml) apple juice

1 cup (145 g) blueberries

½ cup (65 g) raspberries

½ cup (75 g) blackberries

* These gels are called kantens, and they're easy to make. Find nutritious agar flakes, my favorite type, in little baggies in Asian markets and macrobiotic sections of natural food stores. Agar agar also comes in bars and a powder. One bar is about equal to ¼ cup of flakes. The powder has quite a bit more gelling power than the flakes or bar and is also harder to find. I don't use the powder form much because, unlike the other two types, it tastes a little fishy.

HONEYED GINGER PEAR

2 cups (475 ml) apple juice

2 cups (475 ml) water

⅓ cup (115 g) honey*

2 to 3 pears, peeled, cored, and diced

¼ cup (32 g) grated ginger (or you could use crystallized if you're feeling decadent!)

Yield: 4 servings

Per Serving: 39 Calories; trace Fat (1.1% calories from fat); 1g Protein; 10g Carbohydrate; 1g Dietary Fiber; 0mg Cholesterol; 5mg Sodium

* For this one, add the honey once the agar flakes have dissolved, and continue to simmer for 5 minutes longer, stirring often, before adding the fruit and ginger.

FROM CHEF JEANNETTE:

The enzymes and acids in certain raw fruits will cause agar to break down somewhat and not gel properly, so you should use cooked versions of those: pineapple, papaya, peach, and mango. Those enzymes affect conventional animal-based gelatins as well, so anything that won't gel in Jell-O won't gel in a kanten either. One tablespoon (3.6 g) of agar flakes is about the equivalent of one teaspoon of regular gelatin, but with a lot more nutrition.

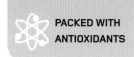
SMOOTH MOVE COMFORTING FRUIT COMPOTE

From Dr. Jonny: Okay, I know it's not a sexy subject, but let's talk constipation. There, I've said it. The truth is, more than 4.5 million people in the United States alone report being constipated most or all of the time, and the number of people who suffer from it intermittently is many times that. Constipation is the most common gastrointestinal complaint in the United States and results in more than 2 million annual doctor visits. The truth is, there's so much you can do to relieve constipation with food—and water, as dehydration is a major cause! And because your immune system is only as good as the nutrients you absorb and digest, if you're not digesting well, your immune system suffers. Here's a gourmet solution to the problem. Even if it wasn't great for digestive issues, it would still be a terrific addition to your diet. The warm prune, apple, and OJ will do the trick. Promise! This is sweet and tart, tastes (and smells!) great, and is good hot or cold. Love Chef Jeannette's great ideas for multiple uses!

---

²/₃ cup (117 g) prunes, chopped

²/₃ cup (87 g) dried apricots, chopped

2 cups (475 ml) water

1½ cups (355 ml) orange juice, fresh squeezed or bottled, not from concentrate

1 tablespoon (15 ml) fresh-squeezed lemon juice

2 tablespoons (40 g) maple syrup

1 teaspoon ground cinnamon

½ teaspoon ground ginger

¼ teaspoon ground cardamom

3 cups (375 g) cooking apples, peeled, cored, and chopped

2 cups (460 g) plain Greek yogurt or cottage cheese, optional

¾ cup (90 g) toasted chopped walnuts or almonds (83 g) or high-quality granola (86 g), optional

In a large saucepan over high heat, combine the prunes, apricots, water, juices, syrup, cinnamon, ginger, and cardamom, and mix well. Once it reaches a boil, reduce the heat to low, cover, and simmer for about 20 minutes or until the fruit is tender. Add the apples and simmer for an additional 10 minutes or until very tender. Purée to desired consistency with an immersion blender or, cooled, in a blender or food processor. Serve as is or spoon yogurt or cottage cheese and nuts over cooled compote.

Yield: about 4–6 generous servings

Per Serving: 51 Calories; 17g Fat (32.1% calories from fat); 12g Protein; 70g Carbohydrate; 8g Dietary Fiber; 15mg Cholesterol; 59mg Sodium

FROM CHEF JEANNETTE:

My Real Food Moms partner Tracee Yablon Brenner, R.D., conceived this compote concept. Jonny and I love a compote as an immune booster because it's so rich in life-enhancing nutrients and so very versatile. Try it as described for dessert, or over pancakes in place of too much sugary syrup, or mixed into cooked oats or amaranth, or even with cooked lean meats such as turkey or ground beef.

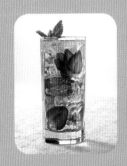

DRINKS

. . . .

Toasted Chai Latte for Long Life
Juicy, Stress-Bustin' Ginseng Ale
Fresh Start Strawberry-Mint Fizz
Green Pineapple Pleaser
The Potassium Powerhouse: Fruit-Potato Juice

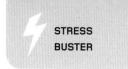

TOASTED CHAI LATTE FOR LONG LIFE

From Dr. Jonny: Okay, what's the point of living long if you can't enjoy any of your favorite foods or drinks, right? Take chai latte, one of life's great pleasures. But first, take a look at the amount of sugar in a vanilla chai latte at Dunkin' Donuts or Starbucks. Both contain 30 or more grams of sugar. Chef Jeannette whipped up a latte that actually tastes better but won't give you a big dose of sugar which, if it doesn't directly shorten your life, as many health professionals believe, certainly doesn't extend it! And excess sugar depresses immune function. There are only 13 grams of sugar per mug in this recipe, but it's all from raw honey, and you can reduce that to zero if you use stevia! So enjoy. Tea is enjoyed by some of the longest-lived cultures on Earth. This version tastes amazing and will make your house smell like a spice market in tropical Grenada.

1½ tablespoons (9 g) whole cardamom pods (about 23)

¼ teaspoon whole black peppercorns

1 teaspoon whole cloves

2 cinnamon sticks (or ½ teaspoon ground cinnamon)

2 star anise pods (or ¾ teaspoon whole fennel seeds)

6 cups (1.5 L) water

¼ cup (32 g) grated ginger

3 tablespoons (60 g) honey (or 4 drops liquid stevia for sugar free)

½ cup (120 ml) unsweetened evaporated skim milk, unsweetened vanilla soy, or almond milk

4 high-quality black tea bags (pure Ceylon or Darjeeling work well)

Toast all spices except ginger in small dry skillet over medium heat for about 5 minutes or until spices are very fragrant. Remove the cinnamon sticks and grind the remaining spices coarsely in a spice grinder (or dedicated coffee grinder), about 9 short pulses (if you don't have a spice grinder, you can grind them by hand with a mortar and pestle, but it's hard work!).

Add the ground spices, cinnamon sticks, plus 6 cups (1.5 L) water and ginger to a medium pot over high heat. Bring the water to a boil and lower the heat to a low simmer for 10 minutes, uncovered. Add the tea bags and continue to simmer for 5 minutes. Reduce the heat to low to end the simmer and add the evaporated cow's milk, if using. Continue to heat for 5 minutes. (If using vegan milk, lower the heat but don't add the milk until the last minute to prevent curdling or separation.)

Strain the tea twice through a double-mesh sieve, stir in sweetener, and enjoy.

Yield: 4 mugs

Per Serving: 116 Calories; 2g Fat (12.0% calories from fat); 2g Protein; 27g Carbohydrate; 7g Dietary Fiber; 0mg Cholesterol; 12mg Sodium

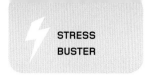
JUICY, STRESS-BUSTIN' GINSENG ALE

From Dr. Jonny: Ginseng is categorized as an *adaptogen*, meaning it helps your body increase its resistance to stress, which in turn is one of the greatest depressors of immunity on the planet. That alone would make it worth consuming for immunity, but the health benefits of ginseng go well beyond its use as a stress buster. It has strong antioxidant and anti-inflammatory properties. Both Asian and American ginseng contain *ginsenosides*, substances that are thought to give ginseng its medicinal properties. And in one important study at the National Autonomous University of Mexico it was judged to be a "promising dietary supplement" when assessed for an increase in quality of life.

2 cups (475 ml) apple cider

2 gingerroot tea bags

4 ginseng root tea bags

2 tablespoons (40 g) honey, or to taste (or xylitol)

3 tablespoons (45 ml) ginger juice, or to taste (peel, grate, and hand-squeeze juice, run root through a juicer, or use prepared, such as from The Ginger People)

2 tablespoons (28 ml) lemon juice, or to taste

1 to 2 cups (235 to 475 ml) ice cold sparkling mineral water (or seltzer)

Yield: 4 servings

Per Serving: 96 Calories; trace Fat (1.2% calories from fat); trace Protein; 25g Carbohydrate; trace Dietary Fiber; 0mg Cholesterol; 5mg Sodium

In a small saucepan, bring the cider to a boil. Lower the heat, add the tea bags, cover, and simmer for 2 minutes. Remove from the heat and let steep for 5 minutes, covered. Remove the tea bags and stir in the honey until dissolved. Stir in the ginger juice and chill in the fridge for at least 30 minutes. Stir in the lemon juice, adjust the sweetness, tartness, and ginger to taste (it should be strong), then add cold sparkling water and serve as is (use 2 cups, or 475 ml, sparkling water), or over ice (use 1 cup, or 235 ml, sparkling water).

FROM CHEF JEANNETTE:

You can spice this up for cold weather, if you like, by adding a few star anise, cinnamon sticks, or cardamom pods to the cider before heating. Just strain out before drinking and serve hot (add 2 cups or 475 ml, hot water) or cold.

We use apple cider in this recipe, great for immune-boosting vitamin C, but Jonny had another healthful suggestion: Add a couple of tablespoons of raw apple cider vinegar to the mix. You will hardly notice the slight bite of the vinegar, and raw apple cider vinegar helps keep your body in a healthy, alkaline state (as opposed to acid, where colds and viruses tend to thrive!). Raw apple cider vinegar has all kinds of antibacterial properties and is rich in nutrients.

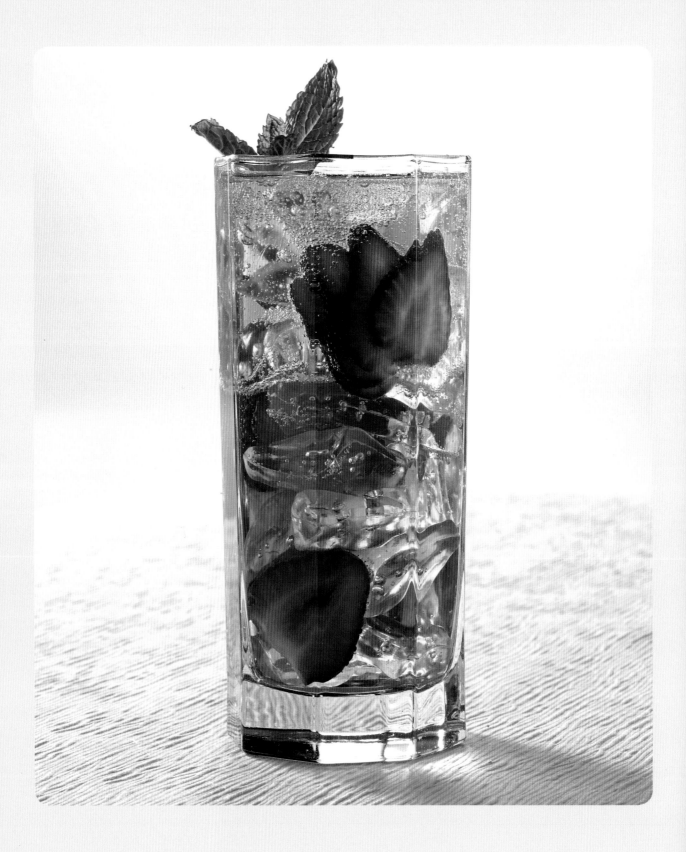

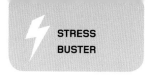

FRESH START STRAWBERRY-MINT FIZZ

From Dr. Jonny: Eating a half pound of strawberries or spinach can be just as good as taking a large dose of vitamin C when it comes to helping the body defuse oxygen radicals that damage cells, according to research from the U.S. Department of Agriculture's Human Research Center on Aging at Tufts University. This delicious fizz may not contain a whole pound of strawberries, but it sure beats the alcohol- and sugar-soaked versions of "fizzes" we used to drink in college bars! And it tastes as fresh as a summer morning.

2 cups (475 ml) water

2 ounces (55 g) fresh peppermint leaves, plus extra for garnish, washed

2 to 3 tablespoons (40 to 60 g) raw honey, to taste (or substitute 4 drops liquid stevia)

12 large strawberries, washed, stemmed, and cut into fans

2 cups (475 ml) sparkling mineral water

Bring the water to a quick boil. Place the mint leaves in a teapot and pour boiling water over all. Cover and steep for 10 minutes. Strain the leaves out through a fine-mesh sieve and stir in the honey to dissolve. Chill for 1 hour in the fridge.

Place the prepared strawberries in the sparkling water and chill for 1 hour in the fridge. Gently combine the tea and sparkling water with the strawberries in a pitcher. Serve garnished with a few mint leaves.

Yield: 4 servings

Per Serving: 66 Calories; trace Fat (3.1% calories from fat); 1g Protein; 17g Carbohydrate; 2g Dietary Fiber; 0mg Cholesterol; 5mg Sodium

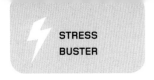

GREEN PINEAPPLE PLEASER

From Dr. Jonny: One way to get your vitamin C is with a supplement. Another is with the perfectly named Green Pineapple Pleaser. Loaded with vitamin C from the apples and pineapple, this tangy drink has the added benefit of detoxifying chlorophyll from the barley grass. Chlorophyll is to plants what blood is to humans. It even has a similar chemical structure, except that red blood cells have an atom of iron in their center whereas cholorophyll has an atom of magnesium. A derivative of cholorophyll called *chlorophyllin* has been found to prevent damage to DNA by carcinogenic substances such as aflatoxins. It's a great blood purifier, helping the body get rid of nasty microbes that can make you sick. And while vitamin C may not exactly prevent colds, it stimulates the production of white blood cells, the army of soldiers your immune system sends out to attack foreign invaders such as bacteria. The hint of mint adds to the cleansing feeling you get with this refreshing drink.

4 apples, unpeeled, quartered

¼ cup (24 g) fresh mint

1 cup (165 g) fresh or frozen pineapple (thawed),
  cut into chunks

2 cups ice cubes or to taste

2 teaspoons young barley grass powder*

* Barley grass powder is probably the mildest tasting of the green drink
  powders. Find it in natural food stores and larger whole foods grocers.
  You may also substitute wheat grass powder, spirulina, chlorella, or
  thawed wheat grass juice. For a less frosty drink, omit the ice cubes
  and juice a cucumber with the apples to increase the liquid quantity
  without increasing the sugar content too much.

Juice the apple and pour the fresh juice into a blender. Add the mint and pineapple and blend until smooth. Add the ice cubes and blend to desired consistency. Add the barley powder and blend briefly on low just to combine. Serve immediately.

Yield: 2 glasses

Per Serving: 89 Calories; 1g Fat (5.4% calories from fat); 1g Protein; 48g Carbohydrate; 9g Dietary Fiber; 0mg Cholesterol; 4mg Sodium

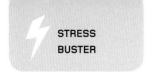

STRESS
BUSTER

THE POTASSIUM POWERHOUSE: FRUIT-POTATO JUICE

From Dr. Jonny: Full confession: When I first read this recipe I was flummoxed—potato juice? You're kidding! So I went downstairs and actually made it. All I can say is don't laugh till you try it. Not only is it incredibly (okay, surprisingly!) good, but it's an antioxidant buffet with vitamin C, vitamin A, and more potassium than a banana. The ginger gives it just the right edge of sharpness. This might be my new favorite drink.

---

1 white grapefruit, peeled

1 large apple, unpeeled (your choice)

1 large pear, unpeeled (your choice)

1 small sweet potato or yam, unpeeled

1 piece ginger (1 inch, or 2.5 cm), unpeeled

Scrub everything well (especially the sweet potato), cut into portions to fit through your juicer, juice, mix gently, and serve.

Yield: 1 large or 2 small glasses

Per Serving: 205 Calories; 1g Fat (4.3% calories from fat); 3g Protein; 50g Carbohydrate; 7g Dietary Fiber; 0mg Cholesterol; 9mg Sodium

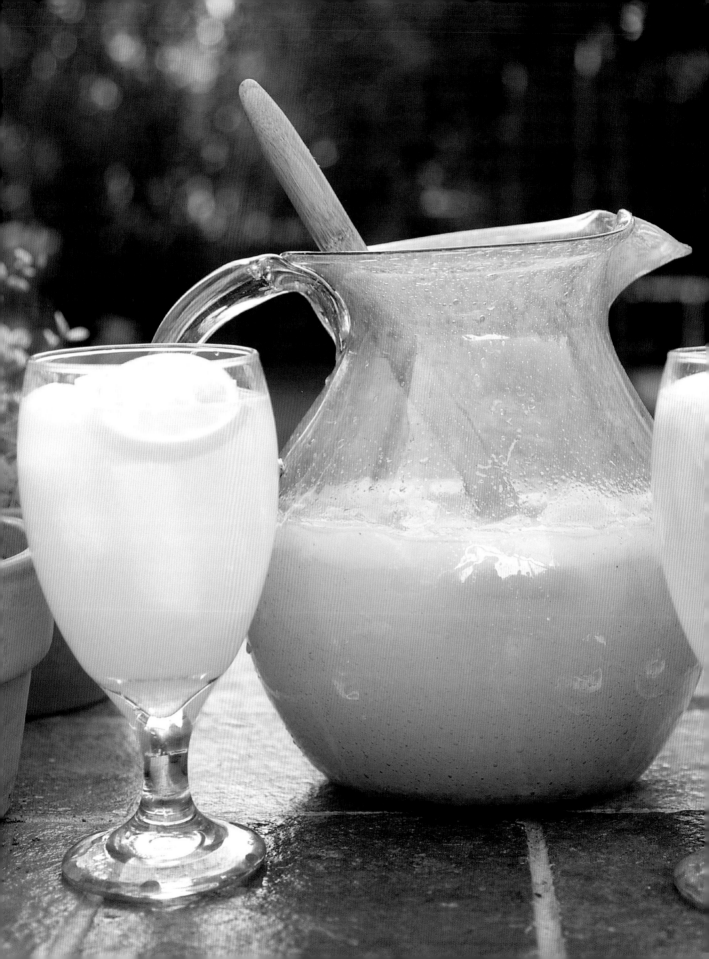

Chapter V
Help Your Liver Deep-Six the Toxins
. . . .

I know this isn't a weight-loss book, but bear with me for a minute while I talk about belly fat.

It's a great way to introduce our next subject, the liver.

Stay with me now, because this is a fascinating story that not only has implications for health and longevity, but also for weight loss.

Though most people might not be aware of it, fat on your body actually comes in two flavors: visceral and subcutaneous. We all know (and hate) the subcutaneous kind, which is the type that makes your thighs push against each other in your jeans and causes you to ask the dreaded question: "Do I look fat in these?" But basically that annoying subcutaneous fat isn't really dangerous, it's just unsightly.

Visceral fat, however, is another matter.

Visceral fat is the stuff around the middle, the kind of fat that gives you what's known as an "apple" shape. This kind of belly fat is actually the most dangerous because it's the most metabolically active, gushing out nasty little chemicals and hormones that shorten your life. In fact, researchers writing in the November 12, 2008, issue of the *New England Journal of Medicine* reported a study that followed 360,000 Europeans for more than ten years and found that those with the most belly (visceral) fat had double the risk of dying compared to people with the least amount of belly fat. Let me repeat that: *double* the risk of dying. And that's on top of previous research showing an association between visceral fat and a host of other diseases including some cancers, diabetes, and even dementia.

So, what does this have to do with the liver?

Everything.

WORKING ITS DETOXIFICATION MAGIC

Belly fat correlates with something that's becoming increasingly prevalent, although at the moment it's kind of flying under the radar. It's called nonalcoholic fatty liver disease (NAFLD), and it refers to the accumulation of fat in the liver that is not caused by drinking alcohol. As the liver is the main organ of detoxification in the body, fat accumulation can damage overall health and well-being. If you think of the fat coming through the liver as traffic going through a tollbooth, you can think of NAFLD as what would happen if none of those cars had E-Z Pass and the traffic got jammed up for miles.

Fat accumulated in the liver is a particular concern for other reasons: It can easily cause both inflammation and scarring in the liver. "At its most severe, nonalcoholic fatty liver disease can progress to liver failure," according to the Mayo Clinic.

A recent study of middle-aged Dallas residents showed that 34 percent of this population had liver fat accumulation. This disease isn't restricted to adults. An autopsy study in San Diego revealed that 12 percent of adolescents who died from accidents already had liver fat accumulation, and those who were overweight had much greater buildup of fat around their livers.

Clearing fat from the liver is essential to getting rid of life-shortening belly fat.

See, the liver is like the Rodney Dangerfield of the body. It doesn't get any respect. But it ought to. Every single minute almost 2 quarts of blood pass through the liver, whose job is to filter out everything that doesn't belong, such as toxins, chemicals, pesticides, and medicines. And each day the liver manufactures about a quart of bile, which carries out many of the toxic substances and dumps them into the intestines.

Fiber binds up much of this bile together with its toxic load, and the whole mess is excreted. This is one reason fiber is so important for liver health, and it's why you'll see high-fiber foods used throughout this section (as well as throughout this book).

Having a toxic, overburdened body is not a good prescription for long life.

But I digress.

The liver works its detoxification magic through a two-phase system of enzymatic reactions. Phase 1 generally converts a toxic chemical into a somewhat less harmful chemical. But during this process, the body produces free radicals that, in excessive amounts, can damage the liver. If antioxidants are lacking, these toxic chemicals can become far more dangerous. My good friend, nutritionist Robert Crayhon, M.S., uses the analogy of a hand grenade. Phase 1 detoxification pulls out the pin, but if phase 2 isn't working properly, you now have an active grenade on your hands!

Getting the grenade out of the house is where phase 2 comes in. If phase 2 isn't working properly, those intermediate substances (like the pinless hand grenade) can do substantial damage, including initiating carcinogenic (cancer-forming) processes. Proper functioning of the liver's entire detoxification system is extremely important for the prevention of cancer. Research has found that some antioxidants, such as the powerful *sulforaphane* found in cruciferous vegetables, actively stimulate phase 2 detoxification.

This complicated machinery of detoxification is all fueled by nutrients. These nutrients literally provide the metabolic gas that allows the liver to do its essential work, both in getting rid of fat (as in NAFLD) and in getting rid of toxins. These nutrients literally help the liver take out the trash. When the liver is unable to do this properly, the trash accumulates and results in a toxic, overburdened body, which is not a good prescription for long life.

The army of enzymes that allow the liver to do this work is collectively known as the cytochrome P450 enzymes. When cytochrome P450 metabolizes a toxin, it chemically transforms it to a less-toxic form, makes it water soluble, or—and this is the kicker—occasionally turns it into a more chemically active and potentially more dangerous form, like the grenade with the now-missing pin. Turning it into a more chemically active form actually makes it easier to be metabolized by the phase 2 enzymes, assuming, of course, that they're working properly.

So, a highly efficient liver detoxification system is absolutely necessary for health and vitality, and this means it's essential that you include key nutrients in your diet. B vitamins play a major role because they act as cofactors for many enzyme systems, including the ones in the liver. Depletion of vitamin C may impair the whole operation. Vitamin C also helps prevent the free-radical damage that can occur in phase 1. And a ton of amino acids, which are found in protein-rich foods such as seafood, chicken, beef, lamb, and tofu, play important roles in phase 2 detoxification.

The liver is also a storehouse of vitamins, especially the fat-soluble ones—vitamins A, D, E, and K. "Damage to the liver has profound effects on numerous body processes, including digestion, absorption, storage, and use of vitamins and minerals," says nutritionist Elizabeth Somer, M.A., R.D.

So, to make a long story short: A healthy liver is essential to a healthy—and long—life.

Period.

REWARD YOUR LIVER WITH THESE RECIPES

In this section, you'll find recipes rich in the nutrients that help support the liver in doing its essential and numerous tasks. Recipes such as Enzyme-Enhancing Cauliflower-Cashew Curry, Brassica Brussels Sprouts and Bacon, and Superfood Wrap: Stuffed Cabbage Rolls all feature liver-protecting cruciferous vegetables. These vegetables, members of the brassica family of vegetable royalty, contain plant compounds called *isothiocyanates*, which literally induce phase 2 detoxification enzymes in the liver, the same detoxification enzymes that work to rid the body of carcinogenic compounds.

You'll find recipes rich in protein (Pure, Protein-Packed Citrus Mint Grilled Lamb Chops, for example), which provide amino acids necessary for phase 2 detoxification. And you'll find recipes such as Toxin Timeout: BBQ Bean Burgers, rich in the fiber that helps bind toxins to bile so they can be excreted out of the body.

The liver is an amazing organ. It's the only organ that can actually regenerate itself, so if you haven't been taking good care of it, this is the perfect time to start.

Reward your liver with the nutrients in these recipes, and it will reward you back by helping to get rid of belly fat, toxins, chemicals, and other life-shortening substances. Take care of your liver and it will repay you with the gift of health.

Your liver will thank you—and so will your taste buds! Enjoy!

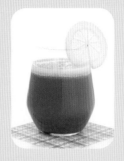

CLEANSING DRINK "TONICS"

A Ginger-Aid for What Ails You
Cranberry Cleanse
Delicious Dandelion Tea
Iron Power Juice
Juicy Liver Tonic

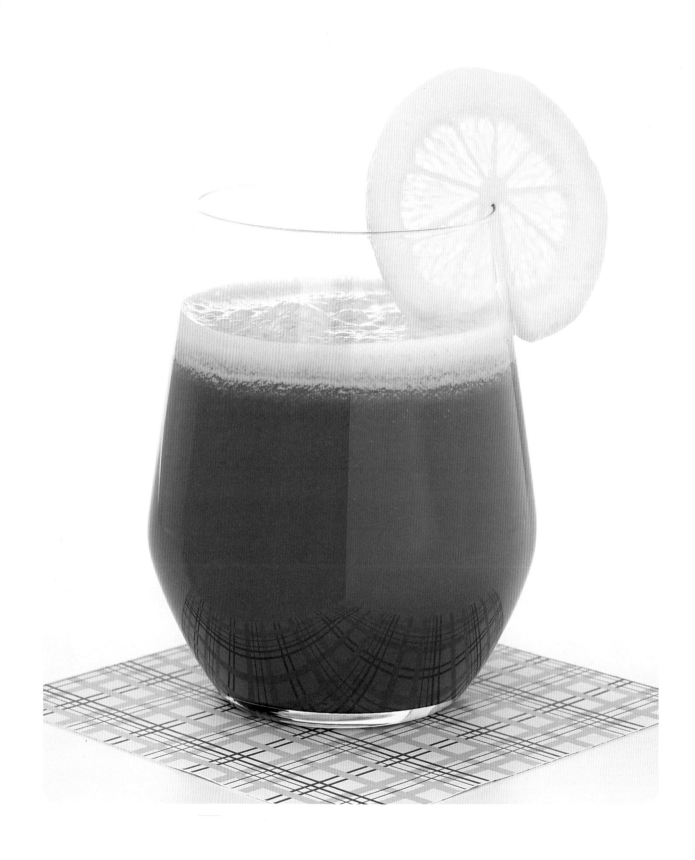

A GINGER-AID FOR WHAT AILS YOU

From Dr. Jonny: Greens are one of the most detoxifying groups of plants in the world, but a lot of people shy away from the flavor, which can sometimes be bitter. This fabulous drink gives you a great way to consume dark, leafy greens with none of the "downside." It tastes fresh and light and gingery, and the sweetness of the apple and sour of the lemon completely mask any bitterness of the mineral-rich kale. So good even the vegetable-phobic teenager in our family didn't notice the green stuff!

1 lemon, peeled

3 leaves of kale or small collards

1 large cucumber, unpeeled

1 sweet apple, unpeeled and stemmed

1 thumb ginger, unpeeled

Wash all produce thoroughly, cut it into large chunks, and run it through a juicer.

Stir gently to combine and drink immediately.

Yield: 1 huge glass or 2 medium glasses

Per Serving: 123 Calories; 1.3g Fat (8% calories from fat); 5g Protein; 30g Carbohydrate; 7.5g Dietary Fiber; 0mg Cholesterol; 50mg Sodium

FROM CHEF JEANNETTE:

An "aid" for what ails you, I'm not sure where this amazing recipe concept originated, but there are several versions floating around in the juicing world. You can use any dark green leafies you happen to have on hand, except maybe arugula or mustard greens, which would be too intense. I've also seen versions that call for a romaine heart in place of the cucumber, but the cucumber is just as light and even juicier. You can also add a pear or another apple to sweeten it further, if desired. This juice makes an excellent a.m. tonic for your liver and will give you the get-up-and-go you need to start your day off right!

CRANBERRY CLEANSE

From Dr. Jonny: I'm a big fan of pure cranberry juice (not the stupid cocktail, which is only about 10 percent juice). I learned about it years ago from my friend and colleague Ann Louise Gittleman, Ph.D., "The First Lady of Nutrition." It's a daily part of her famous Fat Flush Diet, and here's why. It's alkalizing, helps prevent bacteria from adhering to the urinary tract, and it's packed with polyphenols that help support liver health and detoxification in general. (Cranberry polyphenols have been shown to have biological activity against *Streptococcus mutans*, among other nasty microbes.) Add some apple for sweetness, orange for vitamin C (and a killer taste), and fabulous ginger, which not only imparts a nice bite to the drink, but helps with digestion as well! The perfect cleanse!

1½ cups (150 g) fresh or frozen cranberries

1 sweet red apple, stemmed

1 orange, peeled

½ lemon, peeled

1 piece ginger (½ inch, or 1 cm), unpeeled, optional

Scrub everything well, cut into portions to fit through your juicer, juice, mix gently, and drink immediately.

Yield: 1 glass

Per Serving: 241 Calories; 1g Fat (4.4% calories from fat); 3g Protein; 62g Carbohydrate; 14g Dietary Fiber; 0mg Cholesterol; 4mg Sodium

FROM CHEF JEANNETTE:

If this powerhouse tonic is too tart for your liking, try adding another apple for added nutrition, or a few drops of liquid stevia to sweeten things up.

DELICIOUS DANDELION TEA

From Dr. Jonny: Go on any support board for liver ailments such as hepatitis and before you can say "Google," you'll see a million references to dandelion. It's not an accident. This is one of the most healing plants for the liver and is a part of virtually every liver-cleansing formula or liver strengthener I know of. Dandelion root and leaves are used in traditional medicine to treat liver problems, according to the University of Maryland. Dandelion is a rich source of vitamins A, B complex, C, and D, as well as minerals such as iron, potassium, and zinc. And you certainly don't have to have hepatitis to benefit! The root has a bitter, earthy quality that is nicely masked with this warming combination of spices. Drink it hot or keep it cold in the fridge to sip throughout the day!

5 cups (1 L) water

2 cinnamon sticks

2 tablespoons (12 g) dried orange peel

½ teaspoon whole cloves

¼ cup (32 g) fresh grated ginger

3 tablespoons (9 g) dried dandelion root

2 tablespoons (40 g) honey, or to taste (or substitute 4 drops liquid stevia)

In a medium saucepan, add water, cinnamon sticks, orange peel, cloves, and ginger, and bring to a boil over high heat. Reduce the heat, add the dandelion root, cover, and simmer for 15 minutes. Strain out the solids twice with a double-mesh sieve and stir in the honey to taste.

Yield: 4 cups (950 ml)

Per Serving: 81 Calories; 1g Fat (7.4% calories from fat); 1g Protein; 20g Carbohydrate; 5g Dietary Fiber; 0mg Cholesterol; 7mg Sodium

FROM CHEF JEANNETTE:

You can find dried dandelion root in most natural food stores or any herbal shop. If you can't find it loose, substitute 4 tea bags instead. If you can find roasted dried root, use that to add a nice nutty dimension to the flavor. Note: Fresh dandelion greens make a great longevity salad.

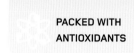
IRON POWER JUICE

From Dr. Jonny: Ask any ten natural health practitioners to give you a recipe for a cleansing liver drink and nine out of ten will include beets and carrots. Although this combo may be a bit high in sugar (and therefore not the perfect drink for people who need to watch their blood sugar carefully), it's a superb liver tonic. Beets and beet tops are a rich source of *betaine*, a natural liver detoxifier and bile thinner. (There's no reason not to throw the nutrient-rich tops into the juicer!) Britain's leading nutritionist, Jane Clarke, says, "eat carrots to liven up your liver," and calls carrots "a great liver tonic." The celery and cucumber provide a refreshing light touch to this rich, full-flavored, liver-lovin' drink. Hint: Throw in a teaspoon or so of high-lignan flaxseed oil, such as Barlean's. The healthy carotenoids in the carrots are best absorbed with some fat!

2 medium beets, unpeeled

2 large carrots, unpeeled

1 stalk celery

1 cucumber, unpeeled

Wash all produce thoroughly, cut it into large chunks, and run through a juicer.

Stir gently to combine and drink immediately.

Yield: 2 glasses

Per Serving: 89 Calories; trace Fat (4.4% calories from fat); 3g Protein; 20g Carbohydrate; 6g Dietary Fiber; 0mg Cholesterol; 110mg Sodium

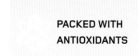

JUICY LIVER TONIC

From Dr. Jonny: You can't do much better for your liver than this light, refreshing tonic of liver-friendly vegetables (unless you add dandelion greens, but that's got its own recipe). I like substituting frozen, prepared wheatgrass juice for spinach because it's a great blood purifier and detoxifier. Even better—use them both! And milk thistle is just about the best and most studied herb for liver support. The acidophilus powder will give a nice boost to your digestive and immune systems.

2 carrots, unpeeled

2 stalks celery

1 cup (30 g) spinach*

1 small cucumber, unpeeled

¼ cup (15 g) parsley

½ teaspoon acidophilus powder

3 drops milk thistle extract

* For a longevity alternative, substitute 1 to 3 teaspoons of fresh or frozen prepared wheatgrass juice for the spinach in this mixture. Fresh wheatgrass requires a special extractor for proper juicing, but you can find it frozen in most natural food stores or high-end natural grocers. Wheatgrass juice has a powerful cleansing effect on the body, so start with small doses, such as 1 teaspoon, and work your way up from there.

Wash all produce and parsley thoroughly, cut veggies into large chunks, and run through a juicer, using the cucumber to help push the parsley and spinach through.

Add acidophilus powder and milk thistle extract, stir gently to combine, and drink immediately.

Yield: 1 large or 2 small glasses

Per Serving: 63 Calories; trace Fat (6.1% calories from fat); 3g Protein; 14g Carbohydrate; 5g Dietary Fiber; 0mg Cholesterol; 79mg Sodium

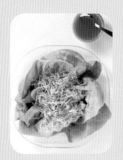

CRUCIFERS and LIVE SALADS

Brassica Brussels Sprouts and Bacon
Superfood Wrap: Stuffed Cabbage Rolls
Enzyme–Enhancing Cauliflower-Cashew Curry
Cleansing Carrot–Parsley Salad
Bloody Mary Sprout Salad

BRASSICA BRUSSELS SPROUTS AND BACON

From Dr. Jonny: Nothing says "love" to the liver like members of the brassica family, or, as I like to call them, "vegetable royalty." If the brassica vegetables—cabbage, broccoli, Brussels sprouts, kale, and cauliflower—were rock stars, they'd be in the Hall of Fame. That's because they're loaded with cancer-fighting *indoles*, phytochemicals that fight inflammation, and nutrients that support liver detoxification. Forget about visions of 1960s casseroles of boiled Brussels sprouts smothered in canned cream of mushroom soup. Pshaw. This recipe is Brussels sprouts brought into the new millennium!

2 to 4 slices turkey or vegan bacon, to taste, optional.

2 tablespoons (28 ml) olive oil

1 small yellow onion, thinly sliced

2 teaspoons (10 ml) apple cider vinegar

1 teaspoon maple syrup

1 pound (455 g) Brussels sprouts, halved, stems trimmed

Salt, to taste

Fresh-ground black pepper, to taste

½ cup (75 g) grated peeled apple

Cook the bacon crisp, according to package directions, if using, and set aside to cool.

Heat the oil in a large skillet over medium heat. Add the onion and sauté for 2 minutes.

Mix the vinegar and syrup together in a small cup and pour over the onions, stirring to combine well. Continue cooking for 5 to 7 minutes until the onions are soft and translucent. Add Brussels sprouts, salt, and pepper to taste and cook for 5 to 7 minutes until the sprouts are bright green and beginning to get tender.

While the sprouts are cooking, break or chop up the bacon into crumbles. Add the grated apple to the Brussels sprouts and cook, stirring to prevent sticking, for about a minute. Sprinkle the bacon crumbles over all to serve.

Yield: 4 servings

Per Serving: 146 Calories; 7g Fat (43.0% calories from fat); 4g Protein; 16g Carbohydrate; 5g Dietary Fiber; 8mg Cholesterol; 242mg Sodium

SUPERFOOD WRAP: STUFFED CABBAGE ROLLS

From Dr. Jonny: Cabbage first came to be recognized as a superfood when researchers acting like Detective Columbo finally identified it as the food in the diet of eastern European women that seemed to be responsible for their remarkably low levels of breast cancer. Since then, multiple studies have confirmed that people eating the most servings of cruciferous vegetables such as cabbage have lower rates of a number of cancers. But remember also that the liver is responsible for an enormous number of metabolic operations, and vegetables such as cabbage offer a wide range of nutrients that are important for these functions to be carried out. Fiber from the bulgur helps bind the toxins that are removed by the liver and helps the body excrete them. This recipe contains probiotics from the yogurt, which also assist with liver functioning. But fair warning: This project is fairly time consuming. However, the preparation time is a labor of love. (And even stress reducing, if you really get into it!) Even after all that, it needs an hour to cook—but believe me, it's worth it. Tender and mild, this is truly a "deep comfort" food, a Middle Eastern twist on a middle European classic.

2 cups (475 ml) boiling water

1 cup (140 g) bulgur (medium or coarse grind)*

1 head green cabbage

2 tablespoons (28 ml) olive oil

1 onion, diced

4 cloves garlic, minced

1 stalk celery, diced fine

1 pound (455 g) lean ground turkey

1½ teaspoons ground cumin

1 teaspoon oregano

1 teaspoon salt

½ teaspoon cracked black pepper, or more, to taste

¼ cup (15 g) fresh parsley

²/₃ cup (100 g) raisins

Juice of ½ lemon

Dash or two of hot pepper sauce, optional

2 cans (14.5 ounces, or 413 g each) diced tomatoes, undrained

1 can (6 ounces, or 170 g) tomato paste

¾ teaspoon garlic powder

¾ teaspoon onion powder

½ teaspoon oregano

¼ teaspoon salt

¼ teaspoon cracked black pepper

Splash red wine vinegar

¹/₃ cup (77 g) yogurt

2 tablespoons (8 g) minced fresh parsley

* If you have a wheat or gluten issue, use 2 cups (330 g) cooked brown basmati rice in place of the bulgur.

In a medium bowl, pour boiling water over bulgur, cover, and soak for 15 minutes. Once soaked, drain in a double-mesh sieve, pressing on grains heavily to remove as much moisture as possible. Set aside.

In the meantime, set a stockpot or large soup pot of salted water to boil.

Core the cabbage and cut away the whole leaves, removing the ends of the hard veins at the bottom, keeping as many intact as possible. In a few batches, boil the leaves for 1 to 3 minutes until tender, and remove with tongs to drain. Drain stockpot, reserving a few cups of the cooking liquid. Set aside.

In a medium sauté pan, heat the oil over medium. Add the onion and sauté 5 minutes or until soft. Add the garlic and celery and sauté 2 minutes.

While the vegetables are cooking, in a large bowl mix together the drained bulgur, raw turkey, cumin, oregano, salt, pepper, parsley, raisins, lemon juice, and hot pepper sauce, if using. When veggie mixture is cooked, stir it into the turkey mixture, mixing well.

Line the bottom of the stockpot with the small or torn cooked leaves from the cabbage. Using the larger leaves, place a generous ¼ cup (23 g)—more for the large leaves—of mixture into each cabbage leaf, folding the bottom up over the mixture, then folding the sides over and rolling from the bottom up. Place the rolls, seam side down, on top of the cabbage layer in the pot, nestling them close together, and stacking them when necessary.

Mix the diced tomatoes with the paste, garlic powder, onion powder, oregano, salt, pepper, and vinegar, and pour over the top, adding enough reserved cabbage stock to just cover the rolls. Heat over high to boil the tomato liquid, then reduce the heat to low and simmer, covered, for 1 hour or until the cabbage is very tender and the meat is cooked through, checking liquid level frequently and adding more stock to keep the level from going too low, if necessary.

In a small bowl, mix the yogurt and parsley with ½ cup (122 g) of the tomato sauce from the pot and spoon over rolls just before serving.

Yield: About 6 servings

Per Serving: 356 Calories; 11g Fat (26.0% calories from fat); 23g Protein; 48g Carbohydrate; 9g Dietary Fiber; 51mg Cholesterol; 953mg Sodium

ENZYME-ENHANCING CAULIFLOWER-CASHEW CURRY

From Dr. Jonny: The liver is Detoxification Central in the human body; it's like a giant E-Z Pass. Just about everything has to go through the liver, including all the toxins, medicines, pesticides, chemicals, and various nasty things we're exposed to on a daily basis. The liver gets rid of these in two phases (aptly named phase 1 and phase 2 detoxification) by using enzymes. And why, you ask, does this matter? Because compounds in cruciferous vegetables such as cauliflower are powerful inducers of phase 2 enzymes. That means they make your detoxification pathways work better. This gentle, soothing curry marries the healing power of cauliflower with the protein and healthy fat of cashews and the spice of turmeric for a flavor trifecta that tastes like a balmy Indian evening. Enjoy.

1 tablespoon (15 ml) olive oil

1 large sweet onion, diced

1 teaspoon curry powder

¾ teaspoon turmeric

½ teaspoon cardamom

⅛ teaspoon red pepper flakes

Pinch ground nutmeg

1 can (15 ounces, or 425 g) light coconut milk

1 head cauliflower, stemmed and cut into small florets
(½ to ¾ inch, or 1 to 2 cm)

½ teaspoon salt

1 cup (130 g) frozen peas

1 cup (135 g) roasted cashews

½ cup (8 g) cilantro, chopped, optional

Heat the oil in a Dutch oven over medium heat. Add the onion and sauté for 5 to 6 minutes until beginning to brown. Add the curry, turmeric, cardamom, red pepper flakes, and nutmeg and sauté, stirring, for 1 minute. Pour in the coconut milk, stirring gently to combine. Add the cauliflower and salt and cook until the cauliflower is tender, 25 to 30 minutes. For the last 10 minutes of cook time, add the peas and cashews, stirring gently to combine. Stir in the cilantro, if using, just before serving.

Yield: 4 to 6 servings

Per Serving: 227 Calories; 17g Fat (61.7% calories from fat); 6g Protein; 17g Carbohydrate; 3g Dietary Fiber; 0mg Cholesterol; 210mg Sodium

CLEANSING CARROT-PARSLEY SALAD

From Dr. Jonny: Just looking at this brightly colored, piquant salad will make you feel all squeaky clean and energized. Eating it's even better. Parsley enriches the liver, nourishing the blood and bodily fluids, according to British holistic nutritionist Gillian McKeith, Ph.D. (host of the hit series *You Are What You Eat*). Sprouts in general are loaded with enzymes, but broccoli sprouts are particularly liver friendly because of their levels of a powerful antioxidant known as *sulforaphane*. More than 300 published studies point to sulforaphane as a powerful health protector. Studies show that it increases the production of enzymes in the liver that help deactivate cancer-causing chemicals. Add to this the cleansing daikon radish and the protein and fiber in garbanzos, and you've got a cleansing salad that truly lives up to its name!

¾ cup (83 g) sliced peeled carrots (about 2 medium carrots)

⅔ cup (160 ml) carrot cooking water

1 can (14 ounces, or 400 g) garbanzo beans, drained and rinsed

1 cup (60 g) loosely packed flat-leaf parsley, lightly chopped

¼ cup (29 g) grated peeled daikon radish

1 cup (50 g) loosely packed broccoli sprouts

4 cups (220 g) baby spring greens (or chopped romaine hearts)

2 tablespoons (28 ml) lemon juice

1 tablespoon (10 g) minced shallot (about 1 small shallot)

2 teaspoons tahini

½ teaspoon ground coriander

¼ teaspoon salt

Pinch cayenne pepper, optional

In a salad bowl, gently toss together the garbanzo beans, parsley, daikon, sprouts, and salad greens.

In a food processor or blender, add the cooled cooked carrots, ⅔ cup (160 ml) reserved cooking water, lemon juice, shallot, tahini, coriander, salt, and cayenne, if using.

Process until very smooth. Dress the salad to taste.

Yield: 4 servings

Per Serving: 167 Calories; 3g Fat (14.4% calories from fat); 8g Protein; 30g Carbohydrate; 8g Dietary Fiber; 0mg Cholesterol; 466mg Sodium

Cook sliced carrots in a small saucepan over high heat with water to cover well. When water begins to boil, lower temperature to keep a good simmer, cover, and cook carrots until they are tender, about 5 to 7 minutes. Once tender, drain the cooking water and reserve ⅔ cup (160 ml). Set the carrots and cooking water aside to cool while you prepare the salad.

FROM CHEF JEANNETTE:

Daikon radish is a mildly flavored Asian radish that looks like a large white carrot. Older daikon can become bitter, so look for fresh young radishes in your natural food store, natural grocer, or Asian market. If you can't find daikon, substitute thinly sliced red radish. You can also add a handful of toasted sunflower seeds to boost longevity-increasing protein and fiber.

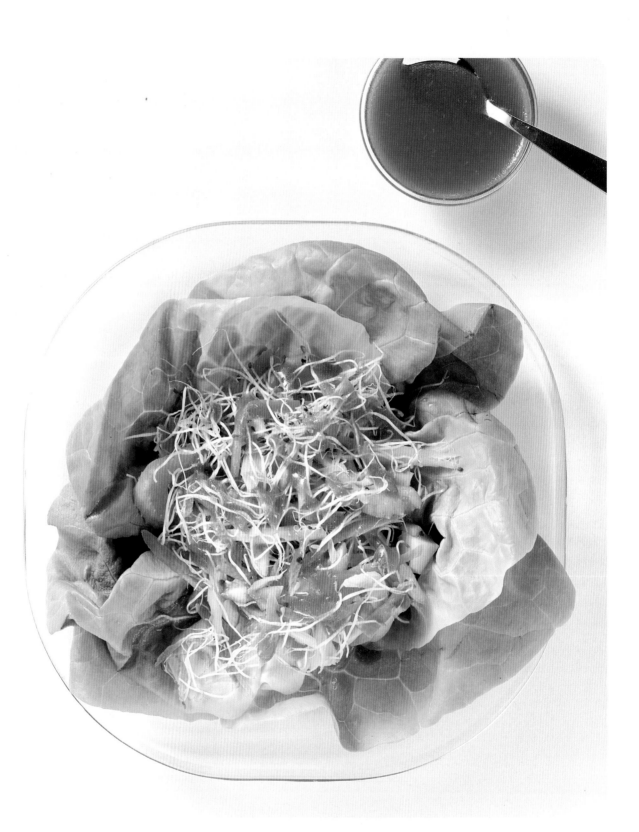

BLOODY MARY SPROUT SALAD

From Dr. Jonny: Who ever heard of eating a Bloody Mary? Well, here's your chance, and you're going to love it. So is your liver. A 2005 study conducted in China found direct evidence that broccoli sprouts, for example, can enhance the body's detoxifying system to help prevent cancer. One reason is that they are a potent source of a compound called *sulforaphane*, which seems to help activate detoxifying enzymes in the liver, helping them to get rid of carcinogens. Live foods such as sprouts also contain chlorophyll, easily one of the most detoxifying substances on the planet and a well-known blood purifier. And the lignans—naturally occurring chemicals found in flaxseed and high-lignan flaxseed oil such as Barlean's brand—have proven anticancer activity. Add to this a nice dose of vitamin C from the tomato-veggie juice, which has been shown to help reduce fatty buildup in the liver. That's an awful lot of reasons this is one liver-healing (versus liver-destroying) version of a Bloody Mary you should definitely be eating!

⅓ cup (80 ml) tomato-veggie juice (we like Knudsen's Very Veggie)

Juice of 1 lime

2 tablespoons (28 ml) high-lignan flaxseed oil (such as Barlean's) or olive oil

½ teaspoon Bragg Liquid Aminos (or tamari), or to taste

½ teaspoon prepared horseradish, or to taste

Sprinkle cayenne pepper, or to taste

2 cups (100 g) sprouts (broccoli, alfalfa, or clover)

1 cucumber, peeled and diced fine or grated (about 2 cups, or 270 g)

2 carrots, peeled and grated (about 2 cups, or 220 g)

4 celery ribs, diced fine (about 2 cups, or 240 g)

2 cups (110 g) shredded, mild lettuce, optional

In a small bowl, whisk together the juices, oil, liquid aminos or tamari, horseradish, and cayenne. Adjust the seasonings to taste.

In a salad bowl, toss together the sprouts, cucumber, carrots, celery, and lettuce, if using. Dress to taste, toss well, and serve.

Yield: 4 servings

Per Serving: 122 Calories; 8g Fat (50.8% calories from fat); 3g Protein; 13g Carbohydrate; 4g Dietary Fiber; 0mg Cholesterol; 155mg Sodium

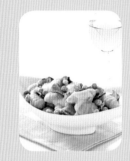

COOKED GREEN LEAFIES

Not Your Average Leek and Potato Soup
Hot Tahini Greens
Healthy Hot Greens and Eggs Pie
Nutritious Gnocchi with Parmesan–Spinach "Cream" Sauce

NOT YOUR AVERAGE LEEK AND POTATO SOUP

From Dr. Jonny: Let me tell you, the liver just loves those dark green leafies. Vegetables such as escarole and leeks (not dark green, but fabulous nonetheless) are just loaded with nutrients that make the metabolic machinery of the liver run smoothly. Leeks, for example, contain vitamin K, which the liver needs to make factors necessary for proper blood clotting. And, anything that strains or impairs liver function, such as alcohol, can seriously deplete antioxidants. You'll find a ton of antioxidants in both the escarole and the leeks. Escarole is often used as a salad green, but Chef Jeannette used it to great effect by cooking it into this soup. This is a creamy and satisfying leek and potato soup without the cream!

2 tablespoons (28 ml) olive oil

Whites and tender greens of 3 small leeks, chopped (see page 256 for info about cleaning leeks)

4 cloves garlic, minced

1 pound (455 g) small baby red or new potatoes, unpeeled and quartered (well scrubbed!)

4 cups (950 ml) unsweetened plain soy milk

¾ teaspoon salt, or to taste

¼ teaspoon white pepper, optional

½ teaspoon cracked black pepper, or to taste

1 head escarole, cored and chopped into bite-size pieces

1 to 2 tablespoons (16 to 32 g) mellow white miso, to taste

¼ cup (35 g) toasted pine nuts, optional, for garnish

Heat the oil in a large soup pot over medium. Sauté the leeks until tender, 5 to 7 minutes.

Add the garlic and potatoes and sauté, stirring well, for about 3 more minutes. Add the soy milk, salt, and peppers. Increase heat and bring just to a boil. Reduce heat, cover, and simmer until potatoes are tender, about 10 minutes, adding more soy milk, if necessary. Using an immersion blender, purée the soup until nearly smooth. Stir in escarole, cook until tender, about 3 to 5 minutes, and remove from the heat. Stir in the miso, blending lightly with an immersion wand to get it to disperse and mix. Adjust the seasonings to taste. Serve garnished with pine nuts, if using.

Yield: 4 to 6 servings

Per Serving: 223 Calories; 10g Fat (40.2% calories from fat); 9g Protein; 26g Carbohydrate; 5g Dietary Fiber; 0mg Cholesterol; 497mg Sodium

FROM CHEF JEANNETTE:

When making a puréed soup, it's more typical to peel the potatoes for smoothness, but I encourage you to leave them—and their nutrients—intact for this life-lengthening version. You can use baby red, new, or baby Yukon gold. Look for potatoes about the size of golf balls.

HOT TAHINI GREENS

From Dr. Jonny: Your liver is ground zero for detoxification in the body, and there's nothing on Earth it loves better than dark green leafy vegetables with their rich assortment of antioxidants, anti-inflammatories, and other liver-friendly nutrients. The creamy nuttiness of the warmed tahini in this recipe mellows the normally sharp, bitter flavor of the greens. This makes a delectable side dish to almost any grilled meat or fish entrée, or stuff it into a baked potato (sweet or white) and top with your choice of toasted nuts to make it a vegan meal.

3 tablespoons (45 g) tahini

2 tablespoons (28 ml) water or vegetable broth

1 tablespoon (15 ml) fresh-squeezed lemon juice

½ teaspoon grated lemon zest

1 teaspoon low-sodium tamari

1 large bunch of dark green leafies (try collards, kale, dandelion, etc.)

1 tablespoon (15 ml) olive oil

½ sweet onion, diced

2 cloves garlic, minced

Bring a large pot of water to a boil over high heat.

In a small bowl mix together the tahini, water, lemon juice, zest, and tamari until smooth (an immersion blender works well for this). Set aside.

Wash the greens very well, stem, and chop them into bite-size pieces. Place the greens into the boiling water and cook for about 2 minutes (3 for kale) until just tender.

Drain well in a colander.

Heat the oil in a large sauté pan over medium heat. Add the onion and sauté for 4 minutes. Add the garlic and sauté for 1 minute. Add the greens and toss with the onions, sautéing for 1 to 2 minutes to desired doneness. Remove from the heat, add the tahini dressing, and stir until well combined.

Yield: 4 servings

Per Serving: 120 Calories; 10g Fat (68.5% calories from fat); 3g Protein; 7g Carbohydrate; 2g Dietary Fiber; trace Cholesterol; 127mg Sodium

HEALTHY HOT GREENS AND EGGS PIE

From Dr. Jonny: I tried this dish for breakfast, and it just might become my go-to morning meal if I can remember to preheat the oven before taking a shower! Seriously, you've got eggs for protein and sulfur (good for the skin and liver). You've got spinach packed with iron, calcium, vitamin A, and a ton of other nutrients, and feta cheese for extra calcium and protein. Your liver will love you, not to mention your heart and brain, too. And here's the best part—the "no-crust" approach to quiche (naked quiche, anyone?) leaves out all the carbs and hydrogenated oils found in typical pie crusts without sacrificing a whit of flavor. Beauty! Good for breakfast, lunch, dinner, or a snack. Tip: It's surprisingly good cold!

Cooking oil spray

1 tablespoon (15 ml) olive oil

1 red onion, diced

1 clove garlic, minced

2 packed cups (60 g) baby spinach

2 packed cups (40 g) baby arugula

6 eggs

½ cup (120 ml) milk (cow's or unsweetened, unflavored soy or almond milk)

¼ cup (10 g) chopped fresh basil (or 1 teaspoon dried)

½ teaspoon salt

½ teaspoon cracked black pepper

½ cup (75 g) feta cheese (or other grated cheese), crumbled

Preheat the oven to 375°F (190°C, or gas mark 5).

Coat a 9-inch (23-cm) pie plate with cooking oil spray.

Heat the oil in a large sauté pan over medium heat. Add the onion and sauté for 5 minutes. Add the garlic and sauté for 1 minute. Add the spinach and arugula, stir to combine, and cover for 2 to 3 minutes or until the greens start to wilt. Lay the wilted greens and onions in the prepared pie plate.

In a medium bowl, beat the eggs. Whisk in the milk, basil, salt, and pepper.

Stir in the feta and pour the mixture over the greens. Cook for 35 to 40 minutes or until the center of the pie is set. If top browns too quickly, cover it lightly with foil at 30 minutes.

Yield: 4 servings

Per Serving: 227 Calories; 16g Fat (63.7% calories from fat); 14g Protein; 6g Carbohydrate; 1g Dietary Fiber; 339mg Cholesterol; 611mg Sodium

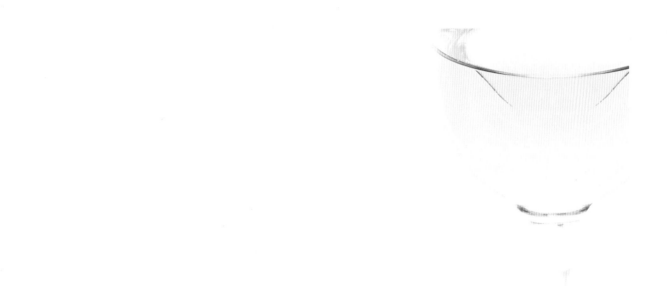
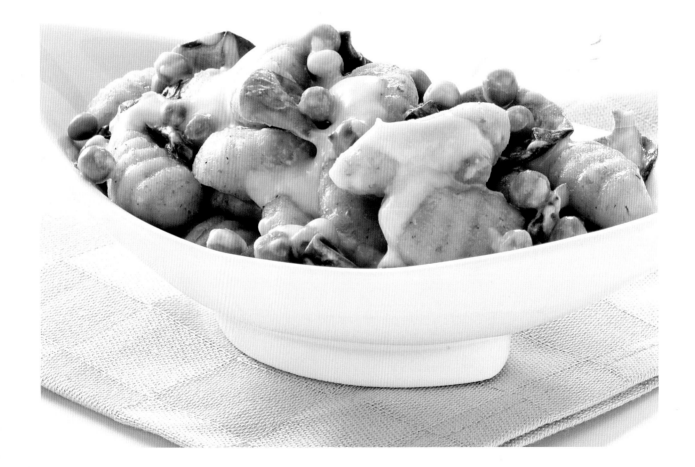

NUTRITIOUS GNOCCHI WITH PARMESAN-SPINACH "CREAM" SAUCE

From Dr. Jonny: You can't give your liver a better gift than the daily consumption of greens. The rich array of nutrients and the overall alkalizing effect of green vegetables help the liver perform its important function of detoxification. Unfortunately, however, most people don't exactly salivate when they think about spinach. Not to worry. This rich-tasting pasta dish is loaded with greens, but with Chef Jeannette's creative use of spices and Parmesan cheese you'll never notice. Instead of cream, she uses silken tofu and unsweetened milk (my fave is almond) for a fraction of the calories and way better taste. Creamy and surprisingly light, the hint of lemon makes this simple liver-friendly dish really "pop"!

1 pound (455 g) whole-wheat gnocchi* (we like Delallo Whole Wheat Potato Gnocchi)

1 container (12.3 ounces, or 340 g) soft silken tofu

¼ cup (60 ml) plain unsweetened milk (cow's, soy, almond, or rice)

⅓ cup (33 g) fresh-grated Parmesan cheese

Zest of 1 small lemon

1 teaspoon fresh lemon juice

¼ teaspoon salt

¼ teaspoon lemon pepper (or cracked black pepper)

1 to 2 dashes hot sauce, to taste

1½ tablespoons (25 ml) olive oil

2 shallots, diced fine

2 cloves garlic, minced

4 cups (120 g) triple-washed baby spinach or one 10-ounce (280-g) box frozen spinach, thawed and well drained**

1 cup (130–150 g) fresh or frozen peas, unthawed

Cook the gnocchi according to package directions.

* If you do not wish to use gnocchi, this dish works equally well with almost any whole-grain pasta cooked al dente.

** To drain thawed frozen spinach, as nutritious as the fresh version, press it up against the walls of a colander or, better, a double-mesh sieve to squeeze out the excess moisture.

Using a blender, immersion blender, or food processor, blend the tofu and milk until smooth and creamy. Stir in the Parmesan, zest, lemon juice, salt, pepper, and hot sauce.

Heat the oil in a large sauté pan over medium heat. Add the shallots and sauté 3 to 4 minutes until they start to become tender. Add the garlic and sauté for 1 minute. Add the spinach and sauté for 2 minutes. Add the tofu mixture and peas, stirring gently to combine thoroughly.

Reduce the heat to low and cook for 5 to 7 minutes until the peas are cooked through and (fresh) spinach is wilted.

Spoon over the gnocchi and serve.

Yield: 4 servings

Per Serving: 346 Calories; 14g Fat (34.5% calories from fat); 17g Protein; 41g Carbohydrate; 6g Dietary Fiber; 9mg Cholesterol; 755mg Sodium

FROM CHEF JEANNETTE:

This dish is a longevity adaption of a recipe concept from www.epicurious.com by Andrea Albin. Blended silken tofu makes a high quality, neutral-flavored "cream" base with enough protein to balance the carb load of pasta (but remember to always choose whole grain for a higher fiber content!).

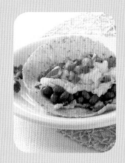

LIVER SUPPORTS

LIVE LIVER HELPER: ARTICHOKE-SPINACH DIP

From Dr. Jonny: It pretty much goes without saying that if we want to live a long time in good health, we need our liver to function properly. The poor organ is overworked—burdened by chemical overload, toxins in the environment and the food supply, pollutants in the air, and medicine in the cabinets. It just can't catch a break. Artichokes can help. Maoshing Ni, Ph.D., a renowned expert in traditional Chinese medicine, calls artichokes "your liver's best friend." Indeed. Artichoke heart extract stars in dozens of liver support formulas, largely because it contains a powerful antioxidant and live helper called *silymarin*. (Silymarin is the active ingredient in milk thistle, the number-one herb for liver support.) You can whip up this easy, no-cook dip for a tangy, fresh-tasting snack anytime, or to serve at the last minute to unexpected company.

DIP

1 bunch fresh spinach, chopped

1 ¼ cups (290 g) plain Greek yogurt

1 jar (6 ounces, or 170 g) artichoke hearts, well drained

2 cloves garlic, minced, or to taste

Juice of ½ lemon

2 teaspoons olive oil

½ teaspoon salt

Fresh-ground black pepper, to taste

CRUDITÉS

4 cups assorted raw or blanched vegetables: grape tomatoes, celery sticks, baby carrots, bell pepper strips, zucchini rounds, broccoli or cauliflower florets, endive spears, haricots verts, and so on.

In 2 batches, add the spinach and a few spoons of the yogurt to a food processor and process until finely chopped, scraping down the sides as necessary. (The yogurt will help the blades catch the spinach leaves and move them down.) Add the artichoke hearts and pulse several times until chopped. Add the remaining yogurt, garlic, lemon juice, olive oil, salt, and pepper and process until well incorporated.

Serve at room temperature with crudités.

Yield: 4 to 6 servings

Per Serving: 61 Calories; 3g Fat (42.6% calories from fat); 3g Protein; 7g Carbohydrate; 2g Dietary Fiber; 6mg Cholesterol; 231mg Sodium

FROM CHEF JEANNETTE:

Play with this basic longevity combination to make it your own, adding more or less lemon and garlic or adding additional fresh herbs or spices, such as a tablespoon (4 g) of fresh chopped dill, chives, or parsley, plus chopped scallions, hot sauce, Parmesan cheese, pesto, sun-dried tomatoes, and so on.

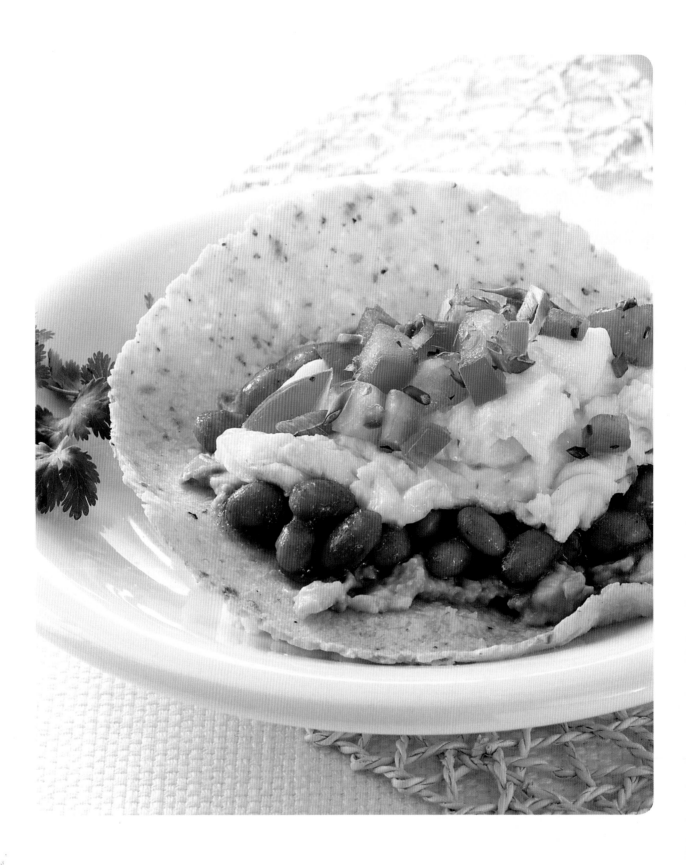

EASY, ANYTIME HUEVOS RANCHEROS

From Dr. Jonny: Nothing supports the liver like sulfur-containing compounds, and this recipe hits the trifecta—eggs, garlic, and onions. What a combo! Plus you've got iron in the blackstrap molasses (my favorite sweetener) and a ton of fiber in the beans. What's not to like? Best of all (for a bachelor like me), this dish comes together easily, but the rich layered flavors make it seem like something you slow-cooked all day long! This great dish works equally well for a nourishing breakfast, lunch, or dinner!

POWER MEXI-BEANS

1 can (15 ounces, or 425 g) kidney or pinto beans, rinsed and drained

3 tablespoons (45 ml) chicken or vegetable stock (or water)

2 tablespoons (28 ml) red wine

2 tablespoons (32 g) tomato paste

2 teaspoons (14 g) blackstrap molasses

1 to 2 cloves garlic, minced

¾ teaspoon ground cumin

1 teaspoon chili powder

¼ teaspoon salt

¼ teaspoon chipotle chile pepper, optional

SASSY HEIRLOOM SALSA

2 large Ugli tomatoes (or any large variety, preferably low-acid heirloom), finely chopped

3 tablespoons (18 g) chopped scallions

1 teaspoon to 1 tablespoon (3 to 9 g) minced jalapeño, to taste (fresh, seeded, and deveined, or jarred)

¼ cup (4 g) chopped cilantro

1 tablespoon (15 ml) fresh-squeezed lime juice

Pinch Sucanat*

¼ teaspoon salt

4 to 8 eggs

4 large sprouted corn or sprouted grain tortillas

1 Hass avocado, peeled, pitted, and mashed with a fork

For the beans: Combine all beans ingredients in a medium saucepan over medium heat and bring to a low simmer. Reduce the heat to medium low and cook, gently stirring occasionally, for 5 to 7 minutes.

Meanwhile, combine all salsa ingredients in a bowl.

Prepare the eggs any style. We like them scrambled soft for this recipe.

Warm the tortillas in a toaster oven or toast them lightly in a dry frying pan for 1 to 2 minutes per side over medium heat. Spread a thin layer of the mashed avocado on each tortilla, spoon equal portions of beans over the avocado, add the eggs, and top with the salsa.

Serve them immediately, open face, or rolled up, seam side down.

Yield: 4 wraps

Per Serving: 110 Calories; 1g Fat (4.6% calories from fat); 6g Protein; 20g Carbohydrate; 4g Dietary Fiber; trace Cholesterol; 671mg Sodium

FROM CHEF JEANNETTE:

To speed the huevos prep time, use a high-quality prepared salsa instead of making your own.

Most huevos rancheros include some type of cheese, but when you're doing any type of liver detox or support protocol, it can be helpful to avoid all but fermented dairy. The avocado more than makes up for the cheese, with a lot more fiber to boot.

* Sucanat is a form of nonrefined cane sugar. The word Sucanat is a trade name derived from "sugar cane natural". As opposed to other forms of sugar derived from the sugar cane, Sucanat retains most of the original nutrient content of the plant, including the naturally occurring molasses. It is granular in form, rather than crystalline, so has a coarser texture than traditional forms of sugar.

ASPARAGUS-POTATO SOUP—THE TOXIN TERMINATOR

From Dr. Jonny: Asparagus for a hangover? Could be. New research suggests that an extract made from the shoots and leaves of the asparagus plant increases enzymatic activity in the liver and improves the breakdown of alcohol. But even if you're a teetotaler like me, there's gold in them thar asparagus hills. The same extract was also found to reduce toxicity in human liver cells that had been exposed to hydrogen peroxide. The researchers believe their results show that *A. officinalis*—that's asparagus to us mortals— helps protect liver cells from "toxic insults." Good enough for me! The use of white potato gives this great soup its creamy texture. Rich and oniony, it works great as a lunch or dinner starter. Tip: Try it with a seafood entrée!

1 medium leek, roots and tough stalk removed

2 tablespoons (28 ml) olive oil

1 medium yellow onion, diced fine

4 cloves garlic, minced

6 cups (1.5 L) vegetable broth

½ teaspoon salt, or to taste

½ teaspoon cracked black pepper

2 pounds (900 g) Yukon Gold potatoes, peeled and cut
into small cubes*

1 pound (455 g) asparagus cut into 1-inch (2.5-cm)
pieces, woody stems removed (about 20 to 25 spears,
depending on thickness)

1 teaspoon tamari

2 tablespoons (28 ml) Marsala wine

1 tablespoon (2.4 g) minced fresh thyme

* If you'd like to keep the potato skins on for the nutrients, use
scrubbed, unpeeled, and quartered baby Yukon Gold potatoes
in place of mature peeled ones.

Cut the prepared leek in half lengthwise and then chop it into 1-inch (2.5-cm) segments. Immerse the pieces in a clean sink or large bowl of water and separate to clean completely, removing all grit. Drain, rinse, and set aside.

In a large soup pot, heat the oil over medium heat. Add the onion and sauté 1 minute.

Add the prepared leek and sauté the onion and leek until soft, about 5 minutes. Add the garlic and sauté for 1 minute. Add the broth, salt, pepper, and potatoes. Increase the heat to high and bring to a boil. Reduce the heat, cover, and keep a low boil for about 20 minutes until the potatoes are tender. Add the asparagus, tamari, wine, and thyme, and simmer on low for 5 to 10 more minutes until the asparagus is tender. Purée with an immersion wand (or, cooled, in a blender) until smooth.

Yield: 6 servings

Per Serving: 366 Calories; 8g Fat (20.9% calories from fat); 11g Protein; 61g Carbohydrate; 7g Dietary Fiber; 3mg Cholesterol; 1923mg Sodium

ROOT AND CABBAGE STEW: LONG-LIVED LIVER

From Dr. Jonny: Rutabagas are believed to be a mutation of wild cabbage and turnips, sort of a mutt, if you will, according to well-known plant and herbal expert Brigitte Mars. She calls rutabagas "liver stimulating," because they provide nutrients that the liver needs for detoxification. Kombu is a sea vegetable rich in minerals that the liver also needs to perform the myriad functions it carries out on a daily basis. And, of course, cabbage contains a wealth of nutrients, one of which provides chemicals that stimulate detoxifying pathways in the liver. Blend them together in a delicious stew such as this one, and you've got a supper that supports liver function. On a personal note, one thing I particularly love about meals such as this is that they are easy on my blood sugar. A stew like this satisfies for a long time without putting you in the kind of blood sugar hell that creates cravings and overeating. This is a hearty, creamy stew with an eastern European feeling. Tip: It's even better the next day!

2-inch (5-cm) piece kombu

2 tablespoons (28 ml) olive oil

1 large onion, chopped

2 cloves garlic, minced

1 celery rib, sliced

2 carrots, peeled and sliced on the bias
(½ inch, or 1 cm thick)

1 medium rutabaga, peeled and diced (or yellow turnip)

½ green cabbage, cut in half lengthwise and sliced into thin ribbons

6 cups (1.5 L) vegetable or chicken broth + more broth or water, if necessary

2 tablespoons (28 ml) tamari

1 tablespoon (15 ml) apple cider vinegar

½ teaspoon salt

½ teaspoon tarragon

½ teaspoon cracked black pepper

¾ cup (150 g) hato mugi (Job's Tears) or use quick-cooking barley*

1 can (15 ounces, or 425 g) garbanzo beans, drained and rinsed

In a small bowl, soak the kombu for 10 minutes in just enough water to cover.

In a large soup pot heat the oil over medium. Add the onion and sauté 5 minutes.

Add the garlic and sauté 1 minute. Add the celery, carrots, and rutabaga and cook for 2 minutes, stirring frequently. Add the cabbage and stir to combine. Pour the broth over all to cover generously. Add the tamari, vinegar, salt, tarragon, and pepper, and mix well. Add the hato mugi, stir gently, and bring to a boil. Add the garbanzos, reduce heat, cover, and simmer for 30 to 40 minutes or until all veggies and hato mugi are tender.

When the kombu is soft (after 10 minutes soaking), pour the soaking water into the stew, dice the kombu finely, and add to the stew. Check the stew occasionally for liquid level, adding more broth or water if needed to cover.

Yield: 6 to 8 servings

Per Serving: 389 Calories; 9g Fat (19.8% calories from fat); 16g Protein; 64g Carbohydrate; 14g Dietary Fiber; 2mg Cholesterol; 1341mg Sodium

* Hato mugi is an Asian heirloom grain that looks like barley on steroids. Unlike barley, it is totally gluten free. It has a soft, chewy texture and is easy to digest. In the macrobiotic world, it is considered to be a mild detoxifier. Look for it in Asian markets (it is also called Job's Tears and yimi in Chinese). I add it to brown rice for added texture. If you can't find it, in this recipe you can substitute quick-cooking pearl barley. Add it for the last 15 to 20 minutes of simmer time.

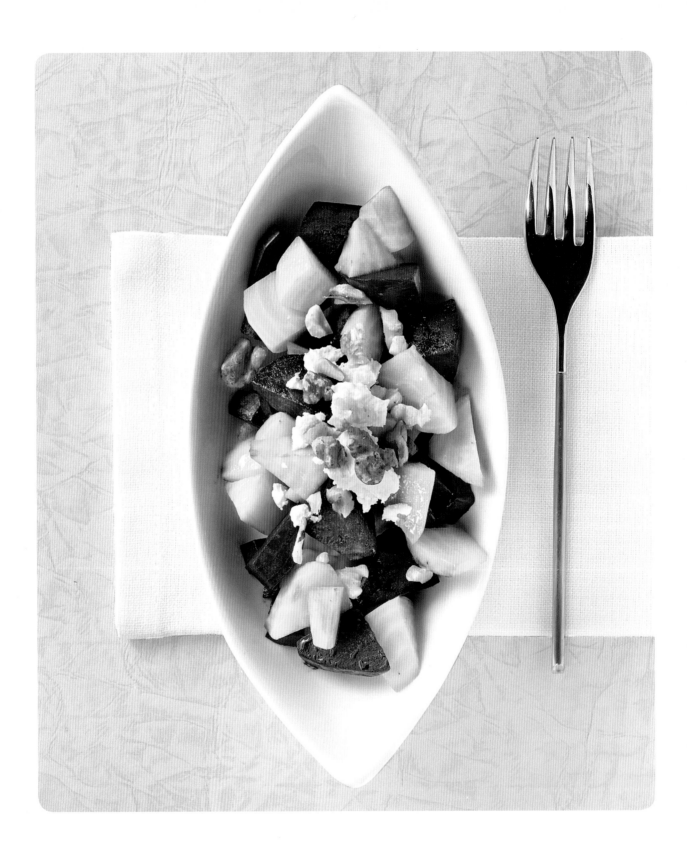

UNBEATABLE ROASTED BEETS WITH GOAT CHEESE

From Dr. Jonny: Goat cheese is one of my favorite cheeses and a terrific source of all those amino acids your liver needs to properly function. Amino acids are needed specifically to make the detoxification pathways work right; they nourish and stimulate the phase 2 detoxification enzymes that help your body get rid of metabolic garbage, such as toxins and chemicals. And the light, tangy taste of goat cheese perfectly complements the sweet taste of the beets (also a great liver tonifier!). Don't freak out if you eat too much of this dish and your pee turns red—you're not dying. It's a scary but harmless side effect of the beet's natural pigmentation.

6 small or 4 medium red or yellow beets, peeled, ends trimmed

3 tablespoons (45 ml) olive oil, divided

Sprinkle salt

2 tablespoons (28 ml) walnut oil

2 tablespoons (28 ml) balsamic vinegar

1 teaspoon Dijon mustard

1 teaspoon finely minced shallot

½ teaspoon orange zest, optional

Salt, to taste

Fresh-ground black pepper, to taste

¼ cup (38 g) chèvre

⅓ cup (40 g) coarsely chopped toasted walnuts

Preheat the oven to 400°F (200°C, or gas mark 6).

Drizzle the beets with 1 tablespoon (15 ml) olive oil and sprinkle with salt. Place whole in a roasting pan and roast for 25 to 35 minutes or until fork tender (cooking time depends on the size of the beets).

At the end of the cooking time, in a small bowl whisk together the walnut oil, remaining 2 tablespoons (28 ml) olive oil, vinegar, mustard, shallot, zest, if using, salt, and pepper (or you can use an immersion blender).

Quarter the cooked beets and stack in a pile on a shallow plate. Spoon the chèvre into the middle, dress to taste, and top with walnuts.

Yield: 4 servings

Per Serving: 262 Calories; 24g Fat (78.0% calories from fat); 5g Protein; 10g Carbohydrate; 3g Dietary Fiber; 3mg Cholesterol; 106mg Sodium

FROM CHEF JEANNETTE:

If they are in season, look for beets with the nutritious greens still attached and add them to the dish. Remove from the roots, clean, chop, and steam or sauté them lightly in a little olive oil. Make a bed of the hot greens under your beets.

Also, to make peeling easier you can steam-roast unpeeled beets by adding a small amount of water to the roasting pan or sealing the pan tightly with aluminum foil. Once they are slightly cooled, just slip the skins off with your fingers. But watch out, the juice stains!

CHOCO-BANANA CREAM DREAM

From Dr. Jonny: Nutritional yeast is the deactivated form of the yeast *Saccharomyces cerevisiae*. (I know, you really needed to know that, didn't you?) It's got eighteen amino acids and about fifteen different minerals in it and has long been believed to improve liver health and function. Meanwhile, whey protein remains one of the most absorbable and high-quality protein sources around, providing its own array of liver-supporting amino acids as well. The omega-3s in flaxseed are anti-inflammatory and the coconut milk, one of my faves, gives it a creamy, decadent feel. Want to bump up that hint of coconut? Try throwing in a couple of tablespoons (about 9 g) of dried coconut as well!

3 cups (710 ml) milk (cow's, unsweetened vanilla almond, or soy)

⅔ cup (160 ml) light coconut milk (or regular)

2 large frozen bananas

⅓ cup (40 g) whey protein powder

¼ cup (32 g) nutritional yeast, or to taste

3 tablespoons (15 g) raw cacao powder (or 2½ tablespoons [12 g] cocoa or carob powder)

3 tablespoons (20 g) ground flaxseed (or wheat germ or oat bran)

½ teaspoon ground cinnamon

¼ teaspoon ground nutmeg

Ice cubes, to taste

Honey or stevia drops, to taste, optional

Add all ingredients to a blender and blend until smooth.

Yield: 4 servings

Per Serving: 295 Calories; 11g Fat (32.0% calories from fat); 22g Protein; 31g Carbohydrate; 6g Dietary Fiber; 26mg Cholesterol; 161mg Sodium

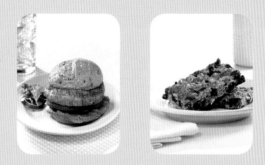

FIBER BLAST

. . . .

Get-Up-and-Go-the-Distance Banana Breakfast Bars
Liver-Loving Nutty Butter Drops
Fiber-Rich Bulgur-Bean Salad with Crunch
Autumnal Fruit, Fiber, and Nut Crumble
Toxin Timeout: BBQ Bean Burgers

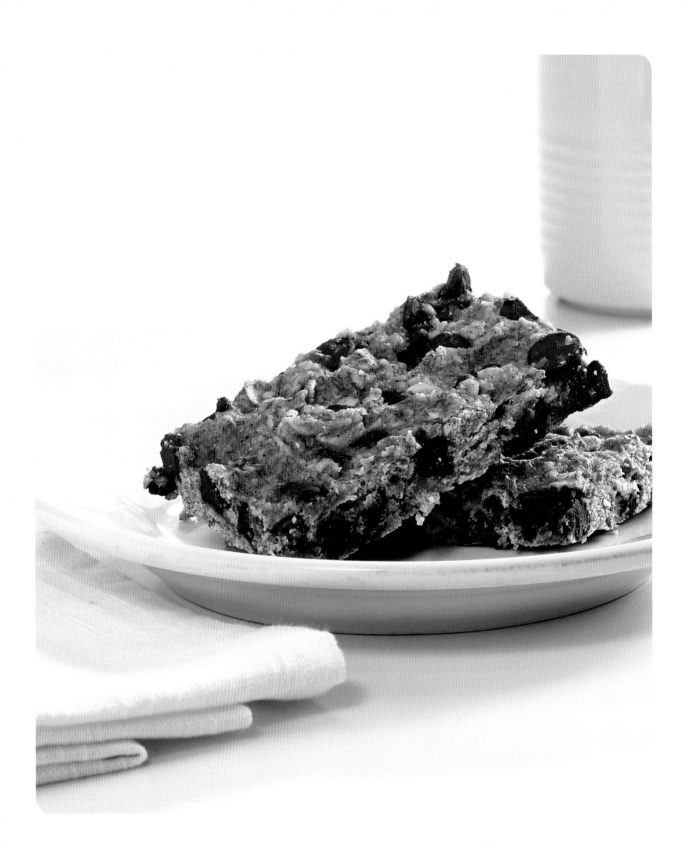

ANTIOXIDANTS

GET-UP-AND-GO-THE-DISTANCE BANANA BREAKFAST BARS

From Dr. Jonny: The first thing to notice about this breakfast bar is what's missing: flour! The second thing to notice is the taste! This bar is healthier than anything you're likely to find at the store, with twice the nutrition and none of the artificial ingredients or hidden trans fats that so often wind up in commercial energy bars. There's not a life-shortening ingredient in this baby, and it still tastes terrific. I still don't know how Chef Jeannette manages to make anything this delicious without any of the traditional ingredients such as flour and sugar, but here it is. These bars are loaded with potassium, they have no added sweetener, they've got protein, and they're high in fiber. Beats any breakfast bar I've ever seen in the store!

Cooking oil spray

3 large ripe bananas

1 teaspoon vanilla extract

¼ cup (60 ml) coconut oil, melted

¾ cup (96 g) whey protein powder

2 cups (160 g) rolled oats

¼ cup (25 g) oat bran

¼ cup (25 g) ground flaxseed

¼ cup (30 g) almond meal (ground almonds or "almond flour")

1 teaspoon baking powder

1 teaspoon ground cinnamon

½ teaspoon ground nutmeg

½ teaspoon salt

1 cup (175 g) dark chocolate chips, preferably grain sweetened

Preheat the oven to 350°F (180°C, or gas mark 4). Lightly coat a 9 x 13-inch (23 x 33-cm) pan with cooking oil spray (glass works well).

In a large bowl, mash the bananas with a fork until they form a smooth paste. Add the vanilla and oil and mix until well combined.

In a separate bowl, whisk together the protein powder, oats, oat bran, flaxseed, almond meal, baking powder, cinnamon, nutmeg, and salt.

Pour the dry ingredients into the wet and stir until well combined. Fold in the chocolate chips.

Scoop the mixture into a prepared pan and flatten it evenly (wet or oiled fingers work best for this).

Bake for about 25 minutes or until the edges are lightly browned. Remove from the oven and immediately make 6 even cuts across the pan (short way) and 2 even cuts the long way to create 21 bars. Allow to cool and solidify in the pan for at least 10 minutes before removing.

Yield: 21 bars

Per Serving: 142 Calories; 7g Fat (40.4% calories from fat); 7g Protein; 16g Carbohydrate; 2g Dietary Fiber; trace Cholesterol; 103mg Sodium

FROM CHEF JEANNETTE:

If the chocolate is a bit much for you at breakfast time, try substituting ¾ cup dried berries for the chips. Either makes a great flourless high-fiber, high-protein bar.

LIVER-LOVING NUTTY BUTTER DROPS

From Dr. Jonny: Quick, name a treat that has protein, fiber, healthy fat, and an all-star collection of liver-friendly nutrients—but tastes like cookie dough. Give up? Look below. These delicious nutty, buttery drops will have you fighting over who gets to lick the bowl. Raw almond butter, macadamia nuts, and walnuts provide an outstanding selection of liver-friendly minerals, the flaxseed adds lignans and fiber, and the whey powder gives you a nice dose of protein. Cherries and blueberries—my two favorite fruits—add anti-inflammatory agents and a ton of nutrients, not to mention great taste. Best of all these nutty treats are a cinch to whip up on a moment's notice!

²/₃ cup (173 g) raw almond butter

¼ cup (85 g) raw honey

½ teaspoon vanilla

²/₃ cup (80 g) vanilla whey protein powder (you can substitute hemp protein powder, but hemp has a strong taste and heavy texture, so make sure you like it before making a big batch!)

¹/₃ cup (45 g) macadamia nuts, raw or roasted, crushed

¼ cup (30 g) walnut pieces, raw or roasted, crushed (or pistachio meats, crushed)

2 tablespoons (13 g) ground flaxseed

2 tablespoons (16 g) raw or toasted sesame seeds

1 ½ cups (90 g) dry cereal (unsweetened, whole-grain "rice crispy"-style cereal or any unsweetened, whole-grain corn or fiber flakes cereal)

¼ cup (31 g) dried cherries

¼ cup (38 g) dried blueberries

¾ teaspoon ground cinnamon

Add all ingredients to a food processor and pulse about 20 times, frequently scraping down the sides, and then process steadily for 30 to 45 seconds or until mixture forms a cohesive "dough." Leave the dough in the food processor for about 15 minutes to give the ingredients time to meld. Press and roll the mixture into inch (2.5 cm)-size balls and store in the refrigerator or freezer. When packing for refrigeration, avoid crowding or balls will stick together. Use sheets of parchment paper to separate layers.

Yield: about 35 drops

Per Serving: 83 Calories; 5g Fat (49.1% calories from fat); 4g Protein; 8g Carbohydrate; 1g Dietary Fiber; trace Cholesterol; 42mg Sodium

FROM CHEF JEANNETTE:

To prevent sticking and for extra nutrients, you can roll the balls in toasted and crushed nuts or seeds of your choice, or in unsweetened cocoa or raw cacao powder.

FIBER-RICH BULGUR-BEAN SALAD WITH CRUNCH

From Dr. Jonny: It's hard to overstate the importance of fiber to the liver. Here's why: Let's say your liver wants to get rid of a toxin. First thing it does is dump it into the digestive tract. If there's enough fiber hanging around, the toxin takes the "A" train right out of the body during your next trip to the bathroom. But what if there's not enough fiber around? Well then, Houston, we have a problem. Without transportation, the toxins will have to be reabsorbed into the bloodstream, where eventually the poor liver will once again have to deal with them. This is probably one reason why traditional folk wisdom has always relied on high-fiber vegetables and fruits for liver-cleansing diets. And nothing provides fiber better than beans, unless perhaps it's a whole grain such as bulgur wheat. Or even corn. Put them all together and you give your liver some real ammunition when it comes to dealing with the molecules that have no business hanging around your body. Bonus points: Bulgur is a simple grain to prepare! And if you have the time to leave it in the fridge to marinate overnight, you'll be rewarded with a particularly rich and satisfying blend of flavors.

---

2 cups (475 ml) vegetable broth

1 cup (140 g) bulgur (fine or medium grind)

1½ cups (150 g) lightly blanched green beans, cut into ½-inch (1-cm) pieces*

1 cup (130 g) crisp corn, fresh, steamed, and cut from the cob (or frozen, thawed)

¾ cup (75 g) scallions, sliced thin

3 plum tomatoes, seeded and diced

¼ cup (15 g) chopped parsley

1 teaspoon lemon zest

1½ tablespoons (25 ml) fresh-squeezed lemon juice, or more, to taste

1 to 2 cloves garlic, finely minced, to taste

½ teaspoon mustard powder

¼ teaspoon salt, or to taste

Pinch Sucanat

1 tablespoon (15 ml) high-lignan flaxseed oil (such as Barlean's)

1 tablespoon (15 ml) olive oil

½ cup (55 g) sliced toasted almonds (or coarsely chopped walnuts [60 g])

Bring the broth to a boil and pour over the bulgur. Soak 7 minutes for fine grind and 15 for medium grind, and drain excess liquid (or follow package directions for cooking). In a large bowl, gently mix together the bulgur, green beans, corn, scallions, tomatoes, and parsley.

In a small bowl, whisk together the zest, lemon juice, garlic, mustard powder, salt, Sucanat, flaxseed oil, and olive oil. Pour the dressing over all and chill in the fridge for at least 1 hour to overnight to allow the flavors to combine. Toss with nuts just before serving.

Yield: about 4 servings

* To blanch beans, place them (stemmed and whole) into a large pan of boiling salted water for 1 to 2 minutes or until bright green and tender-crisp. Drain and plunge into a large bowl of ice water for a couple of minutes to stop the cooking process. Drain and cut to size.

FROM CHEF JEANNETTE:

To make this recipe a meal and for additional, liver-friendly fiber, add 1 can (15 ounces, or 425 g) of drained and rinsed garbanzo beans. (Garbanzos have 12.5 grams of fiber per cup!)

To refresh leftovers the next day, add a few squeezes of fresh lemon juice before serving.

If you have a wheat or gluten issue, make this dish with 2 cups (370 g) of cooked quinoa.

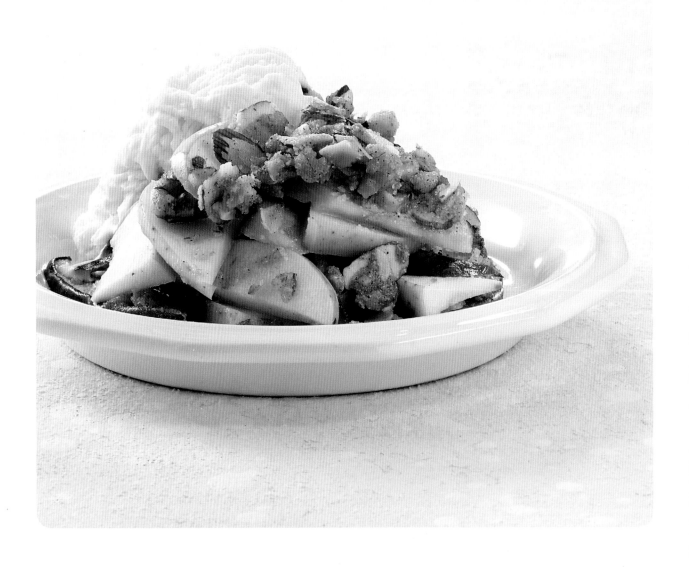

AUTUMNAL FRUIT, FIBER, AND NUT CRUMBLE

From Dr. Jonny: Next time anyone tells you that healthy food doesn't taste great, whip them up one of these babies. You'll think it's dessert. Which, come to think of it, it is, except it's life extending instead of life shortening. You've got fiber from the oats, nuts, apples, and pears, not to mention a panoply of antioxidants and phytochemicals from the fruit. Jeannette used the best "starch" I know of—kudzu—which contains important isoflavones that are anti-inflammatory and antimicrobial. And man, does this dish smell great in the oven! (Hint: Bake it up whenever you need to sell your house!) Bonus: It tastes absolutely great the next day. Trust me, I know.

Cooking oil spray

FILLING

½ cup (120 ml) apple juice concentrate, melted

2 teaspoons kudzu

½ teaspoon vanilla

1 tablespoon (6 g) minced ginger

1 tablespoon (15 ml) fresh-squeezed lemon juice

Zest of 1 lemon

3 large baking apples (Mutsu*, Golden Delicious, or
   Cortland all work well), cored and chopped, unpeeled

3 large pears (Bosc or Bartlett work well), cored and
   chopped, unpeeled

TOPPING

1 cup (110 g) sliced almonds or pecans (110 g)

1 cup (120 g) walnuts, coarsely chopped

1½ cups (120 g) rolled oats (not instant)

½ cup (59 g) brown rice flour (or whole wheat pastry
   flour)

½ teaspoon ground cinnamon

¾ teaspoon ground ginger

⅓ cup (78 ml) maple syrup

⅓ cup (80 ml) almond or walnut oil (refined for medium
   heat)

½ teaspoon vanilla extract

Preheat the oven to 350°F (180°C, or gas mark 4).
Lightly coat an 9 x 13-inch (23 x 33-cm) baking pan with
cooking oil spray.

In a large bowl, whisk together the juice concentrate,
kudzu, vanilla, ginger, lemon juice, and zest until the
kudzu dissolves. Add the sliced apples and pears and
gently stir to coat. Pour into the prepared baking pan.

In a medium bowl, mix together the nuts, oats, flour,
cinnamon, ginger, syrup, oil, and vanilla extract until
it forms a crumbly mixture. Spoon the topping evenly
over the fruit and cover with foil. Bake for 25 minutes,
remove the foil, and continue baking, uncovered, for
another 10 to 15 minutes or until the fruit is soft and
bubbly and the topping just begins to brown.

Yield: about 9–12 servings

Per Serving: 372 Calories; 20g Fat (50.8% calories from
fat); 8g Protein; 37g Carbohydrate; 5g Dietary Fiber;
0mg Cholesterol; 5mg Sodium

* Mutsu apples are also known as Crispin apples.

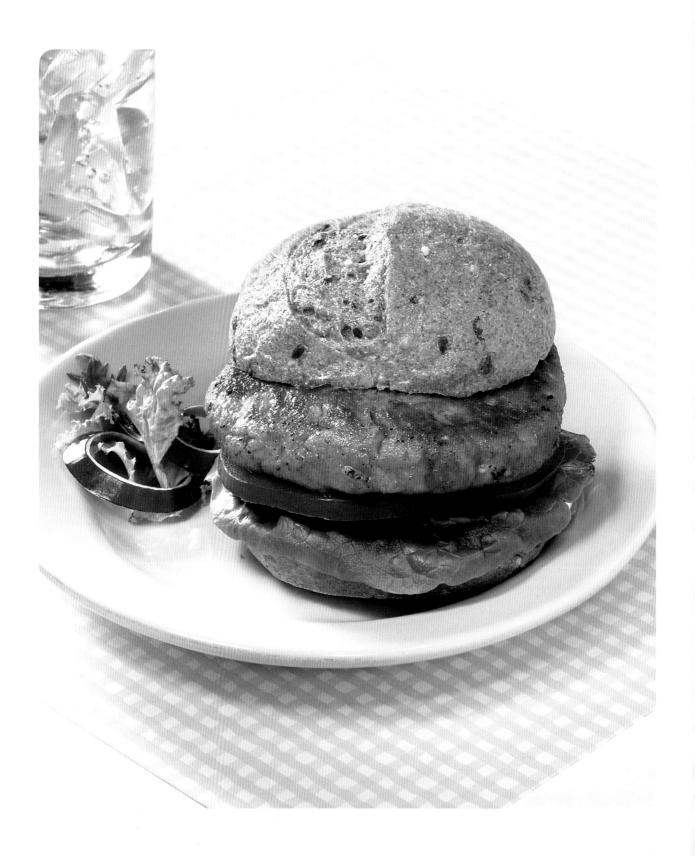

TOXIN TIMEOUT: BBQ BEAN BURGERS

From Dr. Jonny: To really give your liver a much-needed rest from toxins, skip the commercial, supermarket meat and try this fiber-rich bean burger instead. The pintos and oats (there's an unusual combo!) are loaded with fiber, the carrots and tomatoes are loaded with antioxidants, and the whole dish is loaded with flavor. The spicy, tangy barbecue flavor will make you forget all about the local rib joint, where I guarantee you they don't serve grass-fed meat. Come to think of it, these "burgers" will make you forget Mickey D's!

Olive oil cooking spray

1 tablespoon (15 ml) olive oil

1 small sweet onion, diced

2 cloves garlic, minced

½ cup (55 g) grated carrots

2 cans (15 ounces, or 425 g, each) pinto beans, drained and rinsed

1 tablespoon (16 g) tomato paste

2 tablespoons (30 g) tomato sauce or high-quality, low-sugar ketchup

1 ½ tablespoons (25 ml) apple cider vinegar

1 tablespoon (15 ml) Worcestershire sauce

1 teaspoon molasses

1 teaspoon prepared horseradish

1 teaspoon Dijon mustard

1 teaspoon soy sauce

½ teaspoon cracked black pepper

¼ teaspoon cayenne or chipotle pepper

½ teaspoon salt

1½ cups (120 g) whole rolled oats

Heat the oil over medium heat in a medium sauté pan. Add the onion and sauté for 5 minutes.

Add the garlic and sauté for 2 minutes. Add the carrots and sauté for 5 minutes, stirring frequently to prevent burning or sticking. Remove from the heat and set aside.

Partially mash the beans with a potato masher or fork in a mixer bowl.* Add the tomato paste, sauce, vinegar,

Worcestershire sauce, molasses, horseradish, mustard, soy sauce, peppers, and salt. Mix on low until a paste begins to form, then switch to high and mix until most of the beans are mashed and incorporated, scraping down the sides frequently, about 20 seconds, off and on. Add the sautéed onion and carrot and mix briefly until well incorporated. Add the oats and mix briefly until well incorporated.

Form into 6 even patties.

Heat a large frying pan or griddle over medium-low heat and liberally spray with olive oil. Fry the patties for 8 to 10 minutes per side until they develop a lightly browned "crust" on each side.

Yield: 6 patties

Per Serving: 231 Calories; 4g Fat (15.7% calories from fat); 10g Protein; 40g Carbohydrate; 8g Dietary Fiber; 0mg Cholesterol; 917mg Sodium

FROM CHEF JEANNETTE:

You can serve these burgers the usual way—with a pile of lettuce, tomato, and a pickle on a sprouted-grain bun or wrap, or break them up and serve them over salad. They taste great with Dijon mustard, ketchup or barbecue sauce. My husband likes them with a thin slice of smoked Cheddar cheese, but that does add a little saturated fat.

If you want to sweeten them up, try adding ⅓ cup (55 g) thawed frozen corn to the onion/carrot mixture 1 minute before the end of the carrot cooking time.

*If you have a wimpy mixer, it would be better to use a potato masher and do all the mashing and mixing by hand. You don't want to have to overbeat the mix to get the beans to break their skins and form a paste or the patties will seem a little dry.

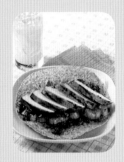

LEAN PROTEINS

· ·

Pure, Protein-Packed Citrus-Mint Grilled Lamb Chops
Grilled Chicken, Tomato, and Pesto Sandwich
Turbocharging Tahini Miso Chicken Salad

PURE, PROTEIN-PACKED CITRUS-MINT GRILLED LAMB CHOPS

From Dr. Jonny: Okay, honestly, when it comes to lamb (and deer) I admit to being more than a little sentimental. But the truth is lamb meat is rarely filled with as much junk (steroids, antibiotics, and hormones) as factory-farmed supermarket meat, is almost always grass-fed, and is a lot better for you. Of all the meats, lamb is one of the highest in omega-3 fatty acids, which benefit you in more ways than I can count. These chops are moist and flavorful. Your mouth will literally water when you smell them grilling. Tip: Like any meat or fish, they shouldn't be grilled on superhigh flames. Those flames look pretty, but they create bad carcinogenic compounds such as *heterocyclic amines*, which you don't want in your body—at least not if you want to live a long time. Keep the flame low, savor the smell, and enjoy the rich taste.

---

3 tablespoons (45 ml) olive oil

¼ cup (60 ml) low-sodium tamari

Juice of 1 lemon

3 cloves garlic, minced

Fresh rosemary leaves from 4 to 5 stalks chopped (about ¼ cup, or 7 g, once stripped)

Fresh thyme leaves from 5 to 6 stalks (about 3 tablespoons, or 7 g, once stripped)

⅓ cup (30 g) mint leaves, chopped

¾ teaspoon salt

1 teaspoon fresh-ground black pepper

4 lamb blade chops (or 8 lamb loin chops)*

In a small bowl, whisk together the olive oil, tamari, and lemon juice. Add the garlic, rosemary, thyme, mint, salt, and pepper and mix thoroughly.

Lay the lamb chops flat in a shallow glass baking dish and pour the marinade over the chops. Cover and marinate for 30 minutes to overnight, flipping several times.

Grill the chops over medium heat for about for 6 to 7 minutes, flip, and grill for 4 to 5 minutes more for medium rare or to desired doneness.

Yield: 4 chops

Per Serving: 88 Calories; 7g Fat (74.2% calories from fat); 5g Protein; 1g Carbohydrate; trace Dietary Fiber; 20mg Cholesterol; 144mg Sodium

* Although loin chops are the leanest cuts of lamb, they are also the priciest. The blade cut, significantly cheaper, is only slightly higher in fat and is very flavorful and tender.

FROM CHEF JEANNETTE:

Try serving hot chops with a sprinkling of feta cheese or a bit of mint jam and rosemary-roasted sweet potatoes. You can double this recipe and slice the other half for cold lamb salad the next day.

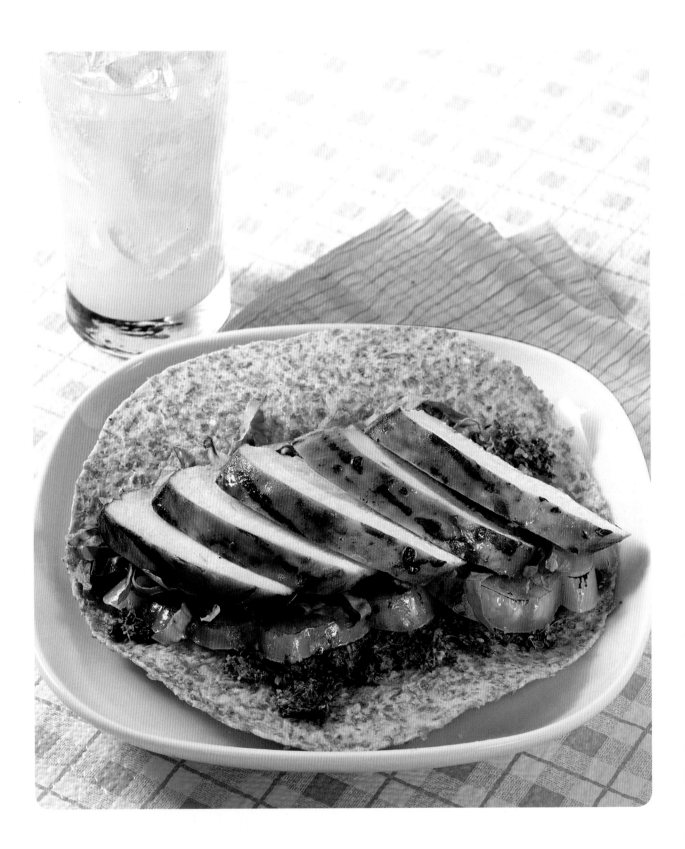

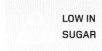
GRILLED CHICKEN, TOMATO, AND PESTO SANDWICH

From Dr. Jonny: I love this "sandwich" as the perfect longevity substitute for traditional fast food fare. It's rich and decadent tasting. Unlike the typical fast food sandwich, the flavor doesn't come from cheap mayonnaise. Replacing the mayo is scrumptious pesto, with unsaturated fat filling in for the usual saturated kind. The mix of honey, macadamia nuts, cilantro, and tomatoes is a genius touch.

CHICKEN

¼ cup (60 ml) fresh-squeezed lime juice

2 tablespoons (30 ml) olive oil

4 cloves garlic, minced

1 tablespoon (20 g) honey

1 teaspoon soy sauce

4 skinless, boneless chicken breast halves (or, for a faster, vegan option, substitute 4 Naked "Chicken" Breasts by Quorn*)

CILANTRO PESTO

1 bunch cilantro, chopped, tougher stems removed

¼ cup (34 g) dry-roasted macadamia nuts or toasted pine nuts (35 g)

1 tablespoon (15 ml) fresh-squeezed lime juice

3 tablespoons (45 ml) olive oil

¼ teaspoon salt

SANDWICH

2 large sliced heirloom tomatoes, roasted (or fresh)**

4 large leaves romaine lettuce, chopped

4 large sprouted grain wraps, warmed or toasted, if desired

Prepare the chicken: In a small bowl, whisk together the lime juice, olive oil, garlic, honey, and soy sauce.

Rinse the chicken and pat dry. Pound each breast to an even thickness, about ½ inch (1 cm). Lay the prepared breasts flat in a pie plate or shallow glass baking pan. Pour the marinade over all and flip the chicken breasts to coat all sides. Cover and marinate for 30 minutes to overnight, turning occasionally.

Make the pesto: In the meantime, prepare the pesto. Add all ingredients to a food processor and process, scraping sides down frequently, until smooth. Drizzle a small amount of extra olive oil if the mixture seems too dry.

Make the sandwich: Preheat the grill to medium.

Grill the breasts for about 6 minutes per side or until cooked through (no pink remaining).

To assemble the sandwiches, slice the grilled breasts on the bias. Spread a generous smear of pesto on each wrap and top with ¼ of the roasted tomatoes. Lay the chopped romaine over the tomatoes and top each with 1 sliced chicken breast. Roll up and serve.

Yield: 4 wraps

Per Serving: 456 Calories; 20g Fat (39.8% calories from fat); 35g Protein; 35g Carbohydrate; 6g Dietary Fiber; 68mg Cholesterol; 377mg Sodium

* To prepare the vegan "chicken" cutlets, place 1 tablespoon (15 ml) olive oil in large skillet and sauté frozen breasts over medium heat for 10 to 12 minutes until lightly browned, flipping as needed. Do not marinate.

** Roasting tomatoes deepens their flavor and brings out extra natural sweetness. If they are in season, choose a large beefy variety. We like heirloom tomatoes because they are less acidic and richer in flavor and nutrients than conventional varieties. But if tomatoes are not in season, look for the Campari variety. They are smaller, so you'll need 7 or 8, but they hold their flavor well, even during colder months.

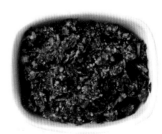

TURBOCHARGING TAHINI MISO CHICKEN SALAD

From Dr. Jonny: I admit it—I'm partial to tahini. If you don't share my love for tahini you may find that you've changed your mind after you taste this incredible chicken salad. Fermented miso, rich in probiotics, coupled with lean protein and cruciferous vegetables, makes this a complete treat for your liver, not to mention your taste buds. The cruciferous vegetables provide superstar antioxidants such as *sulforaphane*, which actually turbocharge the liver's production of detoxifying enzymes, which in turn help your body get rid of carcinogens and other junk! And new research suggests that probiotics may also help fight nonalcoholic fatty liver disease. The toasted sesame seeds and almonds give this nutty, sweet, and salty salad a nice added crunch.

¼ cup (60 g) tahini

¼ cup (60 ml) water

2 tablespoons (32 g) mellow or sweet white miso

1 clove minced garlic

1 teaspoon low-sodium tamari

Pinch cayenne pepper, optional

2 poached skinless, boneless chicken breast halves

⅓ cup (37 g) toasted sliced almonds

2 lightly steamed broccoli crowns, stemmed and cut into bite-size florets

1 small red or yellow bell pepper, seeded and julienne cut

½ cup (55 g) grated carrots

4 cups (360 g) julienned Napa cabbage

1 teaspoon toasted sesame seeds, optional garnish

FROM CHEF JEANNETTE:

Poaching chicken is a healthy, easy way to cook a lean protein that you can batch and use in many different ways. No additional fat or calories are added during the poaching process. Poached chicken is moist and delicious as is, or as an addition to soups, salads, or sandwiches such as this one. To poach 4 skinless, boneless breast halves (about 2 pounds, or 900 g), place them in a medium saucepan over medium-high heat with 3 to 4 cups (710 to 950 ml) of low-sodium chicken broth (to cover), 2 chopped shallots (or half a sweet onion, chopped), a small chopped carrot, a chopped stalk of celery, a bay leaf, and a few grinds of black pepper, to taste. Once the broth begins to boil, reduce the heat and simmer, covered, for 10 minutes. Without uncovering, remove the pan from the heat and set on a cold burner for 30 minutes. Remove the chicken breasts from the mixture, drain well, and they are ready for use.

Thoroughly blend the tahini, water, miso, garlic, and cayenne, if using, in blender, food processor, or, best, in a small bowl with an immersion blender.

Shred or chop the chicken. In a large bowl combine the chicken, almonds, broccoli, julienned pepper, and carrots. Spoon the dressing over and toss to coat all.

Make a bed of julienned cabbage and spoon the chicken salad into the center.

Top with sesame seeds, if using.

Yield: 4 servings

Per Serving: 346 Calories; 15g Fat (36.7% calories from fat); 30g Protein; 30g Carbohydrate; 14g Dietary Fiber; 34mg Cholesterol; 494mg Sodium

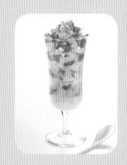

PROBIOTICS

· ·

Tropical Superfruit Parfait
Kickin' Kimchi
Healing Miso–Tahini Spread
Cold Broccoli Salad with Probiotic Dressing

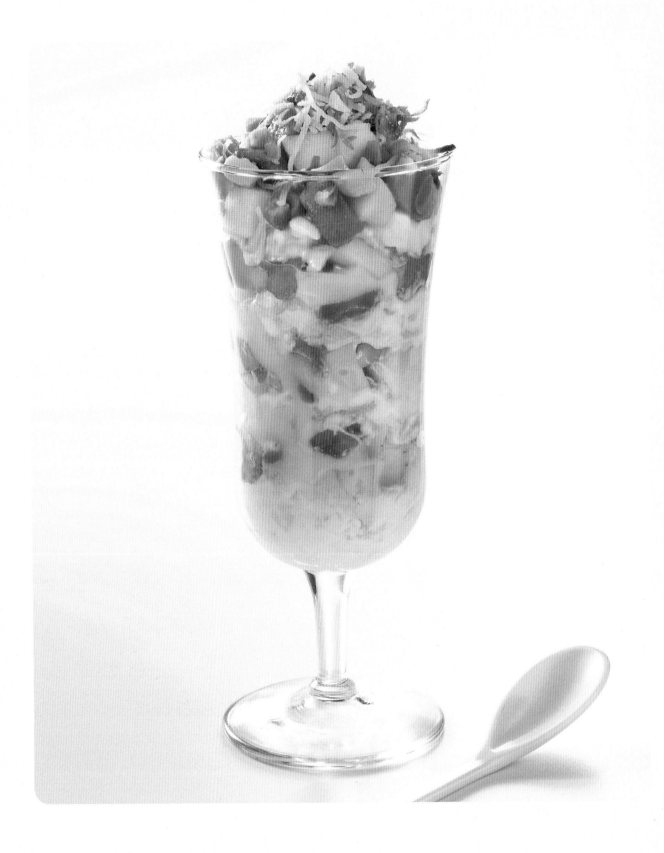

TROPICAL SUPERFRUIT PARFAIT

From Dr. Jonny: You can do a heck of a lot of detoxing naturally by simply giving your liver a ton of nutrients from whole foods, which help it do its primary job of getting rid of riffraff. Compare this tropical blend of fruits, Greek yogurt, whey protein powder, and nuts to the typical life-shortening, empty calorie–laden dessert parfait. No contest, baby! You've got healthy fat and fiber, protein, lots of calcium, and a ton of vitamins A and C. Bonus: A great way to get guava—one of the best-kept secrets in the superfood kingdom—into your diet. (And what makes guava such a superfood, you might ask? Simple: It's high in fiber, vitamin C, vitamin A, and potassium and ridiculously low in calories!) This fabulously luxurious parfait would be right at home on the table at my favorite breakfast restaurant on the beach in St. Martin!

---

1 can (8 ounces, or 225 g) crushed pineapple in water or juice, drained, ¼ cup (60 ml) juice reserved

1 teaspoon orange zest, divided

¼ cup (60 ml) fresh-squeezed orange juice

1 teaspoon lime zest, divided

Juice of 1 lime

1 ripe mango, peeled, pitted, and sliced or cubed (small)

1 small ripe papaya, peeled, seeded, and sliced or cubed (small)

1 ripe guava, peeled, seeded, and sliced (or substitute banana or avocado) or cubed (small)

1 cup (230 g) high-quality plain Greek yogurt (or substitute plain goat, sheep, or soy yogurt)

1 cup (225 g) cottage cheese

¼ cup (32 g) plain or vanilla whey protein powder

1 teaspoon honey, to taste (or a few drops of stevia)

½ teaspoon coconut extract (or orange or vanilla)

SPRINKLES

¼ cup (34 g) roasted macadamia nuts, crushed

2 tablespoons (12 g) toasted coconut

In a medium bowl, whisk together the pineapple juice, ½ teaspoon orange zest, orange juice, ½ teaspoon lime zest, and lime juice. Add prepared fruit slices and toss gently to coat.

Scoop the yogurt into a medium bowl and fold in the drained pineapple, remaining orange and lime zests, cottage cheese, protein powder, honey, and extract, stirring to combine well.

Drain the fruit and build parfaits in 4 parfait glasses (or any tall clear glass) in 4 layers (or 6 if the glasses are very narrow), starting with the yogurt in the bottom of the glass and ending with the fruit and sprinkles of macadamia and coconut on top.

Yield: 4 parfaits

Per Serving: 301 Calories; 11g Fat (31.9% calories from fat); 19g Protein; 35g Carbohydrate; 5g Dietary Fiber; 13mg Cholesterol; 309mg Sodium

FROM CHEF JEANNETTE:

Avocado in a parfait? Might sound weird, but avocado is actually a tropical fruit, not a true veggie. Its creamy texture complements the sweeter fruits and adds a big blast of fiber (about 13 grams in each one!), key to a liver cleanse.

Greek yogurt is strained yogurt with a thicker, stiffer consistency than traditional yogurt. It is rich and creamy and usually has a higher protein content. Adding the whey and cottage cheese increases that protein content even more. To prepare a mango, peel it first, then slice away the chubby "cheeks" of the fruit from the pit. The papaya I prefer to split first, scoop out the seeds with a spoon, and then peel each half with long strokes on the peeler.

KICKIN' KIMCHI

From Dr. Jonny: I gave the traditional Korean dish kimchi a star in my book *The 150 Healthiest Foods on Earth*. Want to know why? Let's start with what it's made from. The most common ingredients are cabbage, onions, garlic, and seafood—all superfoods. Also, kimchi is always, repeat, *always*, fermented. Almost all natural fermented foods are health-promoting because they create healthy bacteria that not only support immunity but are terrific nourishment for the liver, helping it to perform its detoxifying functions. One recent study that looked at the livers of alcoholics found that giving them probiotic supplements for a mere five days significantly improved their liver function. They can do the same for the liver of a nonalcoholic. Kimchi is a also great source of probiotics. Verdict: Kimchi is truly one of the healthiest longevity foods.

6 cups (1.5 L) water

3 tablespoons (57 g) sea salt (avoid table salt)*

1 large Napa cabbage (about 2 pounds, or 900 g), cored and quartered

1 small bunch scallions (about 8), halved lengthwise and sliced into 1-inch (2.5-cm) pieces

¾ cup (87 g) peeled and julienned daikon radish, optional (or ½ cup [58 g] grated)

1 cup (130 g) peeled and julienned carrot, optional (or ¾ cup [83 g] grated)

3 tablespoons (18 g) minced ginger

3 cloves garlic, minced

½ tablespoon red pepper flakes

1 tablespoon (5.3 g) cayenne pepper, or to taste

2 teaspoons sweet paprika

½ teaspoon Sucanat

To make brining water: Boil the water for 20 seconds and remove from the heat. Stir in the salt to dissolve and set aside or in the fridge to cool completely.

Sterilize a 2 ½-quart fermenting crock (or a large glass/enamel bowl and fitted plate), an 8- to 10-pound (3.5- to 4.5-kg) rock, a large colander, a large glass or ceramic

bowl (not aluminum), and a large nonreactive mixing spoon in the dishwasher. Wash your hands thoroughly.

Slice the cabbage quarters widthwise into rectangular strips, approximately 1 x 2 inches (2.5 x 5 cm). Place the sliced cabbage into the crock and pour cooled brine water over all to cover. Mix gently with your hands and cover with top or plate to fit snugly just inside the edges of your crock. Weight with sterile rock or water bag and let it rest for 4 hours to overnight (about 12 hours).** Drain the cabbage in the sterile colander, catching and reserving brining juice in sterile bowl. Return the cabbage to the crock and gently mix in scallions, daikon, and carrot with your hands.

In a small bowl, mix together the ginger, garlic, red pepper flakes, cayenne, paprika, and Sucanat to form a paste. Spoon the paste over the vegetables and mix gently to combine thoroughly. Pour enough brine over the top to cover, mix gently with spoon, and replace cover and weight. Use plastic wrap to seal the entire top and cover with a heavy dish or hand towel.

Allow the mixture to sit, undisturbed, in an area that ranges from 65 to 70 °F (no warmer or your kimchi may spoil), for 4 days. Test for strength at 4 days. For more tartness, re-cover for up to 3 more days. Once kimchi has reached desired strength, store covered but unweighted in its brine in the refrigerator. Serve cold or at room temperature.

Yield: about 6 cups (850 g)

Per Serving: 6.5 Calories; trace Fat (9% calories from fat); .2g Protein; 1.5g Carbohydrate; .4g Dietary Fiber; 0mg Cholesterol; 120mg Sodium

* Regular table salt has added iodine and anticaking agents, which can interfere with the fermentation process. Use unprocessed sea salt, kosher salt, or pickling salt, but use slightly more kosher salt because the crystal is larger.

** If you can't find a heavy rock or other weight, fill a new (clean) gallon-size zip-closure bag ¾ full with reserved and additional brining water. Tightly seal another bag around the first to prevent leakage.

HEALING MISO-TAHINI SPREAD

From Dr. Jonny: If your liver can't do its job properly, your longevity is basically toast! So support your liver with this spread, which is a power pack for that vital organ. Fermented raw miso teems with probiotics for the digestive and immune system and spirulina, an edible blue-green algae that's considered one of the most nutrient-rich foods on earth. Spirulina has long been used as a detoxifier. Nutritional yeast adds a zippy flavor that has been described as somewhere between nutty and cheesy, with a creamy texture. If you like tahini—and who doesn't, once they've tasted it—you'll absolutely love this version!

½ cup (125 g) mellow white miso

½ cup (120 g) tahini

4 cloves garlic, minced

2 tablespoons (30 g) fresh-grated horseradish

2 tablespoons (16 g) nutritional yeast

2 teaspoons spirulina powder

½ teaspoon cayenne pepper

Combine all ingredients in a food processor and process until a smooth paste is formed, scraping down the sides frequently. Store in the refrigerator in a glass jar.

Yield: about 1¼ cups (313 g)

Per Serving: 55 Calories; 3.4g Fat (52% calories from fat); 2.9g Protein; 4.3g Carbohydrate; 1.3g Dietary Fiber; 0mg Cholesterol; 268mg Sodium

FROM CHEF JEANNETTE:

This pungent spread will last for weeks. I usually make a double batch and keep it all winter long. Because of its warming qualities and the antibacterial nature of raw garlic and cayenne pepper, it acts like a kind of winter tonic. I use it at the first sign of any cold-weather bug.

The flavor is very strong, so it should be used sparingly. Spread it thinly over whole-grain crackers or toast, or stir it into hot veggies or any hot grains. You can also spread it thinly on any crudité veggies. You can alter the ingredient amounts according to your personal taste preferences. Keep the miso/tahini base and customize the rest for yourself.

COLD BROCCOLI SALAD WITH PROBIOTIC DRESSING

From Dr. Jonny: We don't ordinarily think of yogurt as the ideal food for liver health, but the probiotics in yogurt may actually help to fight nonalcoholic fatty liver disease, according to my friend Cathy Wong, N.D., about.com's authority on alternative medicine. "In tests on young rats with NAFLD," she told me, "scientists found those that those treated with probiotics had a reduction in inflammatory liver damage." The yogurt in this cold salad is a great source of probiotics, and broccoli is so good for you in so many ways that you could eat it for your health and longevity almost every day. Specifically, broccoli and other cruciferous vegetables contain phytonutrients such as sulforaphane, which is a potent inducer of phase 2 liver detox enzymes. This is a creamy and tangy new presentation that is sure to liven up your regular fare.

2 small bunches broccoli, cut into small florets, stems peeled and sliced (about 5 to 6 cups, or 355 to 426 g)

⅔ cup (154 g) plain yogurt

¼ cup (60 g) vegan mayonnaise (we like Nayonaise or Vegenaise)

1 cup (30 g) baby spinach

Juice of 2 lemons

1 tablespoon (15 g) Dijon mustard

¾ teaspoon curry powder, optional

¼ teaspoon salt

Black pepper, to taste

1 garlic clove, finely minced

¼ cup (25 g) sliced scallions

1 teaspoon lemon zest

In a large pot, steam the broccoli over boiling water for 3 to 4 minutes or until bright green. Shock for 30 seconds in a large bowl of cold water and drain well. Set aside in a medium bowl.

In a food processor, blend together the yogurt, mayo, and spinach until well incorporated and creamy, scraping down the sides as necessary. Add the lemon juice, mustard, curry powder, salt, pepper, and garlic, and pulse until smooth. Pour over the broccoli, add the scallions and zest, and toss lightly to coat.

Yield: 4 to 6 servings

Per Serving: 169 Calories; 15g Fat (74.8% calories from fat); 2g Protein; 9g Carbohydrate; 2g Dietary Fiber; 0mg Cholesterol; 228mg Sodium

Acknowledgements

· ·

Special thanks from both of us to our incredible agent, Coleen O'Shea, for her special combination of creativity, caring, grit, and consummate professionalism; to our favorite editor, Cara Connors, for her slammin' skills, her patience with our process, and the polish and high gloss she brings to our materials; to Tiffany Hill, project manager, for a miraculously smooth and painless (for us!) project flow; to the design team at Fair Winds for the gorgeous photos and sleek look of the book; to Heather Short, recipe designer for Barlean's, www.dining-details.com and www.eatchickpeas.com, for her recipe contributions; and finally, to Will Kiester, for his vision for this book and belief in our work.

In addition, Jeannette would like to extend a warm thank you to her clients and testers for their fine taste and excellent feedback on the recipes, including Barbara Shea, Sharon Lavallee, Leslie Lindeman, and especially, to her Real Food Moms partner, Tracee Yablon Brenner, R.D., for her flawless food advice! Special thanks, too, to Judi Hestnes, triple threat of chef, health counselor, and R.D., for her fabulous family gravalax concept. And, as always, thanks to Aly and John Wood at The Green Grocer in Portsmouth, RI for their wells of wisdom and high quality whole foods.

About the Authors

Jonny Bowden, Ph.D., C.N.S., a board-certified nutritionist with a master's degree in psychology, is a nationally known expert on nutrition, weight loss, and health. A member of the Editorial Advisory Board of *Men's Health Magazine* and a columnist for America Online, he's also written or contributed to articles for dozens of national publications (print and online) including *The New York Times, The Wall Street Journal, Forbes, Time, Oxygen, Marie Claire, W, Remedy, Diabetes Focus, US Weekly, Cosmopolitan, Family Circle, Self, Fitness, Allure, Essence, Men's Health, Weight Watchers, Pilates Style, Prevention, Woman's World, In Style, Fitness, Natural Health,* and *Shape.* He is the author of *The Most Effective Ways to Live Longer, The 150 Most Effective Ways to Boost Your Energy,* and *The 100 Healthiest Foods to Eat During Pregnancy* (coauthored with Allison Tannis, R.D.).

A popular, dynamic, and much sought-after speaker, he's appeared on CNN, Fox News, MSNBC, ABC, NBC, and CBS, and speaks frequently around the country.

In addition to the above, he is the author of award-winning *Living Low Carb: Controlled Carbohydrate Eating for Long-Term Weight Loss, The Most Effective Natural Cures on Earth, The Healthiest Meals on Earth* and *The 150 Healthiest 15-Minute Recipes on Earth* (coauthored with Jeannette Bessinger), and his acclaimed signature best seller, *The 150 Healthiest Foods on Earth.*

You can find his DVDs, *The Truth about Weight Loss* and *The 7 Pillars of Longevity,* his popular motivational CDs, free newsletter, free audio programs, and many of the supplements and foods recommended in this book on his website, www.jonnybowden.com.

He lives in Southern California with his beloved animal companions Emily (a pit bull), and Lucy (an Argentine Dogo).

Jeannette Bessinger, C.H.H.C., owner of Balance for Life, LLC, www.balanceforlifellc.com, is a board-certified holistic health coach, award-winning lifestyle and nutrition educator, and personal whole foods chef.

She is co-author of *The Healthiest Meals on Earth* and *The 150 Healthiest 15-Minute Recipes on Earth* (with Dr. Jonny) and *Simple Food for Busy Families,* and author of *Great Expectations: Best Food for Your Baby and Toddler.* She has written, contributed to, or been interviewed for articles for magazines including *Better Homes and Gardens, Clean Eating, Consumer Reports Health and Fitness Issue, First for Women,* and *Parenting.*

Designer and lead facilitator of a long-running and successful hospital-based lifestyle change program, she is a regular consultant and speaker to public and private organizations and coalitions working to improve the health of schools and cities in the United States.

As co-founder of Real Food Moms® (www.realfoodmoms.com), she provides busy moms with quick answers for how to feed their families well. Follow her and Real Food Moms on Facebook.

She lives in Portsmouth, Rhode Island, with her patient husband, two teenagers, three dogs, and pesky cat.

Index

· · · · · · ·

Note: Page numbers in italics indicate figures and tables.

Note: Page numbers in italics indicate figures and tables.

Note: Page numbers in italics indicate figures and tables.

Hundreds of hours of my personal nutritional research reveals...

7 SUPER FOODS
That Could Change Your Life!

Dr. Jonny Bowden says...

"Do you want to know the best foods to eat to live a longer, healthier, happier, and more energized life?

If so then follow the instructions below and I'll send you the 7 Super Foods audio course...for free!"

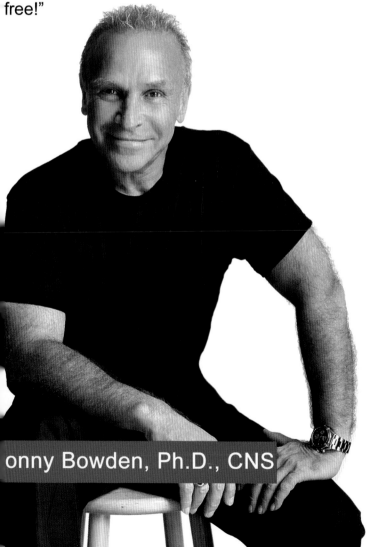

onny Bowden, Ph.D., CNS

This **FREE AUDIO COURSE** reveals the best foods to help you...

- **control weight**
- **look & feel younger**
- **prevent disease**
- **extend your life**
- **increase energy levels**

FREE!

Get started by signing up online now!

Simply go to

http://feelyourpower.com

NOW and enter your name and email address.

It's that easy! And you can rest assured that we will keep your email address private. We will NEVER sell or rent your information.

Change your body. Change your life...with Dr. Jonny Bowden!

Best-selling books by acclaimed nutritionist Jonny Bowden, Ph.D., C.N.S.

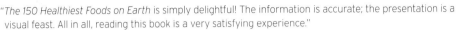

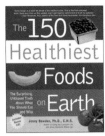

The 150 Healthiest Foods on Earth
The Surprising, Unbiased Truth about What You Should Eat and Why

"*The 150 Healthiest Foods on Earth* is simply delightful! The information is accurate; the presentation is a visual feast. All in all, reading this book is a very satisfying experience."
—CHRISTIANE NORTHRUP, M.D., author of *Mother-Daughter Wisdom*, *The Wisdom of Menopause*, and *Women's Bodies, Women's Wisdom*

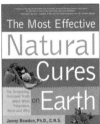

The Most Effective Natural Cures on Earth
The Surprising, Unbiased Truth about What Treatments Work and Why

"I reference this beautifully written and illustrated review of the best cures on the planet so often that it lives on my desk rather than the bookshelf."
—MEHMET C. OZ, M.D., coauthor of *You: The Owner's Manual*

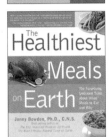

The Healthiest Meals on Earth
The Surprising, Unbiased Truth about What Meals to Eat and Why

"What a simply irresistible book with mouthwatering recipes from all around the world! I plan to use this book as a resource guide and as a gift for all the people I truly care about."
—ANN LOUISE GITTLEMAN, PH.D., C.N.S., author of *The Fat Flush Plan* and *Before the Change*

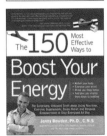

The Most Effective Ways to Boost Your Energy
The Surprising, Unbiased Truth about Using Nutrition, Exercise, Supplements, Stress Relief, and Personal Empowerment to Stay Energized All Day

"Get everyone you love to read my friend Dr. Jonny's brilliance!"
—MARK VICTOR HANSEN, coauthor of *Chicken Soup for the Soul*

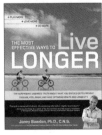

The Most Effective Ways to Live Longer
The Surprising, Unbiased Truth about What You Should Do to Prevent Disease, Feel Great, and Have Optimum Health and Longevity

"A must-read for anyone who wants to live longer! Jonny Bowden takes the lessons we've learned from the world's longest-lived people and offers a research-backed formula for the rest of us to get the most good years out of our lives."
—DAN BUETTNER, author of *The Blue Zones: Lessons on Living Longer from the People Who've Lived the Longest*

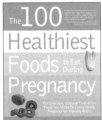

The 100 Healthiest Foods to Eat During Pregnancy
The Surprising, Unbiased Truth about Foods You Should Be Eating During Pregnancy but Probably Aren't

"Another great book from Jonny Bowden! In his signature expert style, Jonny, along with Allison Tannis, recommends the healthiest foods and spices for pregnant women . . . all pregnant women should read this book."
—DEAN RAFFELOCK, D.C.,C.C.N., author of *A Natural Guide to Pregnancy and Postpartum Health*

www.jonnybowden.com